Colorectal Cancer Screening and Computerized Tomographic Colonography

I dedicate this book to my wife, Marianne, and to my children, Madison and Grayson, for their love, patience, and encouragement.

Preface

Computed tomographic colonography, or CTC as we will call it throughout this volume, has come a long way since its conceptual phases in the early 1990s. This colorectal cancer screening modality gained widespread attention in the United States with the 2003 publication of a large, multicenter screening study performed at Navy and Army medical centers that showed excellent comparative results with colonoscopy in average-risk individuals. My interest and involvement in this technology and its potential was somewhat serendipitous as I returned to one of those study sites, the National Naval Medical Center in Bethesda, MD, as a staff gastroenterologist shortly before the publication of the aforementioned study by Perry Pickhardt and colleagues. This also coincided with the departure of Dr. Pickhardt from his position as an active duty Navy radiologist to what would become a highly successful academic career at the University of Wisconsin. Shortly thereafter, our medical center, and the gastroenterology service in particular, were charged with creating an advanced colorectal cancer screening center. On the heels of the successes of CTC, we decided to partner with our radiology colleagues and build the foundation using a combined approach, employing both CTC and colonoscopy individually and reciprocally. The entity that we created, the Colon Health Initiative, was highly successful and continues to this day, serving as an integrated model of excellence and highlighting the potential of CTC as a screening modality.

During the conceptualization of this book and its contents, I tried to take that integrated and collaborative approach with the authors who contributed as well as the subject matter that they discuss. The idea was to provide a source that would appeal to clinicians and radiology personnel, alike. The first chapter of this book provides an overview of the disease and risk factors of colorectal cancer as well as an update of where we have been and where we may be going with regard to colorectal cancer screening tests. This background serves as a critical contextual building block for subsequent discussions of CTC as a screening modality. The middle chapters segue into a discussion specific to the history and development of CTC as both a colorectal imaging and screening modality. Important topics covered in these chapters are practical and realistic discussions of coverage and regulatory decisions surrounding CTC and its widespread deployment as well as very practical guidance regarding the performance, interpretation, and integration of CTC into clinical practice. The book concludes with a review of the controversies, potential pitfalls, and exciting new directions and capabilities inherent in the practice of CTC. These chapters are intentionally filled with high-quality images to better communicate the concepts of this visual modality.

I must also take this opportunity to once again express my utmost gratitude to the experts who contributed to this volume. Without their stalwart support and dedication, what I believe will be a very useful reference and guide would not have come to fruition. This was a complementary effort, bringing together world-renowned gastroenterologists and radiologists for a collaboration to make a whole, echoing the practice of CTC in real life. I am grateful for the opportunity to have been involved in this effort and trust that readers will find this to be a valuable contribution to their library.

Bethesda, MD, USA   Brooks D. Cash, M.D.

Contents

Contributors

Joseph C. Anderson, M.D. Department of Gastroenterology, White River Junction VA Medical Center, White River Junction, VT, USA

Paolo Baldassari, M.D. Department of Radiological, Oncological and Pathological Sciences, "Sapienza" University of Rome, Rome, Italy

Duncan Barlow, M.D. Department of Gastroenterology, Walter Reed National Military Medical Center, Bethesda, MD, USA

Christopher F. Beaulieu, M.D., Ph.D. Department of Radiology, Stanford University Medical Center, Stanford, CA, USA

Darren Boone, M.B.B.S. Centre for Medical Imaging, University College Hospital, London, UK

Steven Carpenter, M.D. Mercer University School of Medicine, Savannah Campus, Savannah, GA, USA

Department of Internal Medicine, Memorial University Medical Center, Savannah, GA, USA

Maria Ciolina, M.D. Department of Radiological, Oncological and Pathological Sciences, "Sapienza" University of Rome, Rome, Italy

Abraham H. Dachman, M.D. Department of Radiology, The University of Chicago Medical Center (UCMC), Chicago, IL, USA

Farid Dahi, M.D. Department of Radiology, The University of Chicago Medical Center (UCMC), Chicago, IL, USA

Steve Halligan, M.B.B.S., M.D. Centre for Medical Imaging, University College Hospital, London, UK

Franco Iafrate, M.D. Department of Radiological, Oncological and Pathological Sciences, "Sapienza" University of Rome, Rome, Italy

Donald W. Jensen, M.D. Department of Gastroenterology, Walter Reed National Military Medical Center, Bethesda, MD, USA

Andrea Laghi, M.D. Department of Radiological, Oncological and Pathological Sciences, "Sapienza" University of Rome, Rome, Italy

Elizabeth G. McFarland, M.D. Department of Radiology, SSM St. Joseph's Hospital, St. Charles, MO, USA

Peter D. Poullos, M.D. Department of Radiology, Stanford University Medical Center, Stanford, CA, USA

Douglas J. Robertson, M.D., M.P.H. Department of Gastroenterology, White River Junction VA Medical Center, White River Junction, VT, USA

Geisel School of Medicine at Dartmouth, Hanover, NH, USA

Don C. Rockey, M.D. Department of Internal Medicine, Department of Medicine, Medical University of South Carolina, Charleston, SC, USA

Stuart A. Taylor, M.B.B.S., M.D. Centre for Medical Imaging, University College Hospital, London, UK

Overview of Colorectal Cancer

Joseph C. Anderson and Douglas J. Robertson

Colorectal cancer (CRC) (adenocarcinoma of the large bowel) arises from a neoplastic process involving the epithelial layer of the intestine. In most CRC, the process begins as a benign polyp or adenoma. The adenoma undergoes a transformation to cancer through a series of molecular changes. Early in the process, the cancer can be treated easily with removal of the adenoma or early stage cancer. Thus, as expected from the nature of this disease, prevention and screening have likely reduced the incidence and mortality rates of this disease. The goal of this chapter is to provide an overview of CRC as well as an understanding of the rational for screening for this cancer.

Epidemiology

In the USA, CRC is the third leading cancer-related death for both males and females [1]. The rate for mortality from CRC has been steadily

J.C. Anderson, M.D. (✉)
Department of Gastroenterology,
White River Junction VA Medical Center,
White River Junction, VT, USA
e-mail: joseph.anderson@dartmouth.edu

D.J. Robertson, M.D., M.P.H.
Department of Gastroenterology,
White River Junction VA Medical Center,
White River Junction, VT, USA

Geisel School of Medicine at Dartmouth,
Hanover, NH, USA

decreasing for the past few decades. However, in the past several years, the mortality rate has decreased at a significantly faster pace, presumably through increased CRC screening [2, 3]. Specifically, whereas the rate was decreasing at 2% per year prior to 2003, the rate decreased by 3% per year in the period from 2003 to 2007 [3]. A recent review of the Surveillance, Epidemiology, and End Result (SEER) mortality database demonstrated that the rates for CRC mortality had decreased to a much greater extent in the Northeastern than in the Southern USA [3]. The authors postulated that the difference in mortality rates between the two geographical regions reflects differences in CRC screening rates, treatment, and risk factors such as smoking and obesity. In addition, the authors attributed the lower screening rates in the southern states to an increased population of poor and uninsured in this region. Furthermore, southern states also have a higher percentage of blacks who have higher rates of CRC mortality than whites [1]. The changes and variation in these mortality rates illustrate the complex factors that can impact the incidence of CRC.

In Europe, CRC is the second commonest cause of cancer-related deaths for males and females [4, 5]. As in the USA, there has been an increase in CRC survival in the past decade [6, 7]. In addition, as observed in the USA, there is a variation in survival trends in Europe [8]. Although Europe has experienced an increase in survival rates for CRC, the improvement has been less pronounced in Eastern

European countries such as Slovakia [8, 9]. Worldwide, CRC incidence rates make this disease the third most common cancer in females and the fourth most common cancer in men [10, 11]. In some countries such as Israel and Japan, the rates have increased [10, 12].

Anatomy and Embryologic Development of the Colon

There are several layers that comprise the wall of the colon. The innermost layer is the mucosa. This layer consists of the epithelial layer, the lamina propria or connective tissue, and a thin muscle layer called the muscularis mucosae. The next layer is the submucosa, comprised of connective tissue, nerves, lymphatics, and blood vessels. The muscle layer, or muscularis propria, is the next layer and is comprised of two bands, a circular and longitudinal. The outermost layer, the serosa, is present from the sigmoid to the cecum and not below the peritoneal reflection. Knowledge of the layers is important with regard to staging, prognosis, and treatment that will be reviewed later in the chapter.

The colon is comprised of two segments, the proximal and distal large bowel. The proximal colon consists of the cecum, the ascending colon, hepatic flexure, and the transverse colon. The distal colon consists of the descending, sigmoid colon, and the rectum. The proximal colon has its embryonic origin in the midgut, while the distal colon originates from the hindgut. The blood supply for the proximal colon derives from the superior mesenteric artery, while the inferior mesenteric artery supplies most of the distal colon [13, 14]. In addition, there are differences in the capillary network surrounding the colon. While the proximal colon is multilayered, the distal colon is single layered [14]. Furthermore, the crypt length in the distal colon is longer than that of the proximal colon [13]. In addition, there are differences between the enteric flora as well as the metabolism of fatty acids in different anatomic regions of the large intestine [15].

The anatomical and physiological differences between the segments of the colon may play a role in the clinical and molecular differences between proximal and distal colorectal neoplasia [13, 16, 17]. While proximal tumors are more likely mucinous and exhibit both microsatellite instability and methylation defects, distal tumors are more likely to have tumors associated with the chromosomal instability pathway, which lacks these features [18, 19]. In addition, proximal neoplasia is associated with female gender and older age [20–22]. Conversely, smoking and alcohol use are associated with distal neoplasia [23–25]. Morphologically, proximal tumors and polyps are more likely to be flat compared to their distal counterparts [26, 27]. Finally, interval neoplasia or lesions diagnosed between regularly scheduled colonoscopies are more likely to be found in the proximal colon. Issues regarding the molecular, clinical, and morphological presentation of colorectal neoplasia will be further discussed elsewhere in this chapter [28].

Adenoma to Carcinoma Sequence

In most cases of CRC, the disease begins as a benign polyp or adenoma that develops into a tumor. This process is accompanied by a sequence of molecular abnormalities that help to facilitate growth and transformation of the adenoma into a more advanced neoplastic lesion. The first model describing this process was published by Fearon and Vogelstein in 1990 [29]. Their model required seven mutations to occur for a cancer to develop from normal mucosa. This includes initial inactivation of the tumor suppressor gene adenomatous polyposis coli (APC) followed by activation of the oncogene KRAS as well as mutations in TP53 and other pathways. This describes the classic "chromosomal instability (CIN) pathway" [30], but there are two other well-described pathways. Additional detail regarding these three pathways will be discussed in a separate section. It has been estimated that 8–15 years are required for normal mucosa to transform into a cancer [31]. This length of time, also known as "polyp dwell time," has been estimated using different methods [32]. The first method compared the mean age of patients with small adenomas to that of patients diagnosed with CRC and observed a difference of 18 years [33]. Koretz used the relationship of prevalence = incidence × duration to conclude that the transformation time from adenoma to carcinoma must be at least 4.8 years, the so-called latent phase [34]. However, since some cancers are detected in asymptomatic patients and some cancers develop de novo from the mucosa, adenoma dwell time is likely longer. The strategy of CRC prevention through adenoma detection and removal is based on this lag time and is the basis for current screening strategies [35].

Molecular Pathways of CRC Development

The development of CRC from normal tissue is a result of an accumulation of multiple genetic mutations. These genetic abnormalities decrease cell death and increase the likelihood of clonal expansion. Although there may be many genetic mutations in a single adenoma, only a small proportion will be responsible for neoplastic transformation. In this section, the three major pathways responsible for CRC will be discussed.

Chromosomal Instability

This pathway was first described approximately 20 years ago by Fearon and Vogelstein and is manifested through the traditional adenoma to carcinoma sequence [29, 36]. The CIN, or suppressor, pathway is characterized by aneuploidy or an abnormal number of chromosomes [37, 38]. The first mutation occurs in the APC gene which is responsible for the APC protein [30]. This protein plays a significant role in cell development and the Wnt signaling pathway by binding to beta-catenin. APC mutations are found in over two-thirds of CRC and most commonly in distally located lesions. In the familial cancer syndrome, familial adenomatous polyposis (FAP), the affected individual has a germline mutation in one copy of the APC gene. Any somatic mutation that inactivates the remaining gene will facilitate the development of adenomas. Mutations of an oncogene, usually

KRAS, are another development that promotes growth of an adenoma. Another important step in the CIN pathway is the inactivation of the TP53 gene, which is responsible for the p53 pathway. The inactivation of this gene occurs as a result of a mutation and a deletion. The loss of this key tumor suppressor aids in the transformation of an adenoma into invasive carcinoma. Other genes involved in this pathway are SMAD2 and SMAD4, which are part of the TGF-beta signaling pathway involved in cell growth, migration, and apoptosis [37]. There is also mutation of the DCC gene that produces a membrane receptor aiding in promoting apoptosis.

Microsatellite Instability

DNA replication errors in the form of mismatched nucleotide base pairs occur frequently in microsatellite regions of DNA and can result in transcription errors and altered gene expression [39]. These errors are collectively known as microsatellite instability (MSI). DNA mismatch repair (MMR) enzymes are responsible for the repair of these erroneous segments. There are seven proteins that are involved in the enzymatic repair process: hMLH1, hMLH3, hMSH2, hMSH3, hMSH6, hPMS1, and hPMS2. Two proteins, hMLH1 and hMSH2, are essential parts of the functioning MMR enzyme [40]. There are several key genes involved in CRC development that contain microsatellite regions particularly susceptible to mismatch errors. These include the following: TGFβ2, β-catenin, IGF-2, APC, MSH3, MSH6, Bax, Caspase 5, and E2F4. Adenomas can develop as a result of these mutations.

There are five standard microsatellite patterns that are used to detect MSI in a tumor: BAT25, BAT26, D5S346, D2S123, and D17S250. If none of these are present, then the tissue is considered to be microsatellite stable (MSS). If one of these patterns is present, then the tissue is MSI-L (low), and if two or more are present, then the tissue is MSI-H [41]. About one in five CRC is MSI-H, but only a fraction of these are in the setting of hereditary nonpolyposis colorectal cancer (HNPCC) syndrome, a familial cancer syndrome that is characterized by colonic adenomas and CRC with high levels of MSI. The majority of MSI-H tumors likely arise from somatic methylation of hMLH1 [42]. Tumors that result from methylation tend to be proximal and less aggressive [39].

CpG Island Methylator Pathway

Methylation of the gene promoter region is associated with epigenetic silencing of gene expression. If there is methylation of CPG promoter regions in genes responsible for hMLH1 and p16, there is an increased risk of CRC [43, 44]. Tumors can be categorized as CIMP+ or CIMP– based on the presence of defined markers: CACNA1G, IGF2, NEUROG1, RUNX3, and SOCS1. CIMP+ tumors present as proximal lesions and occur in older women. CIMP+ tumors that are not MSI-H have a worse prognosis than MSI-H tumors or tumors arising in the setting of the CIN pathway [39, 45]. Since CIMP+/MSI-H tumors are associated with epigenetic silencing of hMLH1, an overlap between the CpG island methylator pathway (CIMP) and the MSI pathway exists in a large proportion of CRC. In some CIMP+ tumors that are not MSI-H, there is a mutation of the oncogene BRAF [46]. These tumors tend to have a poor prognosis [46]. In other CIMP+/non-MSI-H tumors, KRAS mutations are present rather than BRAF mutations [47, 48].

Symptoms and Diagnosis

Presenting complaints for CRC can include rectal bleeding, change in bowel habits such as diarrhea or constipation, abdominal pain, weight loss, and fatigue due to anemia. Many patients with CRC do not have any symptoms. Tenesmus, painful or incomplete defecation, has been associated with rectal cancer. In their review of nearly 200 patients diagnosed with CRC, Majumdar et al. observed that rectal bleeding, abdominal pain, and a change in bowel habits were the most common presenting symptoms [49]. Rectal bleeding and constipation were the strongest independent predictors of distal CRC. Since a delay in diagnosis

in symptomatic patients is a concern in clinical practice, these investigators also examined the duration of symptoms and the stage of cancer at diagnosis. They found no significant association between the duration of symptoms and the stage of the disease. In these studies the overall mean duration of symptoms (or delay to diagnosis) was 14 weeks. The mean patient delay was 26 weeks and 11 weeks for the physician delay.

In a study of 349 patients with CRC, Stapley et al. observed that rectal bleeding was associated with a lower cancer stage and higher survival rates. Anemia was associated with more advanced stages and lower mortality [50]. Duration of symptoms was not associated with the stage of cancer. A study of over 4,000 CRC patients in Norway demonstrated that the duration of symptoms was associated with a less advanced disease stage [51]. The authors explain this paradox by postulating that aggressive tumors may be associated with more worrisome type symptoms than less aggressive cancers. Recently, Adelstein et al. performed a systematic review of 62 articles examining symptoms and the diagnosis of CRC [52]. They observed that rectal bleeding and weight loss were significantly associated with CRC. Other symptoms such as change in bowel habit, constipation, diarrhea, and abdominal pain were not associated with CRC. In summary, it appears that a prudent practitioner would refer for evaluation any patient who presented with new complaints such as rectal bleeding, abdominal pain, or fatigue due to anemia.

Risk Factors

There are many known risk factors associated with colorectal neoplasia although age and family history of CRC are the only ones typically considered when screening for the disease. The recent American College of Gastroenterology CRC screening guidelines introduced the concept of using other factors in selecting patients for screening [53]. Considering other risk factors can allow for both tailoring screening recommendations and/or efforts at modifying them to reduce the risk for CRC. In this section, the risk factors are divided into modifiable and non-modifiable risk factors. In addition, there will be a discussion of the risk factors associated with advanced neoplasia as well as CRC.

Non-modifiable Risk Factors

Age

Age is one of the strongest predictors of colorectal neoplasia in many studies. The high risk observed when examining the association between age and neoplasia likely results at least partially from the number of years of exposure to other factors such as smoking. However, in many studies, the risk remains high even after controlling for many known exposures. The importance of age as a risk factor for CRC is highlighted by the fact that it is used to determine when to start screening. For patients of average risk, the recommended age to start screening is 50 years.

Gender

Most studies of asymptomatic populations have demonstrated an increased risk of developing adenomas and more advanced neoplasia (advanced adenomas) in men [54–56]. A recent meta-analysis by Nguyen et al. found that men were more likely than women to have advanced adenomas (RR = 1.83; 95% CI 1.69–1.97) [57]. While male gender is a significant risk factor for advanced adenomas, the lifetime risk for CRC remains similar for men (5.3%) and women (5.0%) in the USA [1]. The CRC risk for women lags by approximately 5 years that of men such that the risk for a women at 55 is similar to that of a man at 50 years of age [58]. Thus, women have a similar lifetime risk to men with regard to CRC but a substantially lower risk for advanced neoplasia.

This paradox was recently highlighted in review by Bianchi and Roy [59]. They noted that there was a higher rate of interval cancers in women [28]. Interval cancers are lesions that are diagnosed between regularly scheduled colonoscopies, typically every 5 or 10 years. The authors postulated that colonoscopy may be less effective in women than men. They also hypothesized that

women may have a different clinical presentation of CRC due in part to the higher proportion of proximal neoplasia in women, the chemoprotective effect of estrogen, and an increased sensitivity to risk factors such as smoking. One possible explanation that was proposed suggests that women may have a higher rate of adenomas that progress to advanced lesions. The Women's Health Initiative demonstrated a higher rate of metastatic lymph node involvement, but a lower rate of CRC in women who had been treated with estrogen/progesterone [60]. Another explanation was that women may harbor more flat colorectal neoplasia. Recently Johnson et al. observed that adenomas greater than 5 mm in size were more likely to present as flat and proximal in women than men [61]. Despite these observations, there are no differences between screening recommendations for men and women in the current guidelines.

Race

African Americans have a higher rate of CRC incidence and mortality than any other racial or ethnic groups. Disparities in mortality rates from CRC due to racial differences increased from 1960 through 2005, even as the overall CRC mortality rate declined in the same period [62]. Recent data from the SEER database show age- and gender-adjusted CRC incidence and mortality rates to be higher for African American than whites [63]. In addition, African Americans may be diagnosed at a younger age than whites [64]. Reasons for the higher rates in African Americans include lower CRC screening rates [65–67] and higher exposure rates to risk factors such as cigarette smoking or type II diabetes mellitus [67–70]. A recent analysis of the Clinical Outcomes Research Initiative (CORI) database demonstrated an increased prevalence of polyps larger than 9 mm in African Americans compared with that of whites [71]. This relationship was stronger for women than men. In addition, for patients older than 60 years of age, black patients were more likely to have proximal polyps that were larger than 9 mm. The authors concluded that there might be a need to alter the guidelines to screen black patients prior to the age of 50 years.

They did note that this could add to the complexity that exists in the current multi-society guidelines. The American College of Gastroenterology, however, recommends that African Americans begin screening at the age of 45 years of age [53, 72].

Modifiable Risk Factors

Smoking

Tobacco exposure in the form of cigarette smoking has been identified as a major risk factor colorectal neoplasia [24, 27, 73–77]. Smokers may be at an increased risk for MMR defects, and this may play a role in the development of neoplasia in this group [78, 79]. In addition, tobacco exposure may increase the risk for BRAF mutations. An increased association between the point mutation of the oncogene BRAF (V600E) has been seen in people who smoke [80]. BRAF has been shown to be tightly correlated with the CIMP CRC phenotype [81, 82]. Increased methylation defects are the hallmark of a recently described pathway that is also seen in serrated lesions. Accordingly, Anderson et al. observed an increased risk of smoking for sessile serrated adenomas as well as serrated aberrant crypt foci [83].

Smoking may account for 20% of all cancers in the USA [84]. Smoking is associated with as much as 30% increased risk for CRC for men and women [85–90]. In addition, smoking may account for 12% of all CRC-related deaths [91, 92]. Smoking has been observed to be associated with an earlier age of CRC diagnosis than in nonsmokers, and smokers present with a more advanced stage of disease than nonsmokers [93]. A recent study demonstrated an increased mortality in smokers after the diagnosis of CRC [94]. This finding was most pronounced in patients who had tumors with high MSI.

With regard to advanced adenomas, smoking has been consistently associated with an approximately twofold increased risk compared with nonsmokers [95]. Based on colonoscopy findings in nearly 2,500 asymptomatic patients, Anderson et al. concluded that 30 pack years of exposure or more was associated with an increased risk for advanced neoplasia [73]. In a separate gender analysis, they observed that women had an increased risk for advanced neoplasia if they smoked 10–30 pack years [74]. Men required more than 30 pack years to have an increased risk. In addition, while both genders had an increased risk for distal advanced adenomas in smokers, only female smokers had an increased risk for proximal advanced lesions. In this population, there was a distinct difference between men and women with regard to tobacco exposure. The authors postulated that the anatomical differences could be due to increased methylation and MMR defects seen in women [78, 96–98].

Obesity

Obesity is defined as a body mass index (BMI) ≥ 30. An increased waist circumference or waist to hip ratio has been proposed as a more accurate measure of visceral adiposity, which is felt to be important in carcinogenesis. Insulin resistance may play an important role in the development of colorectal neoplasia in obese patients. Elevated insulin levels along with hyperglycemia and increased free insulin-like growth factor (IGF-1) can increase the risk for colorectal neoplasia [99–102]. Insulin resistance can lead to increased cellular proliferation and reduced apoptosis [103–105]. The increased risk of CRC associated with type II diabetes mellitus has been observed in large case control studies [106, 107].

Several studies have demonstrated that obesity is associated with an increased risk for CRC, and the risk appears to be stronger in men than in women [108–112]. In the Health Professionals Follow-Up Study (HPFS), men with the highest BMI had a twofold increased risk compared with the thinnest men [113]. In a comparable study, participants in the Nurses' Health Study (NHS) who were obese were one and a half times as likely to have CRC as the thinnest women [114]. Other longitudinal population studies have observed that an increased risk for CRC is correlated with an increased waist circumference [115].

Obesity is important since it is a modifiable risk factor, and there is data to suggest that weight loss can decrease the risk for colorectal neoplasia [116]. There is an increasing prevalence of obesity in the USA, and it has been shown that obese patients may be less likely to be screened for CRC than nonobese patients [117]. In its 2008 CRC screening guidelines, the American College of Gastroenterology introduced obesity as a potential risk factor that identifies patients who may need screening earlier than age 50 [53]. However, their enthusiasm for this recommendation was tempered by the recognition of the attendant comorbidities associated with obesity that may limit the benefits of screening.

Alcohol

There are several large studies that demonstrate an increased risk for colorectal neoplasia associated with alcohol intake [118–120]. Mechanistically, the increased risk associated with alcohol has been attributed to abnormal DNA methylation and repair, induction of cytochrome p450 enzymes, and altered bile acid composition [121, 122]. The NHS observed a direct increased risk related to alcohol intake of colorectal neoplasia in the colon but not the rectum of women [118]. The HPFS demonstrated an increased risk in men for an intake of 15 grams or more of alcohol per day [123]. One study that combined eight large prospective longitudinal populations observed an increased risk for patients who drank ≥2 alcoholic beverages per day [120]. Most studies have observed an increased risk for all types of alcoholic beverages. However, one study examining CRC [124] and another examining adenomas [23] found a decreased risk associated with wine intake. Overall, it appears that avoiding alcohol would decrease the likelihood of developing colorectal neoplasia.

Diet

Much of the emphasis in the literature regarding diet has focused on the CRC risk associated with red meat consumption and the potential reduction of risk with fiber intake. With regard to red meat consumption, the increased risk of CRC may result through several mechanisms. These included the production of heterocyclic amines, increased animal fat intake, increased heme absorption, and stimulation of insulin [125–127]. In the HPFS study, there was an increased risk of CRC in men who consumed more than five servings of red meat per week [118]. A recent meta-analysis by Alexander et al. observed a modest increased risk for colon cancer and a trend toward an association with the consumption for red meat [128]. The authors concluded that the association was not strong enough to discount potential confounders that may explain any positive correlation.

There are currently conflicting data with respect to fiber intake a risk of CRC. A possible protective effect of fiber intake in the form of fruits and vegetables on the risk for CRC has been examined in many large prospective studies [129, 130]. Some of the proposed mechanisms include increased folate consumption, binding of carcinogens, lower colonic pH, decreased colonic transit time, beneficial effects of micronutrients found in fruits and vegetables, and an increased production of short-chain fatty acids [131, 132]. A meta-analysis of 16 case control studies found a 50% reduction in CRC risks associated with fiber consumption [133]. Randomized controlled studies of fiber in the form of cereal or fruits and vegetables found no effect on the recurrence of colorectal adenomas [134, 135]. In the USA, studies that have examined both male and female health professionals have observed no effect of fiber on CRC risk [136, 137]. One large study did show an increased risk of CRC, but higher amounts of fiber intake did not offer any protective effect [138].

Family History of Colorectal Cancer

In current guidelines [53, 139], a family history of CRC has been used to inform the decision regarding when to start CRC screening. Having a first-degree relative (FDR) with CRC can increase the risk up to three times that of an average risk individual [140]. Johns and Houston performed a meta-analysis of 27 studies regarding CRC risk in patients with relatives with CRC and nine studies of patients with a family history of adenomas [141]. They observed that the relative risk for having an FDR with CRC was 2.25 (95% CI = 2.00–2.53). If a patient had more than one FDR with CRC, the risk was 4.25 (95% CI = 3.01–6.08). If the relative was diagnosed before the age of 45 years, the risk for the affected individual was 3.87 (95% CI = 2.40–6.22). If the relative had a colorectal adenoma, the risk for CRC was 1.99 (95% CI = 1.55–2.55). Although it is well accepted that a family history of CRC significantly increases the risk for CRC, there is less data for a family history of an adenoma. One study by Cottet et al. observed an increased risk of large adenomas or CRC in patients with an FDR with a large adenoma [142]. Based on these data as well the lack of data for small adenomas, the ACG dropped a family history of any adenoma as an indication for earlier screening in its most recent guidelines. Based on available data, patients with second- or third-degree relatives with a history of CRC should receive average risk screening [140, 143].

Familial Syndromes

CRC in the setting of a familial syndrome represents less than 10% of all CRC. However, the identification of patients with these syndromes is important for surveillance of the affected individual as well as for screening of the relatives. Some important clues that an individual may have a familial syndrome include an early age of onset of the CRC, multiple adenomas, more than one affected relative with colorectal neoplasia, and successive generations with colorectal neoplasia. In addition to a family history of colorectal neoplasia, the practitioner should ask the patient about other cancers in first-, second-, and third-degree relatives. The United States Surgeon General's web site has an online tool for patients to collect a family history of diseases including cancer (https://familyhistory.hhs.gov/fhh-web/home.action). In this section we will briefly describe the common syndromes and the colorectal cancer screening guidelines for these patients.

Hereditary Nonpolyposis Colorectal Cancer

This familial syndrome, also known as Lynch syndrome, is responsible for less than 5% of all CRC [144]. The common features of this syndrome include young age of onset and predisposition for proximal tumors. The lifetime CRC risk for patients with the HNPCC mutation is about 50–80% [145]. These tumors are often mucinous, poorly differentiated, and contain infiltrating lymphocytes. The most common extracolonic tumor observed in HNPCC is endometrial cancer with the hMSH6 mutation conferring the greatest risk [146]. Other common sites for tumors include ovaries, small bowel, stomach, brain, skin, pancreas, hepatobiliary system, and the urinary tract. The Muir-Torre variant of HNPCC includes skin lesions such as sebaceous adenomas.

HNPCC occurs in the setting of germline mutations in the MMR genetic code. These genes are responsible for the production of DNA repair enzymes: hMLH1, hMLH3, hMSH2, hMSH3, hMSH6, hPMS1, and hPMS2 [39, 40]. The target of these repair genes is mismatch errors that occur in the microsatellite regions of the genome where there are tandem nucleotide base repeat sequences. When these microsatellite repeats cannot be repaired, MSI ensues.

There are multiple clinical guidelines to assist in the identification of HNPCC. The first set of guidelines was known as the Amsterdam Criteria-I [147]. These guidelines required that an individual have at least three relatives with CRC. One had to be an FDR of the other two with at least two successive generations affected and one individual diagnosed at less than 50 years of age. The second set of guidelines, Amsterdam Criteria-II, was developed to be more sensitive and allowed the relatives to have a diagnosis of an extracolonic HNPCC-associated tumor [148]. The current recommendations are the Revised Bethesda Guidelines for testing CRC for MSI [149]. These criteria recommend MSI testing when any of the following clinical scenarios are present: CRC diagnosed in a patient younger than 50 years, the presence of synchronous or metachronous CRC, the presence of another HNPCC-related tumor, CRC with MSI-related histology in a patient younger than 60 years, CRC diagnosed in an individual with an FDR with an HNPCC-related tumor or CRC less than 50 years of age, and CRC diagnosed in a patient with two or more FDR or second-degree relatives of any age with HNPCC tumors.

Testing for MSI involves a panel of five DNA markers. If two or more of these five markers are present, then an immunohistochemistry (IHC) analysis can be done to confirm the presence of the protein products of the repair genes, which include MSH2, MSH6, MLH1, and PMS2 [150]. Any absence of the proteins in the tumor specimen, when compared to normal cells obtained in a blood sample, suggests that a germline mutation is present. When present, 90% of germline mutations in HNPCC are located in hMSH2 and hMLH1, while hMSH6 and hPMS2 account for the remaining 10% [151]. hMSH6 mutations carry a lower cancer risk than the other abnormalities [152]. A review by Koornstra et al. reported that the risk for endometrial cancer was the highest for hMSH6 and the lowest for hMLH1 [146].

The recommendation for an individual suspected of having HNPCC is a colonoscopy every one to 2 years. In a study by Stupart et al., 129 subjects with an hMLH1 defect underwent surveillance colonoscopy every 2 years until age 30 and then annually after that age, while 49 patients refused surveillance [153]. Patients who refused surveillance had a higher risk of death from CRC as compared to the group who had surveillance. The age recommended to begin screening in HNPCC patients is at 20–25 years of age or 10 years younger than the youngest affected individual with CRC. A flexible sigmoidoscopy is not recommended, given the proximal nature of the colon tumors associated with HNPCC. There is little evidence to support screening for the other HNPCC-related tumors.

Familial Adenomatous Polyposis

Familial adenomatous polyposis (FAP) is an autosomal dominant syndrome that is caused by a genetic mutation of the APC gene on chromosome 5. Unlike HNPCC, the penetrance of FAP is complete and is accompanied by a nearly 100% chance of developing CRC when the genetic mutation is present. APC mutations occur in approximately 1 in 10,000 births [154]. There are two phenotypes of the disease, classic and attenuated FAP. Classic FAP presents with thousands of adenomas in the colorectum by the time an affected individual is 10–12 years of age. The average age at which the individual develops CRC is less than 40 years of age [140]. Most patients with classic FAP will have duodenal

adenomas by their fifth decade [155, 156], and duodenal or peri-ampullary cancer is the leading cause of death after a colectomy is performed [157]. These duodenal adenomas occur in the second portion of the duodenum or around the papilla. Many patients with classic FAP have polyposis of typically benign fundic gland gastric polyps that some studies have demonstrated to have a high rate of dysplasia [158]. Gastric adenomas can occur in less than one-fifth of all FAP patients and are usually located in the antrum [140]. Other manifestations include desmoid tumors, which are usually intra-abdominal. In addition, patients with FAP are at risk for endocrine tumors such as adrenal gland tumors and thyroid papillary carcinoma. Attenuated FAP (AFAP) differs from FAP in that these patients have a later onset of CRC.

The diagnosis of FAP is made by the initial observation of multiple colorectal or duodenal adenomas followed by confirmation with genetic testing for mutation of the APC gene. If the test for the FAP gene is negative, then a test should be performed for the MYH-associated polyposis (MAP) gene. An individual with an APC mutation should have a flexible sigmoidoscopy starting at 10–12 years of age [159–162]. If an adenoma is detected, surgery should be considered in the patient. In AFAP, screening should start at age of 18 years since the disease has a later onset. If an adenoma is detected, the individual should be placed in a yearly colonoscopy surveillance program. With regard to the surveillance of duodenal carcinoma, endoscopy with both forward and side-viewing scopes should begin at the age of 20.

Polyps

Polyps can be classified in several ways that include size, histology, anatomic location, morphology, and degree of dysplasia. In this section, there will be a discussion of traditional adenomas, which are considered neoplastic. In addition, hyperplastic or serrated lesions will be discussed in light of recent data suggesting their prominent role in carcinogenesis.

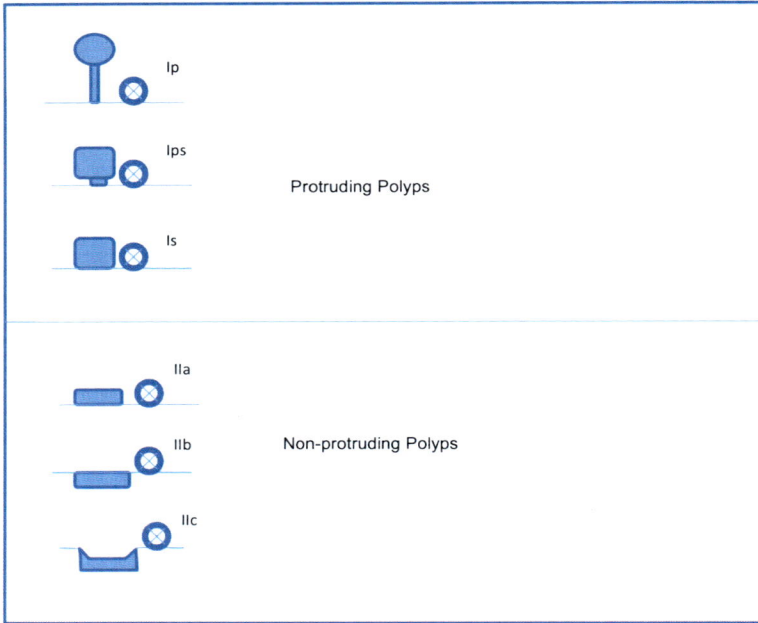

Fig. 1.1 The Paris classification divides polyps into protruding and non-protruding lesions

Traditional Adenomas

Histology

Adenoma histology has classically been described as tubular, villous, or tubulovillous. Over 90% of adenomas will have tubular pathology with less than 10% having some villous elements [55]. The majority of the tubular adenomas will be less than one centimeter in diameter as demonstrated in endoscopic studies of asymptomatic patients [24, 55, 163]. Although the majority of adenomas will be tubular adenomas, villous adenomas are of greater interest with regard to screening. Villous adenomas pose a challenge to the endoscopist since there is great variability to the pathologist's interpretation with regard to presence and extent of villous tissue. Rex et al. suggested that one quality indicator should be that villous adenomas account for less than 10% of all adenomas found [164]. In a study of 3,121 asymptomatic veterans, Lieberman et al. observed that 1,171 patients had adenomas [55]. There were 93 (93/1,171; 7.9%) patients who had adenomas with at least 25% villous elements. The primary importance of villous histology is in its role in defining an advanced adenoma.

Morphology

Adenomas can be classified as flat or protruding, and there are two schemes by which these morphologies can be described. The Japanese Research Society Classification (JRSC) defines flat lesions as those where the height is less than one-half the measured diameter [165–167]. The Paris classification divides lesions into those that are protruding versus those that are non-protruding [168, 169]. This is based on whether the lesion protrudes into the lumen a distance of at least 2.5 mm or the approximate width of a standard snare catheter. Adenomas are categorized into protruding which included pedunculated (Ip), sessile (Is), and mixed (Ips). The non-protruding or flat adenomas include elevated (IIa), flat (IIb), and depressed (IIc). A representation of the Paris classification is shown in Fig. 1.1.

Over the last decade there has been a significant amount of speculation regarding adenoma morphology and its possible association with advanced neoplasia or frank malignancy. Soetikno et al. reported that while less than 15% of 1,819 patients from a veteran's hospital population demonstrated flat adenomas, 6.6% of these lesions had high-grade dysplasia or more ominous features [170]. These data suggested that while only a fraction of adenomas were flat, these lesions had a higher rate of advanced pathology than protruding adenomas. However with the advent of high-definition endoscopy, there are more data to suggest that non-protruding adenomas are common and that among these lesions, depressed morphology is the most important predictor of advanced pathology.

In a study by Kahi et al., there were 780 adenomas found, of which 338 (43.3%) were non-polypoid [171]. Most of the flat lesions were classified as IIa. Among the advanced lesions, only two protruding carcinomas were detected. In an Italian population of 27,400 patients, there were 4,154 patients with adenomas [172]. There were 25.9% of the patients who had non-polypoid adenomas, with a total of 1,121 flat adenomas detected. Among the 176 adenomas with HGD or greater, there was no difference in the prevalence of flat versus polypoid adenomas. The size of the polyp was the most important factor of advanced histology in this study. However, there was a higher rate of HGD or greater in the depressed (IIc) group compared with adenomas that were flat (IIb) or elevated (IIa). In summary, recent data suggests that IIa lesions are the most common morphology and that flat adenomas have high risk of advanced pathology if they present as IIc lesions [173].

Prevalence and Location of Adenomas

Adenomas can be located throughout the colon in at least 20% of all patients older than 50 years. However, there can be great variation with regard to anatomical location and prevalence. With regard to anatomic location, two separate studies examining female and male veterans observed that women [56] were more likely to have proximal neoplasia than men [55]. Anderson et al., in a study of nearly 2,000 screening patients, observed that age greater than 60 years, smoking, and a family history of CRC increased the

likelihood of isolated proximal neoplasia [174]. This is neoplasia that would not have been detected on flexible sigmoidoscopy because it was proximally located and had no index distal lesion that would have prompted a full colonoscopy.

With regard to the prevalence of adenomas, there is also great variation. Although the quality benchmark for the percentage of patients with adenomas detected on a screening exam is 20% [164], many recent studies using high-definition colonoscopy have demonstrated higher detection rates. For example, in their study comparing white light to narrow band imaging, Rex and Heilbig found that over 50% of screening patients had adenomas [175]. In their study of over 600 asymptomatic patients, Kahi et al. examined the difference between white light high-definition colonoscopy versus high-definition colonoscopy plus chromoendoscopy with indigo carmine [171]. The percentage of patients with at least one adenoma detected was 55.5% for the chromoendoscopy arm and 48.4% for the white light-only group. Another recent study of 600 asymptomatic patients demonstrated an adenoma detection rate of approximately 40% [176].

Advanced Features

Advanced adenomas are lesions that have been identified as important targets with regard to screening. Adenomas with features such as size equal to or exceeding one centimeter, containing villous histology, high-grade dysplasia, and/or adenocarcinoma can qualify as an advanced adenoma. These lesions are important due to their malignant potential as well as their association with future neoplasia. Good evidence to support the role of advanced adenomas in the development of CRC can be found in a British study that followed 1,618 patients [177]. Patients who had polyps that were large (>1 cm) or had villous tissue were more likely to develop CRC than the general population (OR=3.6; 95% CI: 2.4–5.0). Recently, Lieberman et al. examined the 5-year follow-up after a baseline screening examination in 3,121 male veterans [178]. This study examined the risk for developing an advanced adenoma depending on the baseline findings. The relative

Table 1.1 Prevalence of advanced adenomas in screening populations

Study	Year	Country	Population	Advanced adenomas
VA 380 [55]	2000	USA	3,121 male veterans aged 50–75 years	10.5% (329/3,121)
University of Navarra [186]	2003	Spain	Asymptomatic patients ($n=2,210$) older than 40 years	7.0% (156/2,210)
Eli Lilly [163, 188]	2003	USA	Asymptomatic patients ($n=3,025$) older than 50 years	6.0% (181/3,025)
CONCeRN [56]	2005	USA	1,463 asymptomatic female veterans aged 50–79 years	4.9% (72/1,463)
Tel Aviv Sourasky Medical Center [187]	2006	Israel	1,177 people aged 40–80	6.3% (74/1,177)
Rockford Gastroenterology [183]	2006	USA	2,053 patients with no previous screening	5.2% (107/2,053)
Maria Sklodowska-Curie Memorial Cancer Center[185]	2006	Poland	50,148 patients ages 40–66. Those less than 50 had a family history of CRC	5.6% (2,796/50,148)
University of Wisconsin [184]	2007	USA	Study compared screening with CTC ($n=3,120$) and OC ($n=3,163$)	CTC: 3.2% (100) OC: 3.4% (107)
CORI [71]	2008	USA	Asymptomatic patients from 17 sites ($n=11,854$)	5.9% avg risk 5.7% Fam Hx CRC or adenoma

risk in patients was 6.40 (95% CI: 2.74–14.94) with tubular adenomas at least 10 mm in size, 6.05 (95% CI: 2.48–14.71) for villous adenomas, and 6.87 (95% CI: 2.61–18.07) for adenomas with high-grade dysplasia. Conversely, the risk was only 1.92 (95% CI: 0.83–4.42) with one or two tubular adenomas <10 mm in size. One corollary was that the risk of CRC in patients with three or more tubular adenomas <10 mm in size was almost as high as the advanced adenomas (RR=5.01; 95% CI: 2.10–11.96). Many other trials such as the National Polyp Study [35, 179], the pooled chemoprevention trials [180], and European calcium trial [181] have reported that adenoma multiplicity is a strong predictor of advanced neoplasia on follow-up exam [182]. Thus although they are not considered an advanced adenoma, the presence of multiple (at least 3) adenomas of any size is an important predictor of future advanced neoplasia.

With regard to the prevalence of advanced adenomas, there are several factors that can affect these rates. These include age, gender, family history of CRC, as well as other lifestyle factors such as smoking and BMI. The overall rates can vary from 3 to 10% [55, 56, 71, 81, 163, 183–188]. Screening studies provide the most reliable data

for prevalence of these lesions, and results from some of the more notable studies are shown in Table 1.1. It is important to note that most of these studies do not comment on sessile serrated adenomas.

Size

Size is an important characteristic for adenomas as the risk for high-grade dysplasia is directly related to this measurement. Although, there are many endoscopists who measure polyp size with an open forceps method, there is data to suggest that the pathologist's measurement is more accurate [189]. Muto et al. observed that the rate of high-grade dysplasia in polyps <1 cm in size was 1.1% compared with larger polyps that had a rate of greater than 10% [190]. One analysis from the National Polyp Study found that the prevalence of high-grade dysplasia was 1.1% in adenomas less than 5 mm in size, 4.6% in patients with 5–9 mm adenomas, and 20.6% in patients with adenomas at least 1 cm in size [191]. Butterly et al. examined 1,933 adenomas resected from 3,291 colonoscopies for evidence of advanced pathology defined by the presence of villous elements, high-grade dysplasia, or adenocarcinoma [192]. In that analysis, they observed that the rate of advanced pathology was 1.7% for adenomas 4 mm or smaller and 10.1% for adenomas that were 5–10 mm.

A similar study was performed by Tsai and Strum on adenomas resected from nearly 5,000 patients who had received a screening colonoscopy [193]. In that population, there were 930 patients with at least one adenoma, 248 with advanced adenomas, and 8 with adenocarcinoma. With regard to size, there were 89 polyps one centimeter or larger, and 76 (85%) had advanced pathology. In this study, advanced pathology is defined as the presence of villous tissue, high-grade dysplasia, or adenocarcinoma. Among the 6–9 mm polyps, 67 (27%) were advanced and 105 (10%) of 1,025 polyps ≤ 5 mm had advanced histology. These rates of advanced pathology are much higher than previous studies. In Table 1.2, the results of other selected studies demonstrating the risk of advanced histology relative to adenoma and polyp size are shown.

Size is not only important with regard to the risk of malignancy. The increasing detection rate of diminutive polyps (<5 mm) may force endoscopists to alter how they treat these small lesions in the course of colon cancer screening. As previously noted, studies that have employed high-definition colonoscopes [27, 171, 175, 176, 191] have yielded adenoma detection rates in screening populations that are much higher than in previously published studies [24, 55, 56, 163]. Resection of these polyps can be associated with complications and substantial pathology costs. Therefore, the benefit from removal is small given the low risk of malignancy. In response to these issues, some experts have recommended a "resect and discard" policy which is designed to decrease cost while maintaining the efficacy of cancer prevention with colonoscopy [196]. While this recommendation appears to address the concern of cost, there are other concerns such as patient acceptance of this policy that require further examination. Another issue is how to deal with multiple polyps. Specifically, while it is recognized and accepted that small adenomas individually pose a small risk with regard to malignant potential and metachronous lesions [178], multiple adenomas have been shown to be

predictive of future adenomas [197, 198]. Although discarding one or two small polyps is unlikely to change surveillance recommendations for the patient, detection of more than two adenomas may change the interval of surveillance by several years. Thus, histologic confirmation by a pathologist may be needed for patients with multiple polyps. Finally, with an increasing detection rate for these small adenomas, we may want to consider raising the threshold for shorter surveillance intervals from three adenomas to a higher number. Thus, more studies evaluating these issues are required.

A study by Rex et al. demonstrates the significance of lesions less than one centimeter in size [195]. In that study, they examined the "high-risk adenoma" rates in patients who underwent an endoscopic examination. High-risk adenomas were defined as advanced adenomas and multiple adenomas. Of the 10,034 patients, there were 5,079 who had at least one adenoma and 1,001 patients with high-risk adenomas. Among patients with high-risk adenomas, 293 (29%) had three adenomas less than 5 mm ($n = 267$) or advanced pathology ($n = 26$). Of the 774 patients with one or two adenomas 6–9 mm in size, 184 (18%) had multiple adenomas ($n = 149$) or had an adenoma with advanced pathology ($n = 35$). This study reinforces that adenomas less than 1 cm can have significant pathology. However, this study also demonstrates the number of patients with multiple adenomas that are either less than 9 mm (18% of the 1,001 high-risk patients) or less than 5 mm (27%).

Serrated Pathway

In 1990, Longacre and Fenoglio-Preiser published data on polyps that had features of both hyperplastic polyps and adenomas [199]. The authors believed that these polyps represented a variant of a villous polyp rather than two separate polyps juxtaposed together. These polyps were denoted serrated adenomas because of the pattern of the architecture.

Since their initial description, these polyps have gained a great deal of interest because of the many challenges that they pose. The first challenge lies in the rapidly changing nomenclature

Table 1.2 Prevalence of advanced histology as a function of adenoma and polyp size

Study	0–5 mm		6–9 mm		≥10 mm	
	Adenomas	Polyps	Adenomas	Polyps	Adenomas	Polyps
Butterly et al. [192]	2.7% (35/1,305)	N/A	8.2% (40/487)	N/A	25.8% (35/141)	N/A
Lieberman et al. [194]	2.5% (46/1,880)	1.2% (46/3,744)	7.9% (64/811)	5.3% (64/1,198)	35.2% (274/778)	28.9% (274/949)
Rex et al. [195]	1.9% (79/4,211)	0.9% (79/8,798)	9.9% (68/689)	5.3% (68/1,282)	N/A	N/A
Tsai et al. [193]	16.0% (105/656)	10.2% (105/1,025)	3.4% (67/198)	27.1% (67/247)	59.2% (45/76)	50.1% (45/89)

of these lesions. Recently, these lesions have been divided into hyperplastic polyps (HP), sessile serrated adenomas (SSA), and traditional serrated adenomas (TSA) [200]. Another recognized, but less commonly used, category is the "mixed polyp" with adenomatous tissue juxtaposed next to hyperplastic tissue. Another challenge lies in the pathologic interpretation of serrated polyps as there are several studies that have demonstrated significant variability among pathologists in interpreting and classifying these lesions [201, 202].

The classification of HP can be divided into two subgroups: the microvesicular serrated polyps (MVSP) and the goblet cell serrated polyps (GCSP), which are primarily located in the distal colon [203]. The GCSP have enlarged distended crypts with many goblet cells in the upper half of the crypts and prominent tufting of the epithelium. Conversely, the MVSP have long funnel-shaped crypts with prominent serration in the upper portion of the crypt. The MVSP appear to have similar molecular abnormalities to SSA and may evolve into these more advanced lesions. On the other hand, it is not known if GCSP progress to SSA or another advanced lesion. An excellent study that demonstrates this divergence is an examination by Rosenberg et al. of the molecular profile of aberrant crypt foci (ACF). ACF are small lesions, one or two crypts in size, that were used by this group as models of carcinogenesis. In this study, Rosenberg et al. observed that ACF with distended crypts were more likely to have KRAS abnormalities, while serrated ACF were more likely to have BRAF mutations. The KRAS lesion is mutually exclusive with BRAF mutations and rarely found in SSA [204].

Sessile serrated adenomas (SSA) are characterized by similar features to MVSP in the upper crypts, but irregularity of the architecture of the lower crypts. This gives the crypts the appearance of an upside "L" or "T." With regard to molecular abnormalities, SSA have BRAF mutations and are CIMP-H lesions [205, 206]. SSA are often proximally located and are often difficult to detect as they often present as flat (IIb) or superficially elevated (IIa) lesions [207]. They frequently can be detected by the presence of a yellowish mucous cap covering the polyp [208].

SSA usually exhibit a type II pit pattern or stellate-shaped pattern due to their serrated crypt formation. In addition, some SSA may develop dysplasia and therefore exhibit a type III or IV pit pattern seen in adenomas.

Another important feature of SSA is their strong association with advanced neoplasia. A few studies have demonstrated that large serrated polyps are likely to have synchronous advanced neoplasia [209, 210]. Hyperplastic polyposis syndrome (HPS) is characterized by multiple HP throughout the colon. In SSA that are adjacent to carcinoma, the transition zone is dysplastic. In addition, Goldstein et al. examined eight serrated polyps with a focus of malignancy [211]. They observed that these serrated polyps averaged 8.3 mm in size, that the carcinoma in these polyps averaged 2.8 mm in size, and that it invaded the submucosa without spreading laterally. Thus SSA appear to have a proclivity to become advanced lesions and could be considered precursors of CRC.

Another group of serrated lesions is TSA which are characterized by serration and a uniform population of dysplastic cells which are columnar with eosinophilic cytoplasm. These polyps tend to be protuberant, unlike SSA which are typically flat. TSA are believed to be a separate entity from SSA with dysplasia, despite both having serration and dysplasia. One important distinguishing factor between the two histologic types is the observation that ectopic crypts are found in TSA. These are crypts whose bases are adjacent with the muscularis mucosa [212].

Another challenge that endoscopists face is the difficulty in detecting serrated polyps. As previously noted, serrated polyps are often proximally located and flat in morphology. A recent study by Kahi et al. observed a marked variation of 1–18% for the prevalence of serrated lesions in nearly 7,000 patients undergoing colonoscopy [213]. Furthermore, the detection rate of serrated lesions correlated with the detection rate of traditional adenomas. The authors concluded that successful detection of serrated polyps is likely dependent on adherence to quality indicators in the performance of colonoscopy.

Interval Cancer

Recently published data have suggested an anatomical difference with regard to the protective effect from colonoscopy. While the risk for distal advanced neoplasia and CRC is reduced in patients who have received a colonoscopy, the risk for proximal CRC is not reduced [214, 215]. Interval CRC is diagnosed between regularly scheduled screening or surveillance colonoscopies. Many studies have demonstrated a proximal proclivity for interval tumors. A study by Bressler et al. demonstrated that older age and female gender are risk factors for interval cancers [28].

There have been several explanations proposed to explain interval neoplasia. Interval CRC may arise from previously resected polyps. Cancers arising from inadequate resection of adenomas may account for a large percentage of interval cancers. Another possibility includes the potential differences in the biology between right- and left-sided neoplasia. The methylation pathway may provide an answer with regard to biological explanations given the proximal location, accelerated path to advanced pathology, and difficulties in detection of interval CRC. One study by Arain et al. observed that interval CRC has a higher rate of CIMP than non-interval cancers [216]. As previously discussed, this molecular abnormality is the hallmark of SSA.

Missed lesions are also likely to play an important role in interval CRC. Major reasons for missing lesions during colonoscopy involve technical performance issues that limit intubation and visualization of the right bowel. The study by Bressler et al. observed that factors affecting performance of colonoscopy can be associated with interval CRC [28]. These include the presence of diverticular disease or pelvic surgery in women [217, 218]. Furthermore, these investigators also observed that having a colonoscopy in an office or performed by an internist or by a family practitioner is also an independent risk factor for interval CRC.

Other factors may result in missed lesions even when the cecum is intubated. Inadequate preparation of the colon as well as quick withdrawal time may result in colorectal neoplasia going undetected. Rex has published multiple papers recommending quality indicators to maximize adenoma detection during colonoscopy [173, 219, 220]. These included adequate withdrawal time, adequate preparation time, and a minimum cecal intubation rate of 90%. Following these recommendations should result in overall adenoma detection rate (ADR) of 20%. Adenoma detection rate is the percentage of all patients in whom an adenoma was detected and is considered the main benchmark with regard to quality of colonoscopy. The importance of two of these quality indicators was validated in landmark colonoscopy studies. The first was an analysis by Barclay et al. of the adenoma detection rate in a population of nearly 8,000 patients who had an endoscopy by one of 12 experienced gastroenterologists [183]. They compared the adenoma detection rate between the endoscopists who used more than 6 min to withdraw the colonoscope versus those who used less than 6 min. Compared with endoscopists with shorter withdrawal times, those with longer withdrawal times had higher rates of detection of any neoplasia (28.3% vs. 11.8%, $P<0.001$) and more importantly of advanced neoplasia (6.4% vs. 2.6%, $P=0.005$). A second study was performed by Kaminski et al. in a population of over 45,000 patients who received a screening colonoscopy [221]. There was a higher rate of interval CRC among endoscopists with an ADR of less than 20%. Thus, one could conclude that better technique such as longer withdrawal time should result in a higher ADR and subsequently lower interval CRC rate.

Pohl and Robertson designed a novel analysis to estimate the frequency of missed interval cancers [222]. They calculated the proportion of missed lesions that resulted from missed adenomas at baseline. Key assumptions based on the literature included published adenoma miss rates, adenoma prevalence rates, and adenoma–carcinoma transition rates. Their analysis demonstrated that the rate for interval CRC within 5 years of screening could range from 0.5/1,000 interval CRC for the lowest adenoma miss rates to 3.5/1,000 for the highest adenoma miss rates.

Staging of CRC

The Dukes' classification was the earliest form of CRC staging. Originally published in 1929, the Dukes' classification has been the most widely used and accepted CRC staging scheme. This classification used intraoperative findings and was based on patients who had undergone a potentially curative resection [223, 224]. The first stage was A for any tumor confined to the submucosa or the muscularis propria. Stage B was for any tumor that penetrated the muscularis propria and invades directly into the peri-colorectal tissue, the surface of visceral peritoneum or adjacent organs or structures. The modified Astler–Coller classification was different in that it subcategorized the Dukes' stages (ABC) into numbered categories to differentiate tumor penetration levels. In addition, tumors penetrating the muscularis propria were taken out of the "A" category and classified as B2. Since this classification, the TNM or tumor-node-metastasis classification

has been used by the Union Internationale Contre le Cancer (UICC) and the American Joint Committee on Cancer (AJCC) [225]. The most important aspect of the staging for CRC pertains to the treatment, which will be discussed in the next section. In the TNM classification, the N category is divided into N0, N1, and N2 depending upon the number of positive lymph nodes. The M category is categorized by the number of organs that the tumor has involved.

The following is the breakdown for the T staging:

- Tis: Tumor confined to the mucosa.
- T1: Tumor extends through the muscularis mucosa into the submucosa.
- T2: Tumor extends through the submucosa into the muscularis propria.
- T3: Tumor extends through the muscularis propria into serosa but not through the bowel wall.
- T4a: Tumor extends through the serosa.
- T4b: Tumor extends though the wall of the colon and invades nearby structures/organs.

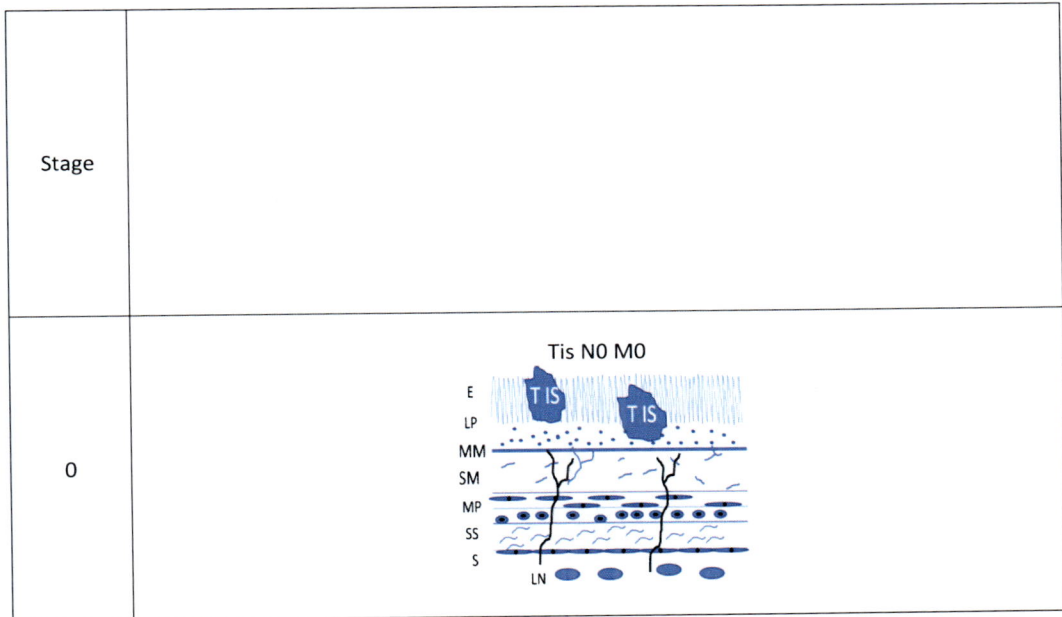

Fig. 1.2 A representation of the stages for colorectal cancer according to the American Joint Committee on Cancer (AJCC)

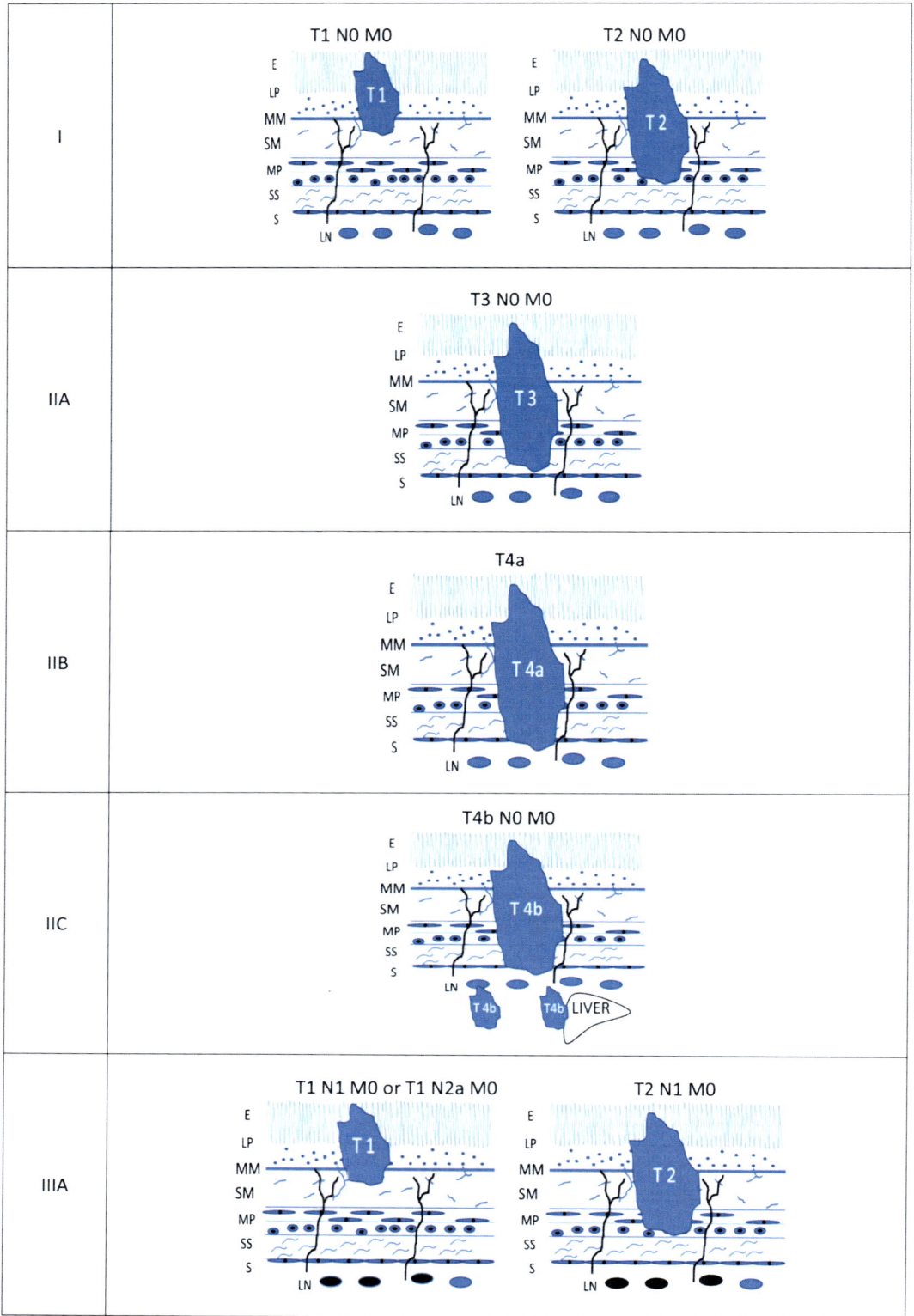

Fig. 1.2 (continued)

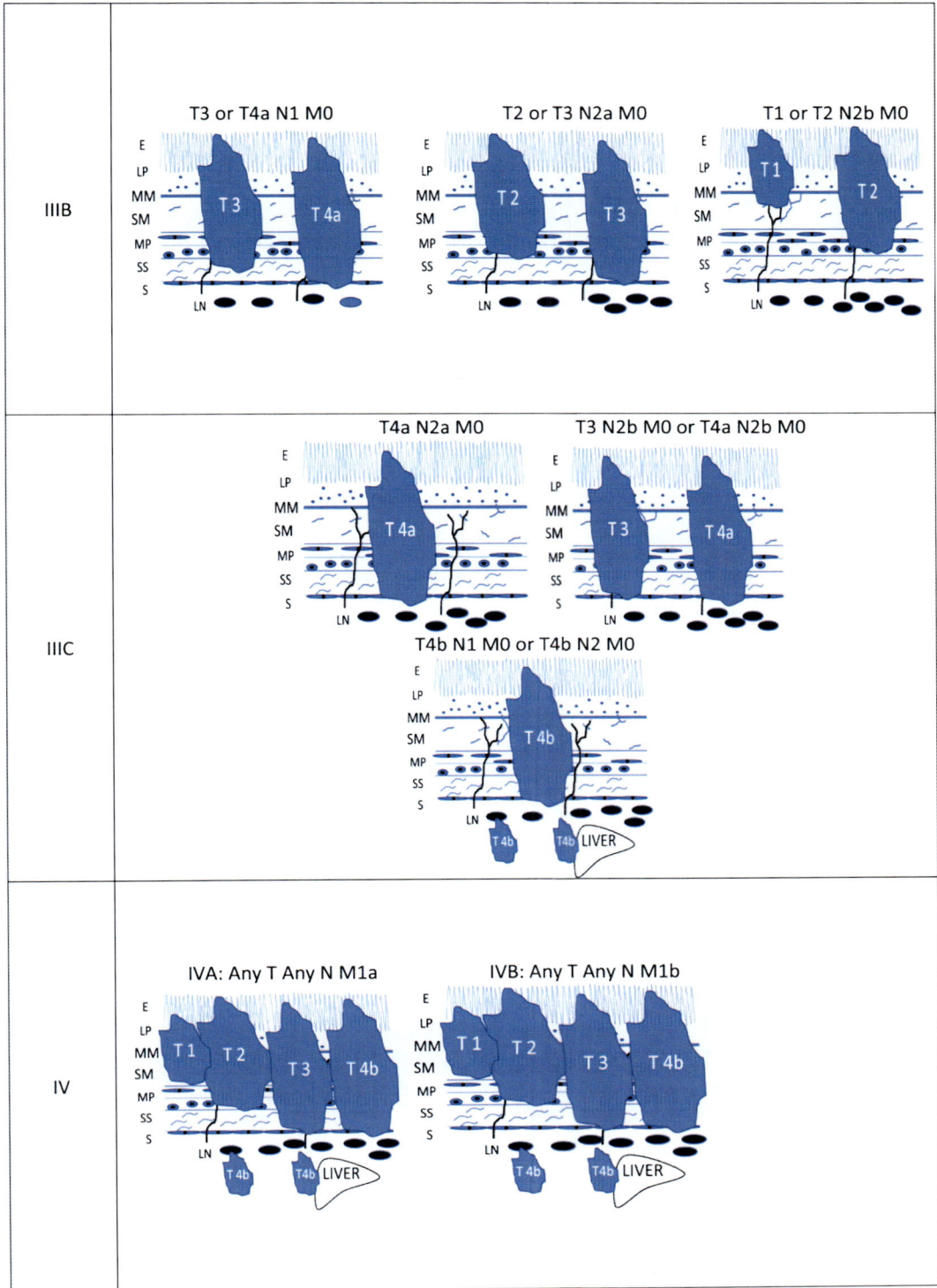

Fig. 1.2 (continued)

The stages of CRC (Figs. 1.1 and 1.2) according to the AJCC guidelines are the following:

- Stage 0: Tis, N0, M0
- Stage I: T1 or T2, N0, M0
- Stage IIA: T3, N0, M0
- Stage IIB: T4a, N0, M0
- Stage IIC: T4b, N0, M0
- Stage IIIA: T1 or T2, N1, M0
- Stage IIIB: T3 or T4a, N1, M0; T2 or T3, N2a, M0; T1 or T2, N2b, M0
- Stage IIIC: T4a, N2a, M0; T3 or T4a, N2b, M0; T1 or T4b, N1 or N2, M0
- Stage IVA: Any T, any N, M1a
- Stage IVB: Any T, any N, M1b
This is shown in Fig. 1.2.

Thus, when a tumor is resected, the following factors need to be reported for staging:

- Grade of the cancer
- Depth of penetration (T)
- Number of lymph nodes evaluated and number that are positive (N)
- Status of proximal, distal, and radial margins
- Presence of lymphovascular invasion
- Presence of perineural invasion
- Presence of extranodal tumor deposits

Treatment of CRC

The treatment of CRC depends on the stage of disease, with colon and rectal cancers having different recommendations from the National Comprehensive Cancer Network (NCCN). The recommendations are usually surgery with or without adjuvant therapy in the form of chemotherapy or radiation. With regard to colon cancer, Stage I can be treated with surgery and does not require adjuvant therapy. Stage II can be treated with surgery, and adjuvant therapy may be used for patients with risk factors that indicate a high rate of recurrence. These factors include tumor grade of 3 or 4, the presence of lymphatic/vascular invasion, bowel obstruction or perforation, or close/indeterminate surgical margins. Adjuvant therapy can be in the form of chemotherapy with 5-FU/leucovorin/oxaliplatin or other chemotherapy agents such as capecitabine. Stage III colon cancer can be treated with surgery and chemotherapy in the form of one of several agents. The treatment of Stage IV colon cancer is dependent on whether the metastases are resectable. For example, if there is a single liver metastasis, then treatment is the surgical removal of both the primary tumor and liver lesion and chemotherapy.

The major difference between rectal and colon cancer is that the former has a higher rate of recurrence partly due to anatomic difficulty of resection in the pelvis [226]. Therefore, Stage II and III rectal cancers require adjuvant therapy in the form of chemoradiation therapy after curative resection. Neoadjuvant preoperative chemoradiation may improve outcomes by shrinking the tumor and increasing the success rate of surgery [227, 228].

Surgical Resection of CRC

Surgical resection of CRC is the cornerstone of treatment in this cancer. For colon cancer, a preoperative CT scan of the abdomen and pelvis as well as data from the colonoscopy provides the information that dictates the extent of the surgery. In rectal cancer, an endoscopic ultrasound and or pelvic MRI can aid in the staging of the cancer [229]. Currently, carcinoembryonic antigen (CEA) and histology or grade of the tumor do not play a role in determining the resection approach. Lymphatic drainage and blood supply are the main factors that dictate the extent of resection. In addition, the AJCC recommends the removal of at least 12 lymph nodes that drain the region of the cancer [225]. When the cancer is located above the peritoneal reflection, the main factor for the amount of colon resected is the mesenteric vasculature [229]. For right-sided cancer, a right hemicolectomy is performed which includes the appendix, cecum, ileocecal valve, ascending colon, hepatic flexure, and a portion of the proximal transverse colon. The resection line distally is the main trunk of the middle colic artery, which is left intact to preserve the blood supply to the remaining transverse colon. With regard to left-sided lesions, the colon is resected from the splenic flexure to just above the peritoneal reflection.

Rectal cancer differs from colon cancer because resection is technically more difficult. One of the main concerns in resecting rectal cancer is the preservation of a functional anal sphincter. The original approach to rectal cancer was a radical resection of the distal rectum and perineum. This method resulted in a permanent colostomy and had a high perineal wound complication rate [230]. The use of the low anterior approach has resulted in better sphincter preservation, but a technique known as total mesorectal excision (TME) has resulted in low recurrence rates [231]. TME involves the total surgical removal of the pelvic nodal tissue with the rectal tumor through sharp dissection. One of main factors that will help a surgeon decide between a sphincter-preserving approach and a more radical resection is the rectal examination. If there is sufficient length between the anal verge and the tumor, then a surgical approach with a colon-anal anastomosis will be considered.

Surveillance for Resected CRC

The recommendations by the NCCN for surveillance after resection of CRC include office visits, periodic CEA, chest/abdomen/pelvic CT, and colonoscopy. The intervals for these examinations are dependent on the stage of the tumor. With regard to colonoscopy, the multi-society task force recommends that a repeat exam be performed in 1 year if the initial colonoscopy was considered a complete evaluation [232]. If there was an obstructing mass or any other reason for incomplete visualization of the colon, then a complete colonoscopy 3–6 months after the surgery is recommended. On the surveillance examination, if there is an advanced lesion, then a repeat colonoscopy is recommended in 1 year. If that second exam is normal, then another colonoscopy should be performed in 3 years. If that exam is normal, then a repeat is recommended in 5 years.

References

1. Jemal A, Siegel R, Xu J, Ward E. Cancer statistics, 2010. CA Cancer J Clin. 2010;60:277–300.
2. Edwards BK, Ward E, Kohler BA, et al. Annual report to the nation on the status of cancer, 1975-2006, featuring colorectal cancer trends and impact of interventions (risk factors, screening, and treatment) to reduce future rates. Cancer. 2010;116: 544–73.
3. Naishadham D, Lansdorp-Vogelaar I, Siegel R, Cokkinides V, Jemal A. State disparities in colorectal cancer mortality patterns in the United States. Cancer Epidemiol Biomarkers Prev. 2011;20:1296–302.
4. Ferlay J, Autier P, Boniol M, et al. Estimates of the cancer incidence and mortality in Europe in 2006. Ann Oncol. 2007;18:581–92.
5. Ferlay J, Parkin DM, Steliarova-Foucher E. Estimates of cancer incidence and mortality in Europe in 2008. Eur J Cancer. 2010;46:765–81.
6. La Vecchia C, Bosetti C, Lucchini F, et al. Cancer mortality in Europe, 2000-2004, and an overview of trends since 1975. Ann Oncol. 2010;21:1323–60.
7. Karim-Kos HE, de Vries E, Soerjomataram I, et al. Recent trends of cancer in Europe: a combined approach of incidence, survival and mortality for 17 cancer sites since the 1990s. Eur J Cancer. 2008;44:1345–89.
8. Brenner H, Bouvier AM, Foschi R, et al. Progress in colorectal cancer survival in Europe, from the late 1980s to the early 21st century: the EUROCARE study. Int J Cancer. 2012;131(7):1649–58.
9. Bosetti C, Levi F, Rosato V, et al. Recent trends in colorectal cancer mortality in Europe. Int J Cancer. 2010;129:180–91.
10. Center MM, Jemal A, Ward E. International trends in colorectal cancer incidence rates. Cancer Epidemiol Biomarkers Prev. 2009;18:1688–94.
11. Parkin DM, Bray F, Ferlay J, Pisani P. Global cancer statistics, 2002. CA Cancer J Clin. 2005;55:74–108.
12. Gellad ZF, Provenzale D. Colorectal cancer: national and international perspective on the burden of disease and public health impact. Gastroenterology. 2010;138:2177–90.
13. Iacopetta B. Are there two sides to colorectal cancer? Int J Cancer. 2002;101:403–8.
14. Skinner SA, O'Brien PE. The microvascular structure of the normal colon in rats and humans. J Surg Res. 1996;61:482–90.
15. McBain AJ, Macfarlane GT. Ecological and physiological studies on large intestinal bacteria in relation to production of hydrolytic and reductive enzymes involved in formation of genotoxic metabolites. J Med Microbiol. 1998;47:407–16.
16. Distler P, Holt PR. Are right- and left-sided colon neoplasms distinct tumors? Dig Dis. 1997;15:302–11.
17. Nawa T, Kato J, Kawamoto H, et al. Differences between right- and left-sided colon cancer in patient characteristics, cancer morphology and histology. J Gastroenterol Hepatol. 2008;23:418–23.
18. Miyakura Y, Sugano K, Konishi F, et al. Extensive methylation of hMLH1 promoter region predominates in proximal colon cancer with microsatellite instability. Gastroenterology. 2001;121:1300–9.
19. Okamoto M, Kawabe T, Yamaji Y, et al. Flat-type early colorectal cancer preferentially develops in

right-sided colon in older patients. Dis Colon Rectum. 2005;48:101–7.

20. Cooper GS, Yuan Z, Landefeld CS, Johanson JF, Rimm AA. A national population-based study of incidence of colorectal cancer and age. Implications for screening in older Americans. Cancer. 1995;75:775–81.

21. Jass JR. Subsite distribution and incidence of colorectal cancer in New Zealand, 1974-1983. Dis Colon Rectum. 1991;34:56–9.

22. Slattery ML, Friedman GD, Potter JD, et al. A description of age, sex, and site distributions of colon carcinoma in three geographic areas. Cancer. 1996;78:1666–70.

23. Anderson JC, Alpern Z, Sethi G, et al. Prevalence and risk of colorectal neoplasia in consumers of alcohol in a screening population. Am J Gastroenterol. 2005;100:2049–55.

24. Anderson JC, Attam R, Alpern Z, et al. Prevalence of colorectal neoplasia in smokers. Am J Gastroenterol. 2003;98:2777–83.

25. Poynter JN, Haile RW, Siegmund KD, et al. Associations between smoking, alcohol consumption, and colorectal cancer, overall and by tumor microsatellite instability status. Cancer Epidemiol Biomarkers Prev. 2009;18:2745–50.

26. Anderson JC. Risk factors and diagnosis of flat adenomas of the colon. Expert Rev Gastroenterol Hepatol. 2011;5:25–32.

27. Anderson JC, Stein B, Kahi CJ, et al. Association of smoking and flat adenomas: results from an asymptomatic population screened with a high-definition colonoscope. Gastrointest Endosc. 2010;71:1234–40.

28. Bressler B, Paszat LF, Chen Z, et al. Rates of new or missed colorectal cancers after colonoscopy and their risk factors: a population-based analysis. Gastroenterology. 2007;132:96–102.

29. Fearon ER, Vogelstein B. A genetic model for colorectal tumorigenesis. Cell. 1990;61:759–67.

30. Pino MS, Chung DC. The chromosomal instability pathway in colon cancer. Gastroenterology. 2010;138:2059–72.

31. Saif MW, Chu E. Biology of colorectal cancer. Cancer J. 2010;16:196–201.

32. Winawer SJ, Fletcher RH, Miller L, et al. Colorectal cancer screening: clinical guidelines and rationale. Gastroenterology. 1997;112:594–642.

33. Kozuka S, Nogaki M, Ozeki T, Masumori S. Premalignancy of the mucosal polyp in the large intestine: II. Estimation of the periods required for malignant transformation of mucosal polyps. Dis Colon Rectum. 1975;18:494–500.

34. Koretz RL. Malignant polyps: are they sheep in wolves' clothing? Ann Intern Med. 1993;118:63–8.

35. Winawer SJ, Zauber AG, Ho MN, et al. Prevention of colorectal cancer by colonoscopic polypectomy. The National Polyp Study Workgroup. N Engl J Med. 1993;329:1977–81.

36. Morson B. President's address. The polyp-cancer sequence in the large bowel. Proc R Soc Med. 1974;67:451–7.

37. Grady WM. Genomic instability and colon cancer. Cancer Metastasis Rev. 2004;23:11–27.

38. Rajagopalan H, Lengauer C. Aneuploidy and cancer. Nature. 2004;432:338–41.

39. Boland CR, Goel A. Microsatellite instability in colorectal cancer. Gastroenterology. 2010;138:2073–2087.e2073.

40. Hoeijmakers JH. Genome maintenance mechanisms for preventing cancer. Nature. 2001;411:366–74.

41. Boland CR, Thibodeau SN, Hamilton SR, et al. A National Cancer Institute Workshop on Microsatellite Instability for cancer detection and familial predisposition: development of international criteria for the determination of microsatellite instability in colorectal cancer. Cancer Res. 1998;58:5248–57.

42. Deng G, Chen A, Hong J, Chae HS, Kim YS. Methylation of CpG in a small region of the hMLH1 promoter invariably correlates with the absence of gene expression. Cancer Res. 1999;59:2029–33.

43. Rashid A, Issa JP. CpG island methylation in gastroenterologic neoplasia: a maturing field. Gastroenterology. 2004;127:1578–88.

44. Toyota M, Ahuja N, Ohe-Toyota M, et al. CpG island methylator phenotype in colorectal cancer. Proc Natl Acad Sci USA. 1999;96:8681–6.

45. Issa JP. CpG island methylator phenotype in cancer. Nat Rev Cancer. 2004;4:988–93.

46. Samowitz WS, Sweeney C, Herrick J, et al. Poor survival associated with the BRAF V600E mutation in microsatellite-stable colon cancers. Cancer Res. 2005;65:6063–9.

47. Whitehall VL, Wynter CV, Walsh MD, et al. Morphological and molecular heterogeneity within nonmicrosatellite instability-high colorectal cancer. Cancer Res. 2002;62:6011–4.

48. Nagasaka T, Koi M, Kloor M, et al. Mutations in both KRAS and BRAF may contribute to the methylator phenotype in colon cancer. Gastroenterology. 2008;134:1950–60, 1960.e1951.

49. Majumdar SR, Fletcher RH, Evans AT. How does colorectal cancer present? Symptoms, duration, and clues to location. Am J Gastroenterol. 1999;94:3039–45.

50. Stapley S, Peters TJ, Sharp D, Hamilton W. The mortality of colorectal cancer in relation to the initial symptom at presentation to primary care and to the duration of symptoms: a cohort study using medical records. Br J Cancer. 2006;95:1321–5.

51. Jullumstro E, Lydersen S, Moller B, Dahl O, Edna TH. Duration of symptoms, stage at diagnosis and relative survival in colon and rectal cancer. Eur J Cancer. 2009;45:2383–90.

52. Adelstein BA, Macaskill P, Chan SF, Katelaris PH, Irwig L. Most bowel cancer symptoms do not indicate colorectal cancer and polyps: a systematic review. BMC Gastroenterol. 2011;11:65.

53. Rex DK, Johnson DA, Anderson JC, et al. American College of Gastroenterology guidelines for colorectal cancer screening 2009 [corrected]. Am J Gastroenterol. 2009;104:739–50.

54. Kolligs FT, Crispin A, Munte A, et al. Risk of advanced colorectal neoplasia according to age and gender. PLoS One. 2011;6:e20076.

55. Lieberman DA, Weiss DG, Bond JH, et al. Use of colonoscopy to screen asymptomatic adults for colorectal cancer. Veterans Affairs Cooperative Study Group 380. N Engl J Med. 2000;343:162–8.

56. Schoenfeld P, Cash B, Flood A, et al. Colonoscopic screening of average-risk women for colorectal neoplasia. N Engl J Med. 2005;352:2061–8.

57. Nguyen SP, Bent S, Chen YH, Terdiman JP. Gender as a risk factor for advanced neoplasia and colorectal cancer: a systematic review and meta-analysis. Clin Gastroenterol Hepatol. 2009;7:676–81.e671–3.

58. Lieberman D. Race, gender, and colorectal cancer screening. Am J Gastroenterol. 2005;100:2756–8.

59. Roy HK, Bianchi LK. Differences in colon adenomas and carcinomas among women and men: potential clinical implications. JAMA. 2009;302:1696–7.

60. Chlebowski RT, Wactawski-Wende J, Ritenbaugh C, et al. Estrogen plus progestin and colorectal cancer in postmenopausal women. N Engl J Med. 2004;350:991–1004.

61. Johnson M, Feinn R, Anderson JC. Clinical factors associated with non-polypoid colonic adenomas 6 mm: a prospective study in an asymptomatic population using a high-definition colonoscope. Am J Gastroenterol. 2011;106(11):2018–22.

62. Soneji S, Iyer SS, Armstrong K, Asch DA. Racial disparities in stage-specific colorectal cancer mortality: 1960-2005. Am J Public Health. 2010;100:1912–6.

63. Siegel R, Ward E, Brawley O, Jemal A. Cancer statistics, 2011: the impact of eliminating socioeconomic and racial disparities on premature cancer deaths. CA Cancer J Clin. 2011;61:212–36.

64. Theuer CP, Wagner JL, Taylor TH, et al. Racial and ethnic colorectal cancer patterns affect the cost-effectiveness of colorectal cancer screening in the United States. Gastroenterology. 2001;120:848–56.

65. Ananthakrishnan AN, Schellhase KG, Sparapani RA, Laud PW, Neuner JM. Disparities in colon cancer screening in the Medicare population. Arch Intern Med. 2007;167:258–64.

66. McMahon Jr LF, Wolfe RA, Huang S, et al. Racial and gender variation in use of diagnostic colonic procedures in the Michigan Medicare population. Med Care. 1999;37:712–7.

67. Murphy G, Devesa SS, Cross AJ, et al. Sex disparities in colorectal cancer incidence by anatomic subsite, race and age. Int J Cancer. 2010;128:1668–75.

68. Irby K, Anderson WF, Henson DE, Devesa SS. Emerging and widening colorectal carcinoma disparities between Blacks and Whites in the United States (1975-2002). Cancer Epidemiol Biomarkers Prev. 2006;15:792–7.

69. Weiderpass E, Gridley G, Nyren O, et al. Diabetes mellitus and risk of large bowel cancer. J Natl Cancer Inst. 1997;89:660–1.

70. Hu FB, Manson JE, Liu S, et al. Prospective study of adult onset diabetes mellitus (type 2) and risk of colorectal cancer in women. J Natl Cancer Inst. 1999;91:542–7.

71. Lieberman DA, Holub JL, Moravec MD, et al. Prevalence of colon polyps detected by colonoscopy screening in asymptomatic black and white patients. JAMA. 2008;300:1417–22.

72. Agrawal S, Bhupinderjit A, Bhutani MS, et al. Colorectal cancer in African Americans. Am J Gastroenterol. 2005;100:515–23.

73. Anderson JC, Latreille M, Messina C, et al. Smokers as a high-risk group: data from a screening population. J Clin Gastroenterol. 2009;43:747–52, discussion 514.

74. Anderson JC, Moezardalan K, Messina CR, Latreille M, Shaw RD. Smoking and the association of advanced colorectal neoplasia in an asymptomatic average risk population: analysis of exposure and anatomical location in men and women. Dig Dis Sci. 2011;56(12):3616–23.

75. Giovannucci E, Colditz GA, Stampfer MJ, et al. A prospective study of cigarette smoking and risk of colorectal adenoma and colorectal cancer in U.S. women. J Natl Cancer Inst. 1994;86:192–9.

76. Giovannucci E, Rimm EB, Stampfer MJ, et al. A prospective study of cigarette smoking and risk of colorectal adenoma and colorectal cancer in U.S. men. J Natl Cancer Inst. 1994;86:183–91.

77. Lieberman DA, Prindiville S, Weiss DG, Willett W. Risk factors for advanced colonic neoplasia and hyperplastic polyps in asymptomatic individuals. JAMA. 2003;290:2959–67.

78. Slattery ML, Curtin K, Anderson K, et al. Associations between cigarette smoking, lifestyle factors, and microsatellite instability in colon tumors. J Natl Cancer Inst. 2000;92:1831–6.

79. Yu JH, Bigler J, Whitton J, Potter JD, Ulrich CM. Mismatch repair polymorphisms and colorectal polyps: hMLH1-93G>A variant modifies risk associated with smoking. Am J Gastroenterol. 2006;101:1313–9.

80. Samowitz WS, Albertsen H, Sweeney C, et al. Association of smoking, CpG island methylator phenotype, and V600E BRAF mutations in colon cancer. J Natl Cancer Inst. 2006;98:1731–8.

81. Kambara T, Simms LA, Whitehall VL, et al. BRAF mutation is associated with DNA methylation in serrated polyps and cancers of the colorectum. Gut. 2004;53:1137–44.

82. Weisenberger DJ, Siegmund KD, Campan M, et al. CpG island methylator phenotype underlies sporadic microsatellite instability and is tightly associated with BRAF mutation in colorectal cancer. Nat Genet. 2006;38:787–93.

83. Anderson JC, Pleau DC, Rajan TV, et al. Increased frequency of serrated aberrant crypt foci among smokers. Am J Gastroenterol. 2010;105:1648–54.

84. Giovannucci E. An updated review of the epidemiological evidence that cigarette smoking increases

risk of colorectal cancer. Cancer Epidemiol Biomarkers Prev. 2001;10:725–31.

85. Heineman EF, Zahm SH, McLaughlin JK, Vaught JB. Increased risk of colorectal cancer among smokers: results of a 26-year follow-up of US veterans and a review. Int J Cancer. 1994;59:728–38.

86. Newcomb PA, Storer BE, Marcus PM. Cigarette smoking in relation to risk of large bowel cancer in women. Cancer Res. 1995;55:4906–9.

87. Paskett ED, Reeves KW, Rohan TE, et al. Association between cigarette smoking and colorectal cancer in the Women's Health Initiative. J Natl Cancer Inst. 2007;99:1729–35.

88. Slattery ML, Potter JD, Friedman GD, Ma KN, Edwards S. Tobacco use and colon cancer. Int J Cancer. 1997;70:259–64.

89. Sturmer T, Glynn RJ, Lee IM, Christen WG, Hennekens CH. Lifetime cigarette smoking and colorectal cancer incidence in the Physicians' Health Study I. J Natl Cancer Inst. 2000;92:1178–81.

90. Terry P, Ekbom A, Lichtenstein P, Feychting M, Wolk A. Long-term tobacco smoking and colorectal cancer in a prospective cohort study. Int J Cancer. 2001;91:585–7.

91. Chao A, Thun MJ, Jacobs EJ, et al. Cigarette smoking and colorectal cancer mortality in the cancer prevention study II. J Natl Cancer Inst. 2000;92:1888–96.

92. Colangelo LA, Gapstur SM, Gann PH, Dyer AR. Cigarette smoking and colorectal carcinoma mortality in a cohort with long-term follow-up. Cancer. 2004;100:288–93.

93. Campbell RJ, Ferrante JM, Gonzalez EC, et al. Predictors of advanced stage colorectal cancer diagnosis: results of a population-based study. Cancer Detect Prev. 2001;25:430–8.

94. Phipps AI, Baron J, Newcomb PA. Prediagnostic smoking history, alcohol consumption, and colorectal cancer survival: the Seattle Colon Cancer Family Registry. Cancer. 2011;117(21):4948–57.

95. Botteri E, Iodice S, Raimondi S, Maisonneuve P, Lowenfels AB. Cigarette smoking and adenomatous polyps: a meta-analysis. Gastroenterology. 2008;134:388–95.

96. Wiencke JK, Zheng S, Lafuente A, et al. Aberrant methylation of p16INK4a in anatomic and gender-specific subtypes of sporadic colorectal cancer. Cancer Epidemiol Biomarkers Prev. 1999;8:501–6.

97. Kennelly R, Kavanagh DO, Hogan AM, Winter DC. Oestrogen and the colon: potential mechanisms for cancer prevention. Lancet Oncol. 2008;9:385–91.

98. Haydon AM, Jass JR. Emerging pathways in colorectal-cancer development. Lancet Oncol. 2002;3:83–8.

99. Jee SH, Ohrr H, Sull JW, et al. Fasting serum glucose level and cancer risk in Korean men and women. JAMA. 2005;293:194–202.

100. Nilsen TI, Vatten LJ. Prospective study of colorectal cancer risk and physical activity, diabetes, blood glucose and BMI: exploring the hyperinsulinaemia hypothesis. Br J Cancer. 2001;84:417–22.

101. Saydah SH, Platz EA, Rifai N, et al. Association of markers of insulin and glucose control with subsequent colorectal cancer risk. Cancer Epidemiol Biomarkers Prev. 2003;12:412–8.

102. Ma J, Giovannucci E, Pollak M, et al. A prospective study of plasma C-peptide and colorectal cancer risk in men. J Natl Cancer Inst. 2004;96:546–53.

103. Grimberg A, Cohen P. Role of insulin-like growth factors and their binding proteins in growth control and carcinogenesis. J Cell Physiol. 2000; 183:1–9.

104. Gunter MJ, Leitzmann MF. Obesity and colorectal cancer: epidemiology, mechanisms and candidate genes. J Nutr Biochem. 2006;17:145–56.

105. Sandhu MS, Dunger DB, Giovannucci EL. Insulin, insulin-like growth factor-I (IGF-I), IGF binding proteins, their biologic interactions, and colorectal cancer. J Natl Cancer Inst. 2002;94:972–80.

106. Vinikoor LC, Long MD, Keku TO, et al. The association between diabetes, insulin use, and colorectal cancer among Whites and African Americans. Cancer Epidemiol Biomarkers Prev. 2009;18: 1239–42.

107. Yang YX, Hennessy S, Lewis JD. Type 2 diabetes mellitus and the risk of colorectal cancer. Clin Gastroenterol Hepatol. 2005;3:587–94.

108. Dai Z, Xu YC, Niu L. Obesity and colorectal cancer risk: a meta-analysis of cohort studies. World J Gastroenterol. 2007;13:4199–206.

109. Ford ES. Body mass index and colon cancer in a national sample of adult US men and women. Am J Epidemiol. 1999;150:390–8.

110. Larsson SC, Wolk A. Obesity and colon and rectal cancer risk: a meta-analysis of prospective studies. Am J Clin Nutr. 2007;86:556–65.

111. Moore LL, Bradlee ML, Singer MR, et al. BMI and waist circumference as predictors of lifetime colon cancer risk in Framingham Study adults. Int J Obes Relat Metab Disord. 2004;28:559–67.

112. Pischon T, Lahmann PH, Boeing H, et al. Body size and risk of colon and rectal cancer in the European Prospective Investigation Into Cancer and Nutrition (EPIC). J Natl Cancer Inst. 2006;98:920–31.

113. Giovannucci E, Ascherio A, Rimm EB, et al. Physical activity, obesity, and risk for colon cancer and adenoma in men. Ann Intern Med. 1995;122:327–34.

114. Martinez ME, Giovannucci E, Spiegelman D, et al. Leisure-time physical activity, body size, and colon cancer in women. Nurses' Health Study Research Group. J Natl Cancer Inst. 1997;89:948–55.

115. Wang Y, Jacobs EJ, Patel AV, et al. A prospective study of waist circumference and body mass index in relation to colorectal cancer incidence. Cancer Causes Control. 2008;19:783–92.

116. Yamaji Y, Okamoto M, Yoshida H, et al. The effect of body weight reduction on the incidence of colorectal adenoma. Am J Gastroenterol. 2008;103:2061–7.

117. Ogden CL, Carroll MD, Curtin LR, et al. Prevalence of overweight and obesity in the United States, 1999-2004. JAMA. 2006;295:1549–55.

118. Wei EK, Giovannucci E, Wu K, et al. Comparison of risk factors for colon and rectal cancer. Int J Cancer. 2004;108:433–42.
119. Ferrari P, Jenab M, Norat T, et al. Lifetime and baseline alcohol intake and risk of colon and rectal cancers in the European prospective investigation into cancer and nutrition (EPIC). Int J Cancer. 2007;121: 2065–72.
120. Cho E, Smith-Warner SA, Ritz J, et al. Alcohol intake and colorectal cancer: a pooled analysis of 8 cohort studies. Ann Intern Med. 2004;140:603–13.
121. Choi SW, Stickel F, Baik HW, et al. Chronic alcohol consumption induces genomic but not p53-specific DNA hypomethylation in rat colon. J Nutr. 1999;129:1945–50.
122. Kune GA, Vitetta L. Alcohol consumption and the etiology of colorectal cancer: a review of the scientific evidence from 1957 to 1991. Nutr Cancer. 1992;18:97–111.
123. Thygesen LC, Wu K, Gronbaek M, et al. Alcohol intake and colorectal cancer: a comparison of approaches for including repeated measures of alcohol consumption. Epidemiology. 2008;19:258–64.
124. Park JY, Mitrou PN, Dahm CC, et al. Baseline alcohol consumption, type of alcoholic beverage and risk of colorectal cancer in the European Prospective Investigation into Cancer and Nutrition-Norfolk study. Cancer Epidemiol. 2009;33:347–54.
125. Gerhardssondeverdier M, Hagman U, Peters RK, Steineck G, Overvik E. Meat, cooking methods and colorectal cancer: a case-referent study in Stockholm. Int J Cancer. 1991;49:520–5.
126. Martinez ME, Jacobs ET, Ashbeck EL, et al. Meat intake, preparation methods, mutagens and colorectal adenoma recurrence. Carcinogenesis. 2007; 28:2019–27.
127. Gunter MJ, Probst-Hensch NM, Cortessis VK, et al. Meat intake, cooking-related mutagens and risk of colorectal adenoma in a sigmoidoscopy-based case-control study. Carcinogenesis. 2005;26:637–42.
128. Alexander DD, Weed DL, Cushing CA, Lowe KA. Meta-analysis of prospective studies of red meat consumption and colorectal cancer. Eur J Cancer Prev. 2011;20:293–307.
129. Giovannucci E, Rimm EB, Stampfer MJ, et al. Intake of fat, meat, and fiber in relation to risk of colon cancer in men. Cancer Res. 1994;54:2390–7.
130. Giovannucci E, Stampfer MJ, Colditz GA, et al. Multivitamin use, folate, and colon cancer in women in the Nurses' Health Study. Ann Intern Med. 1998;129:517–24.
131. Kritchevsky D. Epidemiology of fibre, resistant starch and colorectal cancer. Eur J Cancer Prev. 1995;4:345–52.
132. Potter JD. Colorectal cancer: molecules and populations. J Natl Cancer Inst. 1999;91:916–32.
133. Trock B, Lanza E, Greenwald P. Dietary fiber, vegetables, and colon cancer: critical review and meta-analyses of the epidemiologic evidence. J Natl Cancer Inst. 1990;82:650–61.
134. Schatzkin A, Lanza E, Corle D, et al. Lack of effect of a low-fat, high-fiber diet on the recurrence of colorectal adenomas. Polyp Prevention Trial Study Group. N Engl J Med. 2000;342:1149–55.
135. Alberts DS, Martinez ME, Roe DJ, et al. Lack of effect of a high-fiber cereal supplement on the recurrence of colorectal adenomas. Phoenix Colon Cancer Prevention Physicians' Network. N Engl J Med. 2000;342:1156–62.
136. Bingham SA, Day NE, Luben R, et al. Dietary fibre in food and protection against colorectal cancer in the European Prospective Investigation into Cancer and Nutrition (EPIC): an observational study. Lancet. 2003;361:1496–501.
137. Fuchs CS, Giovannucci EL, Colditz GA, et al. Dietary fiber and the risk of colorectal cancer and adenoma in women. N Engl J Med. 1999;340:169–76.
138. McCullough ML, Robertson AS, Chao A, et al. A prospective study of whole grains, fruits, vegetables and colon cancer risk. Cancer Causes Control. 2003;14:959–70.
139. Levin B, Lieberman DA, McFarland B, et al. Screening and surveillance for the early detection of colorectal cancer and adenomatous polyps, 2008: a joint guideline from the American Cancer Society, the US Multi-Society Task Force on Colorectal Cancer, and the American College of Radiology. Gastroenterology. 2008;134:1570–95.
140. Jasperson KW, Tuohy TM, Neklason DW, Burt RW. Hereditary and familial colon cancer. Gastroenterology. 2010;138:2044–58.
141. Johns LE, Houlston RS. A systematic review and meta-analysis of familial colorectal cancer risk. Am J Gastroenterol. 2001;96:2992–3003.
142. Cottet V, Pariente A, Nalet B, et al. Colonoscopic screening of first-degree relatives of patients with large adenomas: increased risk of colorectal tumors. Gastroenterology. 2007;133:1086–92.
143. Winawer S, Fletcher R, Rex D, et al. Colorectal cancer screening and surveillance: clinical guidelines and rationale-Update based on new evidence. Gastroenterology. 2003;124:544–60.
144. Hampel H, Frankel WL, Martin E, et al. Feasibility of screening for Lynch syndrome among patients with colorectal cancer. J Clin Oncol. 2008;26:5783–8.
145. Stoffel E, Mukherjee B, Raymond VM, et al. Calculation of risk of colorectal and endometrial cancer among patients with Lynch syndrome. Gastroenterology. 2009;137:1621–7.
146. Koornstra JJ, Mourits MJ, Sijmons RH, et al. Management of extracolonic tumours in patients with Lynch syndrome. Lancet Oncol. 2009;10:400–8.
147. Vasen HF, Mecklin JP, Khan PM, Lynch HT. The International Collaborative Group on Hereditary Non-Polyposis Colorectal Cancer (ICG-HNPCC). Dis Colon Rectum. 1991;34:424–5.
148. Vasen HF, Watson P, Mecklin JP, Lynch HT. New clinical criteria for hereditary nonpolyposis colorectal cancer (HNPCC, Lynch syndrome) proposed by

the International Collaborative group on HNPCC. Gastroenterology. 1999;116:1453–6.

149. Umar A, Boland CR, Terdiman JP, et al. Revised Bethesda Guidelines for hereditary nonpolyposis colorectal cancer (Lynch syndrome) and microsatellite instability. J Natl Cancer Inst. 2004;96:261–8.

150. Hampel H, Frankel WL, Martin E, et al. Screening for the Lynch syndrome (hereditary nonpolyposis colorectal cancer). N Engl J Med. 2005;352: 1851–60.

151. Lynch HT, de la Chapelle A. Hereditary colorectal cancer. N Engl J Med. 2003;348:919–32.

152. Bonadona V, Bonaiti B, Olschwang S, et al. Cancer risks associated with germline mutations in MLH1, MSH2, and MSH6 genes in Lynch syndrome. JAMA. 2011;305:2304–10.

153. Stupart DA, Goldberg PA, Algar U, Ramesar R. Surveillance colonoscopy improves survival in a cohort of subjects with a single mismatch repair gene mutation. Colorectal Dis. 2009;11:126–30.

154. Bisgaard ML, Fenger K, Bulow S, Niebuhr E, Mohr J. Familial adenomatous polyposis (FAP): frequency, penetrance, and mutation rate. Hum Mutat. 1994;3:121–5.

155. Spigelman AD, Williams CB, Talbot IC, Domizio P, Phillips RK. Upper gastrointestinal cancer in patients with familial adenomatous polyposis. Lancet. 1989;2:783–5.

156. Burke CA, Beck GJ, Church JM, van Stolk RU. The natural history of untreated duodenal and ampullary adenomas in patients with familial adenomatous polyposis followed in an endoscopic surveillance program. Gastrointest Endosc. 1999;49:358–64.

157. Bulow S, Bjork J, Christensen IJ, et al. Duodenal adenomatosis in familial adenomatous polyposis. Gut. 2004;53:381–6.

158. Bianchi LK, Burke CA, Bennett AE, et al. Fundic gland polyp dysplasia is common in familial adenomatous polyposis. Clin Gastroenterol Hepatol. 2008;6:180–5.

159. Dunlop MG. Guidance on gastrointestinal surveillance for hereditary non-polyposis colorectal cancer, familial adenomatous polyposis, juvenile polyposis, and Peutz-Jeghers syndrome. Gut. 2002;51 Suppl 5:V21–7.

160. Burke W, Petersen G, Lynch P, et al. Recommendations for follow-up care of individuals with an inherited predisposition to cancer. I. Hereditary nonpolyposis colon cancer. Cancer Genetics Studies Consortium. JAMA. 1997;277:915–9.

161. Vasen HF, Moslein G, Alonso A, et al. Guidelines for the clinical management of familial adenomatous polyposis (FAP). Gut. 2008;57:704–13.

162. Winawer SJ. Screening sigmoidoscopy: can the road to colonoscopy be less traveled? Ann Intern Med. 2003;139:1034–5.

163. Imperiale TF, Wagner DR, Lin CY, et al. Risk of advanced proximal neoplasms in asymptomatic adults according to the distal colorectal findings. N Engl J Med. 2000;343:169–74.

164. Rex DK, Bond JH, Winawer S, et al. Quality in the technical performance of colonoscopy and the continuous quality improvement process for colonoscopy: recommendations of the U.S. Multi-Society Task Force on Colorectal Cancer. Am J Gastroenterol. 2002;97:1296–308.

165. Kudo S, Kashida H, Tamura T. Early colorectal cancer: flat or depressed type. J Gastroenterol Hepatol. 2000;15(Suppl):D66–70.

166. Kudo S, Lambert R, Allen JI, et al. Nonpolypoid neoplastic lesions of the colorectal mucosa. Gastrointest Endosc. 2008;68:S3–47.

167. Kudo S, Tamura S, Hirota S, et al. The problem of de novo colorectal carcinoma. Eur J Cancer. 1995;31A:1118–20.

168. The Paris endoscopic classification of superficial neoplastic lesions: esophagus, stomach, and colon: November 30 to December 1, 2002. Gastrointest Endosc. 2003;58:S3–43.

169. Update on the Paris classification of superficial neoplastic lesions in the digestive tract. Endoscopy. 2005;37:570–8.

170. Soetikno RM, Kaltenbach T, Rouse RV, et al. Prevalence of nonpolypoid (flat and depressed) colorectal neoplasms in asymptomatic and symptomatic adults. JAMA. 2008;299:1027–35.

171. Kahi CJ, Anderson JC, Waxman I, et al. High-definition chromocolonoscopy vs. high-definition white light colonoscopy for average-risk colorectal cancer screening. Am J Gastroenterol. 2010;105:1301–7.

172. Bianco MA, Cipolletta L, Rotondano G, et al. Prevalence of nonpolypoid colorectal neoplasia: an Italian multicenter observational study. Endoscopy. 2010;42:279–85.

173. Rex DK. Preventing colorectal cancer and cancer mortality with colonoscopy: what we know and what we don't know. Endoscopy. 2010;42:320–3.

174. Anderson JC, Alpern Z, Messina CR, et al. Predictors of proximal neoplasia in patients without distal adenomatous pathology. Am J Gastroenterol. 2004; 99:472–7.

175. Rex DK, Helbig CC. High yields of small and flat adenomas with high-definition colonoscopes using either white light or narrow band imaging. Gastroenterology. 2007;133:42–7.

176. Stein B, Anderson JC, Rajapakse R, et al. Body mass index as a predictor of colorectal neoplasia in ethnically diverse screening population. Dig Dis Sci. 2010;55:2945–52.

177. Atkin WS, Morson BC, Cuzick J. Long-term risk of colorectal cancer after excision of rectosigmoid adenomas. N Engl J Med. 1992;326:658–62.

178. Lieberman DA, Weiss DG, Harford WV, et al. Five-year colon surveillance after screening colonoscopy. Gastroenterology. 2007;133:1077–85.

179. Winawer SJ, Zauber AG, Ho MN, et al. The National Polyp Study. Eur J Cancer Prev. 1993;2 Suppl 2:83–7.

180. Robertson DJ, Greenberg ER, Beach M, et al. Colorectal cancer in patients under close colonoscopic surveillance. Gastroenterology. 2005;129:34–41.

181. Bonithon-Kopp C, Piard F, Fenger C, et al. Colorectal adenoma characteristics as predictors of recurrence. Dis Colon Rectum. 2004;47:323–33.
182. Winawer SJ, Zauber AG, Fletcher RH, et al. Guidelines for colonoscopy surveillance after polypectomy: a consensus update by the US Multi-Society Task Force on Colorectal Cancer and the American Cancer Society. Gastroenterology. 2006;130:1872–85.
183. Barclay RL, Vicari JJ, Doughty AS, Johanson JF, Greenlaw RL. Colonoscopic withdrawal times and adenoma detection during screening colonoscopy. N Engl J Med. 2006;355:2533–41.
184. Kim DH, Pickhardt PJ, Taylor AJ, et al. CT colonography versus colonoscopy for the detection of advanced neoplasia. N Engl J Med. 2007;357:1403–12.
185. Regula J, Rupinski M, Kraszewska E, et al. Colonoscopy in colorectal-cancer screening for detection of advanced neoplasia. N Engl J Med. 2006;355:1863–72.
186. Betes M, Munoz-Navas MA, Duque JM, et al. Use of colonoscopy as a primary screening test for colorectal cancer in average risk people. Am J Gastroenterol. 2003;98:2648–54.
187. Strul H, Kariv R, Leshno M, et al. The prevalence rate and anatomic location of colorectal adenoma and cancer detected by colonoscopy in average-risk individuals aged 40-80 years. Am J Gastroenterol. 2006;101:255–62.
188. Imperiale TF, Wagner DR, Lin CY, et al. Using risk for advanced proximal colonic neoplasia to tailor endoscopic screening for colorectal cancer. Ann Intern Med. 2003;139:959–65.
189. Schoen RE, Gerber LD, Margulies C. The pathologic measurement of polyp size is preferable to the endoscopic estimate. Gastrointest Endosc. 1997;46:492–6.
190. Muto T, Bussey HJ, Morson BC. The evolution of cancer of the colon and rectum. Cancer. 1975;36:2251–70.
191. O'Brien MJ, Winawer SJ, Zauber AG, et al. The National Polyp Study. Patient and polyp characteristics associated with high-grade dysplasia in colorectal adenomas. Gastroenterology. 1990;98:371–9.
192. Butterly LF, Chase MP, Pohl H, Fiarman GS. Prevalence of clinically important histology in small adenomas. Clin Gastroenterol Hepatol. 2006;4:343–8.
193. Tsai FC, Strum WB. Prevalence of advanced adenomas in small and diminutive colon polyps using direct measurement of size. Dig Dis Sci. 2011;56:2384–8.
194. Lieberman D, Moravec M, Holub J, Michaels L, Eisen G. Polyp size and advanced histology in patients undergoing colonoscopy screening: implications for CT colonography. Gastroenterology. 2008;135:1100–5.
195. Rex DK, Overhiser AJ, Chen SC, Cummings OW, Ulbright TM. Estimation of impact of American College of Radiology recommendations on CT colonography reporting for resection of high-risk adenoma findings. Am J Gastroenterol. 2009;104:149–53.
196. Hassan C, Pickhardt PJ, Rex DK. A resect and discard strategy would improve cost-effectiveness of colorectal cancer screening. Clin Gastroenterol Hepatol. 2010;8:865–9, 869.e861–3.
197. van Stolk RU, Beck GJ, Baron JA, Haile R, Summers R. Adenoma characteristics at first colonoscopy as predictors of adenoma recurrence and characteristics at follow-up. The Polyp Prevention Study Group. Gastroenterology. 1998;115:13–8.
198. Winawer SJ, Zauber AG, O'Brien MJ, et al. Randomized comparison of surveillance intervals after colonoscopic removal of newly diagnosed adenomatous polyps. The National Polyp Study Workgroup. N Engl J Med. 1993;328:901–6.
199. Longacre TA, Fenoglio-Preiser CM. Mixed hyperplastic adenomatous polyps/serrated adenomas. A distinct form of colorectal neoplasia. Am J Surg Pathol. 1990;14:524–37.
200. Leggett B, Whitehall V. Role of the serrated pathway in colorectal cancer pathogenesis. Gastroenterology. 2010;138:2088–100.
201. Farris AB, Misdraji J, Srivastava A, et al. Sessile serrated adenoma: challenging discrimination from other serrated colonic polyps. Am J Surg Pathol. 2008;32:30–5.
202. Sandmeier D, Seelentag W, Bouzourene H. Serrated polyps of the colorectum: is sessile serrated adenoma distinguishable from hyperplastic polyp in a daily practice? Virchows Arch. 2007;450:613–8.
203. Huang CS, Farraye FA, Yang S, O'Brien MJ. The clinical significance of serrated polyps. Am J Gastroenterol. 2011;106:229–40, quiz 241.
204. Rosenberg DW, Yang S, Pleau DC, et al. Mutations in BRAF and KRAS differentially distinguish serrated versus non-serrated hyperplastic aberrant crypt foci in humans. Cancer Res. 2007;67:3551–4.
205. Chan AO, Issa JP, Morris JS, Hamilton SR, Rashid A. Concordant CpG island methylation in hyperplastic polyposis. Am J Pathol. 2002;160:529–36.
206. Wynter CV, Walsh MD, Higuchi T, et al. Methylation patterns define two types of hyperplastic polyp associated with colorectal cancer. Gut. 2004;53:573–80.
207. Anderson JC, Rangasamy P, Rustagi T, et al. Risk factors for sessile serrated adenomas. J Clin Gastroenterol. 2011;45(8):694–9.
208. Rex DK, Rahmani EY. New endoscopic finding associated with hyperplastic polyps. Gastrointest Endosc. 1999;50:704–6.
209. Li D, Jin C, McCulloch C, et al. Association of large serrated polyps with synchronous advanced colorectal neoplasia. Am J Gastroenterol. 2009;104:695–702.
210. Schreiner MA, Weiss DG, Lieberman DA. Proximal and large hyperplastic and nondysplastic serrated polyps detected by colonoscopy are associated with neoplasia. Gastroenterology. 2010;139:1497–502.
211. Goldstein NS. Small colonic microsatellite unstable adenocarcinomas and high-grade epithelial dysplasias in sessile serrated adenoma polypectomy specimens: a study of eight cases. Am J Clin Pathol. 2006;125:132–45.

212. Torlakovic EE, Gomez JD, Driman DK, et al. Sessile serrated adenoma (SSA) vs. traditional serrated adenoma (TSA). Am J Surg Pathol. 2008;32:21–9.
213. Kahi CJ, Hewett DG, Norton DL, Eckert GJ, Rex DK. Prevalence and variable detection of proximal colon serrated polyps during screening colonoscopy. Clin Gastroenterol Hepatol. 2011;9:42–6.
214. Baxter NN, Goldwasser MA, Paszat LF, et al. Association of colonoscopy and death from colorectal cancer. Ann Intern Med. 2009;150:1–8.
215. Brenner H, Hoffmeister M, Arndt V, et al. Protection from right- and left-sided colorectal neoplasms after colonoscopy: population-based study. J Natl Cancer Inst. 2010;102:89–95.
216. Arain MA, Sawhney M, Sheikh S, et al. CIMP status of interval colon cancers: another piece to the puzzle. Am J Gastroenterol. 2010;105:1189–95.
217. Anderson JC, Gonzalez JD, Messina CR, Pollack BJ. Factors that predict incomplete colonoscopy: thinner is not always better. Am J Gastroenterol. 2000;95:2784–7.
218. Anderson JC, Messina CR, Cohn W, et al. Factors predictive of difficult colonoscopy. Gastrointest Endosc. 2001;54:558–62.
219. Rex DK. Colonoscopy turning the focus on quality. Dig Liver Dis. 2002;34:831–2.
220. Rex DK. Speeding up cecal intubation: its role in the efficiency of colonoscopy delivery. Am J Gastroenterol. 2002;97:6–8.
221. Kaminski MF, Regula J, Kraszewska E, et al. Quality indicators for colonoscopy and the risk of interval cancer. N Engl J Med. 2010;362:1795–803.
222. Pohl H, Robertson DJ. Colorectal cancers detected after colonoscopy frequently result from missed lesions. Clin Gastroenterol Hepatol. 2010;8:858–64.
223. Chapuis PH, Chan C, Dent OF. Clinicopathological staging of colorectal cancer: evolution and consensus-an Australian perspective. J Gastroenterol Hepatol. 2011;26 Suppl 1:58–64.
224. Dukes CE. The etiology of cancer of the colon and rectum. Dis Colon Rectum. 1959;2:27–32.
225. American Joint Committee on Cancer. AJCC cancer staging manual. 7th ed. New York: Springer; 2010.
226. Adam IJ, Mohamdee MO, Martin IG, et al. Role of circumferential margin involvement in the local recurrence of rectal cancer. Lancet. 1994;344: 707–11.
227. Roh MS, Colangelo LH, O'Connell MJ, et al. Preoperative multimodality therapy improves disease-free survival in patients with carcinoma of the rectum: NSABP R-03. J Clin Oncol. 2009;27: 5124–30.
228. Sauer R, Becker H, Hohenberger W, et al. Preoperative versus postoperative chemoradiotherapy for rectal cancer. N Engl J Med. 2004;351: 1731–40.
229. Wilkinson N, Scott-Conner CE. Surgical therapy for colorectal adenocarcinoma. Gastroenterol Clin North Am. 2008;37:253–67, ix.
230. Yeatman TJ, Bland KI. Sphincter-saving procedures for distal carcinoma of the rectum. Ann Surg. 1989;209:1–18.
231. Stewart DB, Dietz DW. Total mesorectal excision: what are we doing? Clin Colon Rectal Surg. 2007;20:190–202.
232. Rex DK, Kahi CJ, Levin B, et al. Guidelines for colonoscopy surveillance after cancer resection: a consensus update by the American Cancer Society and the US Multi-Society Task Force on Colorectal Cancer. Gastroenterology. 2006;130:1865–71.

Colorectal Cancer Screening Tests and Recommendations

Don C. Rockey

Overview

While colorectal cancer (CRC) is currently the second leading cause of cancer death in the US [1], it is believed to be a highly preventable cancer. In the USA, it is now recommended that all asymptomatic persons over the age of 50 undergo screening of the colon and rectum. This review will focus only on the methods and evidence for screening asymptomatic individuals— patients with gastrointestinal symptoms fall into another, typically more aggressive diagnostic algorithm category. Despite the fact that excellent screening tests are available, the compliance rate with current screening recommendations in the USA varies between 35 and 65% and is influenced by a multitude of factors [2, 3]. There are many controversial aspects surrounding the assertion that screening for colon cancer in the USA is less than ideal.

It is currently believed that the most accurate method of CRC screening is by colonoscopy. However, prospective clinical trial data demonstrating incidence and mortality benefits from CRC screening currently only exist for fecal occult blood testing (FOBT) and sigmoidoscopy. Additionally,

there is little question that colonoscopy is the CRC screening test that is associated with the greatest procedural risk, including perforation, bleeding, and even death. New methodologies, including novel endoscopic methods, CT colonography (also known as virtual colonoscopy), capsule endoscopy, fecal DNA testing, and, most recently, blood testing (SEPTN9), offer promise that new approaches will be attractive enough to entice a larger proportion of people to undergo CRC screening.

Pathogenesis of Colorectal Cancer

The current view of the pathogenesis of CRC holds that it transitions from a precancerous lesion to cancer over many years. The usual scenario is that an abnormal focus of cells develops into a recognizable lesion, most often a "polyp," and then, some polyps undergo additional mutations to eventually develop into malignant lesions. This is the so-called adenoma–carcinoma sequence [4, 5]. The different types of polyps (flat, serrated, pedunculated) and their histology (hyperplastic, adenomatous) have been well described [4–10]. There are three major types of colorectal adenomas: tubular, villous, and tubulovillous. Hyperplastic polyps are thought to have no increased risk of cancer while adenomas are the precursors of CRC. The likelihood of malignancy in an adenomatous polyp or that it will develop into a CRC depends on its size, histologic type, degree of dysplasia, and likely other

D.C. Rockey, M.D. (✉)
Department of Internal Medicine, Department of Medicine, Medical University of South Carolina, Charleston, SC, USA
e-mail: rockey@musc.edu

B.D. Cash (ed.), *Colorectal Cancer Screening and Computerized Tomographic Colonography: A Comprehensive Overview*, DOI 10.1007/978-1-4614-5943-9_2, © Springer Science+Business Media New York 2013

Table 2.1 Environmental risk factors for development of colon cancer

Diet (low fiber)
Cigarette smoking
Physical inactivity
The metabolic syndrome, diabetes mellitus
Obesity
Industrialized countries
Alcohol
Medications
Other

Table 2.2 Critical features of CRC screening in average-risk individuals

Offer screening to men and women aged 50 years and older
Stratify patients by risk
Options should be offered
Follow-up of positive screening test with diagnostic colonoscopy
Appropriate and timely management is required once cancer is detected
Follow-up surveillance required after polypectomy and surgery
Providers must be proficient
Providers should encourage patient participation

Adapted from Winawer S, Fletcher R, Rex D, et al. Colorectal cancer screening and surveillance: clinical guidelines and rationale-update based on new evidence. Gastroenterology. 2003;124:544–60

unknown factors. It is noteworthy that the prevalence of polyps in the general population varies dramatically but is usually in the 15–25% range (if only adenomas are considered). From a clinical standpoint, a key concept is that small lesions develop into larger lesions and that some of these lesions eventually transform into CRC. Such a transformation is a rare event on a per-polyp basis, but, due to the high prevalence of adenomas in the population, is a common event on a per-person basis. The success of colon cancer screening depends on detecting all of these lesions. Identification and removal of both small and large polyps halt the adenoma–carcinoma sequence. Screening has also demonstrated the ability to identify CRC at earlier stages, which increases the opportunity for curative therapy, something that is uncommon with advanced CRC [11].

An enormous body of literature has focused on understanding the pathogenesis of CRC and thus understanding factors that might enhance its prevention. Genetic variables are undoubtedly important, some of which are known and others of which are unknown. Additionally, environmental factors are clearly important in the development of CRC (Table 2.1) [12–17]. For example, it is commonly accepted that diets high in fiber, physical activity, and intake of non-steroidal anti-inflammatory drugs (NSAIDs) including aspirin and calcium protect against the development of CRC. Conversely, low residue "Western diets," obesity, and smoking predispose to colorectal cancer [12, 13, 15–17].

Colorectal Cancer Screening: Overview

A series of general principles underlying screening of patients for CRC can be found in Table 2.2. In general, screening programs should begin by consideration of each person's level of risk. Again, this review focuses on asymptomatic patients at average risk. Those who have symptoms or who are at higher risk should be managed according to their perceived risk [18].

Who Should Be Screened?

Patients who are not at increased risk for CRC based on the presence of symptoms or known familial risk factors are considered to be of average risk for the development of colorectal cancer once they reach the age of 50. In the USA, current guidelines are that any individual above the age of 50 should be offered screening for colorectal cancer. These recommendations are based on multiple factors, including the population prevalence and incidence of CRC, the associated morbidity and mortality, and the costs trade-offs between the burden of the disease and the costs of screening tests and programs. There are, of course, stipulations to this recommendation. For example, patients with underlying serious life-threatening diseases may not be good candidates for screening, not only because the screening test itself could harm the patient (such as with colonoscopy or sigmoidoscopy), but also because the patient's outcome may not be affected by the finding of a CRC should it be identified through screening. Thus, it is imperative that patients and physicians discuss screening risks and benefits. The average risk, otherwise healthy individual should always undergo screening.

Another controversial caveat having to do with screening surrounds age. The US Preventative Services Task Force recently recommended that persons over the 75 years of age not be routinely screened for CRC and that no screening be performed in those older than age 85 [3, 19, 20]. The rationale for this recommendation is that even though CRC risk increases with age (in fact, age itself is one of the most important risk factors for colon cancer), the presence of other comorbidities can increase the risk of screening and the benefits of screening diminish in terms of quality-adjusted health years saved based on lower life expectancies. Simply stated, patients are more likely to die of diseases other than CRC by the time they reach the age of 85. Thus the decision to recommend screening should be individualized at the extremes of age. For example, a healthy 80-year-old patient may be a reasonable candidate for screening, but a younger patient (e.g., 74 year old) with severe comorbidities may not be. The risks and benefits of screening in elderly patients must be discussed between the patient and his/her care providers.

Screening Modalities

A number of professional societies have not only emphasized the importance of screening for CRC but have also made recommendations. The two consensus groups that have made recent recommendations include the Multi-society Task Force on Colorectal Cancer and the US Preventative Services Task Force (USPSTF). Recommendations from the two groups are similar in their advocacy of FOBT, flexible sigmoidoscopy,

Table 2.3 Screening recommendations

Multi-society Task Force	USPSTF
• Guaiac-based FOBT annually	• High-sensitivity FOBT annually
• FIT annually	• Flex sig q 5 years + high-sensitivity FOBT q 3 years
• Fecal DNA testing	• Colonoscopy q 10 years
• Flex sig q 5 years (±FOBT)	
• ACBE q 5 years	
• Colonoscopy q 10 years	
• CT colonography	

and colonoscopy but differ substantially regarding other tests [19, 21]. (Table 2.3) The Multi-society Task Force emphasizes that approaches offering visualization of the colon are preferable to indirect methods as are techniques designed to prevent CRC over techniques designed to detect CRC. For this reason, the Multi-society Task Force recommends more screening tests than the USPSTF, specifically including CT colonography and fecal DNA testing as acceptable options for interested and appropriate patients. Currently, the USPSTF recommends only using FOBT, sigmoidoscopy, or colonoscopy, and it recommends against routine screening for CRC in adults 76–85 years of age and against screening for CRC in adults older than age 85 years. The USPSTF believes that there is insufficient evidence to assess the benefits and harms of CT colonography and fecal DNA testing as screening modalities for CRC and gives both of these screening modalities an "I" rating.

Fecal Occult Blood Testing

The evidence supporting the use of FOBT for CRC screening is better than for any other method. Three large, prospective, randomized, very high-quality trials have each demonstrated that CRC screening using FOBT (guaiac-based tests were used in the studies; current generation FOBT includes high-sensitivity guaiac-based tests as well as immunochemical tests) reduces mortality from CRC [22–24]. Thus, there is convincing evidence that this modality is effective.

However, there are several important issues related to FOBT that must remain in clinical context. First, in order for a FOBT to be positive, the index lesion must bleed at least enough to be detected by the test. Thus, the sensitivity of FOBT varies depending not only on the kind of test used (i.e., whether guaiac or immunochemical) but also on intrinsic features of the lesion that it is meant to detect. In general, the larger the lesion in the colon/rectum, the more sensitive is FOBT for detecting the lesion. Thus, FOBT is better at detecting cancer than detecting polyps. In all primary programs using FOBT, it is recommended that the FOBT be performed annually. The other important issue to consider is that the false-positive rate of guaiac-based FOBT is relatively high. There are also a number of practical considerations important for FOBT, including that stool specimens must be collected properly and processed appropriately and the fact that for guaiac-based tests, patients should be on a specific diet. Evidence suggests that immunochemical FOBT may be highly sensitive and more specific than guaiac-based tests [25, 26]. Further, they may be less subject to patient preparatory factors because they detect only human blood and may require fewer samples. It is important that patients with a positive (any single positive) FOBT undergo colonoscopy to evaluate the entire colon and rectum.

Flexible Sigmoidoscopy

The use of flexible sigmoidoscopy has become somewhat controversial. On one hand, some have argued that flexible sigmoidoscopy evaluates only the left colon. However, the current available evidence suggests that flexible sigmoidoscopy is effective at preventing CRC deaths. At least four case–control studies have shown that flexible sigmoidoscopy is associated with reduced mortality for CRC. Further, in a recent large, high-quality study of subjects between 55 and 64 years of age, 170,432 men and women were randomly assigned to flexible sigmoidoscopy screening or standard care [27]. CRC incidence in the flexible sigmoidoscopy group was reduced by 23% (95% CI, 0.70–0.84) and mortality by 31% (95% CI, 0.59–0.82). The incidence of distal rectum and sigmoid colon cancer was reduced by 50% (95% CI, 0.42–0.59).

There are several issues that must be considered with flexible sigmoidoscopy. First, this examination typically requires either a full bowel preparation, similar to that required for colonoscopy or CT colonography, or several enemas. Second, this exam is usually performed without sedation and is uncomfortable; in fact, available data suggest that it is more uncomfortable than colonoscopy [28]. Additionally, patients who are found to have an adenoma during flexible sigmoidoscopy require some form of follow-up, most often with colonoscopy, to evaluate the colon proximal to the extent of the flexible sigmoidoscopy examination. Factors associated with an increased risk of advanced proximal neoplasia include age over 65 years, villous histology, an adenoma greater than 1 cm in size, and multiple distal adenomas [29]. These patients should generally undergo full colonoscopy. An area of controversy exists for polyps less than 1 cm in size identified at the time of flexible sigmoidoscopy. This is because biopsy may or may not be performed. Biopsy is recommended, because it will distinguish hyperplastic from adenomatous polyps. If adenomatous features are identified, full colonoscopy is recommended. If histology is hyperplastic, particularly in the left colon, evidence suggests that the risk of advanced proximal neoplasia is comparable to the risk in persons with no distal polyp [30–33]. Of note, however, patients with multiple hyperplastic polyps likely have a polyposis syndrome and appear to be at increased risk of cancer [34, 35]. The other important consideration is that there is some risk associated with sigmoidoscopy; perforation occurs in less than 1 per 1,000 patients [3, 36].

Combined FOBT and Flexible Sigmoidoscopy

The combination of FOBT and flexible sigmoidoscopy has not been as rigorously studied as the effect of either test alone but is recommended given the evidence for each individually. Evidence supporting the combination is equivocal with some studies suggesting a modest benefit of the combination [29], but others revealing no significant enhancement [37, 38]. When both tests are used to screen for CRC, FOBT should be performed first because a positive result is an indication for colonoscopy. This would eliminate the need for the flexible sigmoidoscopy examination. A disadvantage of the combined FOBT/flexible sigmoidoscopy strategy is that people incur the inconvenience, cost, and complications of both tests, but we do not definitively know the gain in effectiveness.

Air Contrast Barium Enema

There are little data with which to assess the utility of air contrast barium enema (ACBE) as a CRC screening tool. Nonetheless, the data suggest that the sensitivity of ACBE for polyps (both large and small) is limited [39, 40]. There is good evidence now indicating that CT colonography is more sensitive than ACBE, suggesting that this noninvasive modality might replace ACBE. ACBE does not permit removal of polyps or biopsy of cancers, and patients with an abnormal ACBE require subsequent colonoscopy.

Colonoscopy

In the USA, colonoscopy has become the most commonly recommended CRC screening test and is considered by many to be the gold-standard CRC screening modality. Although data directly examining whether primary screening colonoscopy reduces the incidence or mortality from CRC in average-risk persons is limited, some data support the effectiveness of screening colonoscopy [3, 41, 42]. Since detection of polyps and CRC by colonoscopy is as good, if not better than flexible sigmoidoscopy, it is likely that the data from the flexible sigmoidoscopy screening studies is applicable to colonoscopy. Further, colonoscopy appears to reduce

Table 2.4 Colonoscopy for CRC screening

Advantages	Disadvantages
Accurate	Typically requires sedation
Diagnostic and therapeutic	Highest complication rate
Large experience	Requires bowel preparation
May be comfortable	Expensive
	Highly operator dependent
	Inconvenient for patients
	May be uncomfortable

the incidence of CRC in people with previous adenomatous polyps [43, 44]. A case–control study from Germany demonstrated that colonoscopy in the preceding 10 years was associated with a 77% lower risk for the development of CRC (OR 0.23, 95% CI, 0.19–0.27) [42]. Risk reduction was prominent for all CRC stages and all ages, except for right-sided cancer in persons aged 50–59 years. Although hampered by a retrospective, observational design with potential for residual confounding and selection bias, this study suggested that colonoscopy with polypectomy reduces the risk for CRC.

The use of colonoscopy is controversial on a number of levels [45] (Table 2.4). Although colonoscopy permits detection and removal of polyps and biopsy of cancer throughout the colon, it clearly involves greater cost, risk, and inconvenience to the patient than other screening tests, and not all examinations visualize the entire colon. Colonoscopy is also the most expensive screening modality. Two areas that appear to add cost include the use of anesthesia providers to perform sedation [46] and the current practice of biopsy/removal of diminutive (1–5 mm) polyps [47].

There have also been recent questions about the quality of colonoscopy; it is clear that not all colonoscopies are performed equally [41, 48, 49]. Use of colonoscopy as an effective screening modality requires performance of high-quality exams, and various metrics designed define adequate colonoscopy practice such as intubation of the cecum, adenoma detection rates, bowel preparation adequacy, and time required for scope withdrawal continue to be refined [50].

Surveillance (Follow-up CRC Screening)

Asymptomatic (No Previous Polyps or Cancer)

Recommendations for surveillance after an initial negative examination depend in large part on which screening examination was initially performed [50]. For example, if FOBT was used initially, the recommendation is for follow-up with FOBT annually. If colonoscopy was the initial examination, the recommendation is for a 10-year follow-up. This recommendation has been derived largely empirically since there is little natural history data on either the development of adenomatous polyps or the time required for them to transform into cancer [50, 51].

Previous Adenomatous Polyps

Since a personal history of CRC and/or adenomatous polyps represents one of the most important risk factors for development of CRC, it is imperative that once a patient has been found to have a CRC or adenomatous polyp, they should undergo programmatic and rigorous surveillance. Follow-up examinations accomplish two major goals. First, they can permit the detection and removal of polyps or masses missed on the initial examination. Second, they help determine whether the patient has a tendency to form new adenomas. Interestingly, it is believed that the major benefit of colonoscopy derives from the index polypectomy and that the follow-up colonoscopy may be beneficial primarily in those at highest risk for future advanced adenomas [50]. Thus, there is a critical need for stratification of risk based on index lesions.

The appropriate interval between screening examinations for average-risk people (if the preceding examination is negative) remains an area of controversy [2, 51, 52]. Essentially all current programs recommend that surveillance be performed with colonoscopy in those who have had adenomatous polyps [21, 50]. However, little work has been done in the area of the use of

alternative means of surveillance. Importantly, many studies have revealed that interval screening with repeat colonoscopy is typically performed (inappropriately) too often [52–55].

Those with only one or two small adenomas at index (baseline) examination (typically colonoscopy) appear to be at low risk for future development of advanced adenomas [21, 43, 44, 50]. Those with large adenomas (greater than 1 cm), villous features, or multiple adenomas are at increased risk for future development of advanced adenomas and colorectal cancer [21, 50]. Follow-up colonoscopy after polypectomy (polyp removal) in patients with adenomatous polyps has been shown to reduce subsequent cancer incidence [43, 44]. However, it is clear that the rate of developing adenomas after index colonoscopy and polypectomy is low [43, 44].

A number of special surveillance circumstances exist. One has to do with patients who have a poor preparation at the time of initial colonoscopy. These patients should be handled on an individual basis and require judgment on the part of the colonoscopist. For example, if the colonoscopist cannot rule out the possibility of a large adenoma, then a repeat study is warranted sooner (e.g., within 1 year). If on the other hand, lesions larger than five millimeters can be excluded, it is reasonable for the patient to return to a standard surveillance program [50]. The other special situation is the patient with a large adenoma that may not have been removed entirely. These patients generally require a repeat exam within 3–6 months, particularly if the adenoma has advanced features. Finally, patients with a remote history of adenomatous polyps with an interval normal colonoscopy can usually have a repeat colonoscopic surveillance at a longer interval (5–10 years or perhaps even longer) [21, 50, 56].

A summary of recommendations for follow-up by the US Multi-society Task Force is shown in Table 2.5 [21, 51].

History of Colon Cancer

The incidence of CRC is increased after the index diagnosis (not including recurrence of the

Table 2.5 Surveillance—adenomas

- Data strongly support role of surveillance
- The more advanced the lesion, the shorter the follow-up
- 3 or more adenomas or advanced histology ("high risk")—follow-up colonoscopy in 3 years
- 1 or 2 small tubular adenomas ("low risk")—follow-up colonoscopy in 5–10 years
- Further follow-up depends on the findings

Table 2.6 CTC for CRC screening

Advantages	Disadvantages
Accurate	Diagnostic only
No sedation	Minimal overall experience
Safe	Requires bowel preparation
Convenient for patients	Highly operator dependent
May be comfortable	May be uncomfortable

original cancer) [21, 50, 56, 57]. Since these cancers presumably develop as a result of the adenoma–carcinoma sequence, surveillance should theoretically detect new polyps. It is recommended that patients with a CRC that have been resected (removed) for cure should have a full colonoscopy at the time of initial diagnosis to rule out synchronous neoplasms. If the colon is obstructed preoperatively, colonoscopy should be performed later, generally within 6 months after surgery [21, 50, 56, 57]. In those who have undergone a curative cancer resection, follow-up colonoscopy should be offered after 3 years and then, if normal, every 5 years [21, 50, 56, 57].

New Colon Cancer Screening Modalities

CT Colonography (Virtual Colonoscopy)

CT colonography is one of the newest modalities proposed as a method to screen the colon for cancer. It has a number of attractive features by which it should be considered a potentially important CRC screening examination (Table 2.6). Currently, the test requires a cleansing preparation of the colon but is otherwise noninvasive and does not appear to cause major complications. A limitation of the exam is that if abnormalities are identified, subjects will require (therapeutic) colonoscopy. Additional chapters of this book will provide extensive details about CT colonography preparation, performance, and interpretation and thus are not described in further detail here.

Fecal DNA

CRC is associated with several acquired genetic abnormalities that may be responsible for the transition from normal mucosa to polyp to cancer sequence. Since it is possible to recover analyzable human DNA from the stool, abnormalities can be detected. A number of studies have now demonstrated that neoplastic polyps and cancers can be detected by obtaining DNA samples from the stool (the sensitivity appears to be much greater for cancers than polyps) [58–62]. However, at this point, whether fecal DNA testing is better than FOBT with a highly sensitive FOBT remains controversial. In one study, 4,482 average-risk adults underwent FOBT with Hemoccult and HemoccultSensa (Beckman Coulter, Fullerton, CA) on three stools and a first-generation fecal DNA marker test panel on one stool per patient [59]. The sensitivity for screen-relevant neoplasms was 20% by fecal DNA testing, 11% by Hemoccult ($P=0.020$), and 21% by HemoccultSensa ($P=0.80$), and the sensitivity for cancer plus high-grade dysplasia was the same among the different tests. Specificity was 98%, 96%, and 97%, respectively, for the three tests [59]. A second-generation fecal DNA test had greater sensitivity for both large adenomas and cancers. However, among patients with a normal colonoscopy, the positivity rate was 16% for the fecal DNA test, compared with 4% with Hemoccult ($P=0.010$) and 5% with HemoccultSensa ($P=0.030$). Newer techniques are under active study, consistent with the belief that genetic abnormalities in precancerous and malignant lesions may be detected in the stool [58, 62].

Table 2.7 Colon capsule for CRC screening

Advantages	Disadvantages
Safe	Diagnostic only
No sedation	Requires bowel preparation
No discomfort	Requires specialized capsule
Likely convenient	May be operator dependent
	Minimal overall experience

Capsule Endoscopy

One of the more controversial potential new tools with which to screen the colon is by capsule endoscopy [63–69] (Table 2.7). The colon capsule operates in a similar fashion as the capsule swallowed for evaluation of the upper GI tract but has dual cameras, a total operating time of approximately 10 h, a delay mode (typically 2 h) to allow passage through small bowel, wide-angle optics, sensor array, and standard data recorder connected to the patient. It is capable of obtaining high-quality images from within the colon and can detect polyps [63–69]. Screening the colon of asymptomatic average-risk 50 year olds with capsule endoscopy is attractive, because it is likely to be extremely safe. However, a number of limitations exist, including the accuracy of the test and the fact that if abnormalities are identified, patients will require colonoscopy. An additional challenge for capsule endoscopy includes the technical issue related to timing of bowel preparation with the ingestion of the capsule. A complete bowel preparation is required, and in addition, the capsule must be given soon after the completion of the bowel preparation so that it passes into the colon while cleansed.

Overall, the sensitivity for the detection of polyps with capsule endoscopy has been modest. In two meta-analyses, the sensitivity of the colon capsule for polyps of any size and significant findings was 71 and 73%, while the specificity for polyps of any size was 75 and 89% [68, 69]. While there was substantial heterogeneity in these studies—limiting robust conclusions—these data suggest that capsule endoscopy will require further refinement. It is also noteworthy that capsule endoscopy identified 16 of the 21

cancerous lesions detected by colonoscopy, a level of sensitivity that is probably too low to be considered acceptable [69]. Nonetheless, capsule endoscopy may be useful for certain select groups of patients such as those with medical conditions that make standard colonoscopy risky, those with previously incomplete colonoscopy, or patients not willing to undergo standard colonoscopy.

Serum Tests

The pathogenesis of CRC is complex and involves a number of different pathways and molecules. This complexity suggests that a number of different cytokines or other molecules important in the pathogenesis of CRC could be measured, perhaps in blood. Advances in proteomics have further helped inform this process. While serum levels of carcinoembryonic antigen appear to exhibit a relatively low sensitivity and specificity in early disease, other cytokines, growth factors, and proteins such as IL-8, vascular endothelial growth factor (VEGF), complement C3a des-arg, alpha1-antitrypsin, and transferrin may offer greater sensitivity [70–73]. Additional work in this area is expected, and in particular, a focus on multiplex arrays may prove beneficial.

Summary

CRC is a major cause of morbidity and mortality in the USA and is largely preventable. Extensive work has been done in the area of development of tests and in their deployment, but a major issue contributing to low CRC screening rates in the USA continues to be the unwillingness of a sizable population to accept the costs, processes, discomforts, and risks of some of these tests. Multiple different and effective screening options exist, but programmatic implementation of these modalities continues to be the exception rather than the rule. Clearly increased patient and provider awareness of the importance and options available for CRC screening is needed, as well as the continued efforts to develop additional accurate, acceptable, safe, and cost-effective screening tests.

Key Points

1. Colon cancer is an important, preventable cancer for which screening is important.
2. Colon cancer screening levels are not optimal in the USA; thus, new and better approaches than those currently commonly used are needed.
3. There are multiple risk factors for colon cancer, and screening should take into account these risk factors.
4. Screening should be offered to all healthy average-risk persons over the age of 50.
5. The most commonly used colon cancer modality in the USA is currently colonoscopy.
6. Colonoscopy as a primary colon cancer screening modality is associated with a number of issues, including its cost and safety.
7. Newer approaches including CT colonography, fecal DNA, and capsule endoscopy hold promise and require further evaluation and consideration as screening tests.
8. Regardless of which test is recommended, physicians should actively urge patients to undergo screening.

References

1. Cheng L, Eng C, Nieman LZ, Kapadia AS, Du XL. Trends in colorectal cancer incidence by anatomic site and disease stage in the United States from 1976 to 2005. Am J Clin Oncol. 2011;34(6):573–80.
2. Sonnenberg A, Amorosi SL, Lacey MJ, Lieberman DA. Patterns of endoscopy in the United States: analysis of data from the Centers for Medicare and Medicaid Services and the National Endoscopic Database. Gastrointest Endosc. 2008;67:489–96.
3. Whitlock EP, Lin JS, Liles E, Beil TL, Fu R. Screening for colorectal cancer: a targeted, updated systematic review for the U.S. Preventive Services Task Force. Ann Intern Med. 2008;149:638–58.
4. Mitros FA. Polyps: the pathologist's perspective. Semin Surg Oncol. 1995;11:379–85.
5. Watne AL. Colon polyps. J Surg Oncol. 1997;66: 207–14.
6. Hixson LJ, Fennerty MB, Sampliner RE, McGee DL, Garewal H. Two-year incidence of colon adenomas developing after tandem colonoscopy. Am J Gastroenterol. 1994;89:687–91.
7. Robert ME. The malignant colon polyp: diagnosis and therapeutic recommendations. Clin Gastroenterol Hepatol. 2007;5:662–7.
8. Soetikno RM, Kaltenbach T, Rouse RV, et al. Prevalence of nonpolypoid (flat and depressed) colorectal neoplasms in asymptomatic and symptomatic adults. JAMA. 2008;299:1027–35.
9. Hiraoka S, Kato J, Fujiki S, et al. The presence of large serrated polyps increases risk for colorectal cancer. Gastroenterology. 2010;139:1503–10, 1510.e1–3.
10. Gurudu SR, Heigh RI, De Petris G, et al. Sessile serrated adenomas: demographic, endoscopic and pathological characteristics. World J Gastroenterol. 2010;16:3402–5.
11. Mandel JS, Church TR, Bond JH, et al. The effect of fecal occult-blood screening on the incidence of colorectal cancer. N Engl J Med. 2000;343:1603–7.
12. Boyle T, Fritschi L, Heyworth J, Bull F. Long-term sedentary work and the risk of subsite-specific colorectal cancer. Am J Epidemiol. 2011;173:1183–91.
13. Weinstein SJ, Yu K, Horst RL, Ashby J, Virtamo J, Albanes D. Serum 25-hydroxyvitamin D and risks of colon and rectal cancer in Finnish men. Am J Epidemiol. 2011;173:499–508.
14. Wasif N, Etzioni D, Maggard MA, Tomlinson JS, Ko CY. Trends, patterns, and outcomes in the management of malignant colonic polyps in the general population of the United States. Cancer. 2011;117:931–7.
15. Winzer BM, Whiteman DC, Reeves MM, Paratz JD. Physical activity and cancer prevention: a systematic review of clinical trials. Cancer Causes Control. 2011;22:811–26.
16. Wang L, Wilson SE, Stewart DB, Hollenbeak CS. Marital status and colon cancer outcomes in US Surveillance, Epidemiology and End Results registries: does marriage affect cancer survival by gender and stage? Cancer Epidemiol. 2011;35:417–22.
17. Zhang X, Smith-Warner SA, Chan AT, et al. Aspirin use, body mass index, physical activity, plasma C-peptide, and colon cancer risk in US health professionals. Am J Epidemiol. 2011;174:459–67.
18. Winawer S, Fletcher R, Rex D, et al. Colorectal cancer screening and surveillance: clinical guidelines and rationale-Update based on new evidence. Gastroenterology. 2003;124:544–60.
19. Screening for colorectal cancer: U.S. Preventive Services Task Force recommendation statement. Ann Intern Med. 2008;149:627–37.
20. Zauber AG, Lansdorp-Vogelaar I, Knudsen AB, Wilschut J, van Ballegooijen M, Kuntz KM. Evaluating test strategies for colorectal cancer screening: a decision analysis for the U.S. Preventive Services Task Force. Ann Intern Med. 2008;149:659–69.
21. Levin B, Lieberman DA, McFarland B, et al. Screening and surveillance for the early detection of colorectal cancer and adenomatous polyps, 2008: a joint guideline from the American Cancer Society, the US Multi-Society Task Force on Colorectal Cancer, and the American College of Radiology. Gastroenterology. 2008;134:1570–95.
22. Mandel JS, Bond JH, Church TR, et al. Reducing mortality from colorectal cancer by screening for

fecal occult blood. Minnesota Colon Cancer Control Study. N Engl J Med. 1993;328:1365–71 [published erratum appears in N Engl J Med. 1993;329(9):672] [see comments].

23. Kronborg O, Fenger C, Olsen J, Jorgensen OD, Sondergaard O. Randomised study of screening for colorectal cancer with faecal-occult-blood test. Lancet. 1996;348:1467–71.

24. Hardcastle JD, Chamberlain JO, Robinson MH, et al. Randomised controlled trial of faecal-occult-blood screening for colorectal cancer. Lancet. 1996;348: 1472–7.

25. Allison JE, Tekawa IS, Ransom LJ, Adrain AL. A comparison of fecal occult-blood tests for colorectal-cancer screening. N Engl J Med. 1996;334:155–9.

26. van Rossum LG, van Rijn AF, Laheij RJ, et al. Random comparison of guaiac and immunochemical fecal occult blood tests for colorectal cancer in a screening population. Gastroenterology. 2008;135: 82–90.

27. Atkin WS, Edwards R, Kralj-Hans I, et al. Once-only flexible sigmoidoscopy screening in prevention of colorectal cancer: a multicentre randomised controlled trial. Lancet. 2010;375:1624–33.

28. Kim LS, Koch J, Yee J, Halvorsen R, Cello JP, Rockey DC. Comparison of patients' experiences during imaging tests of the colon. Gastrointest Endosc. 2001;54:67–74.

29. Lieberman DA, Weiss DG. One-time screening for colorectal cancer with combined fecal occult-blood testing and examination of the distal colon. N Engl J Med. 2001;345:555–60.

30. Provenzale D, Garrett JW, Condon SE, Sandler RS. Risk for colon adenomas in patients with rectosigmoid hyperplastic polyps. Ann Intern Med. 1990;113:760–3.

31. Rex DK, Smith JJ, Ulbright TM, Lehman GA. Distal colonic hyperplastic polyps do not predict proximal adenomas in asymptomatic average-risk subjects. Gastroenterology. 1992;102:317–9.

32. Lin OS, Gerson LB, Soon MS, Schembre DB, Kozarek RA. Risk of proximal colon neoplasia with distal hyperplastic polyps: a meta-analysis. Arch Intern Med. 2005;165:382–90.

33. Laiyemo AO, Murphy G, Sansbury LB, et al. Hyperplastic polyps and the risk of adenoma recurrence in the polyp prevention trial. Clin Gastroenterol Hepatol. 2009;7:192–7.

34. Renaut AJ, Douglas PR, Newstead GL. Hyperplastic polyposis of the colon and rectum. Colorectal Dis. 2002;4:213–5.

35. Hyman NH, Anderson P, Blasyk H. Hyperplastic polyposis and the risk of colorectal cancer. Dis Colon Rectum. 2004;47:2101–4.

36. Gatto NM, Frucht H, Sundararajan V, Jacobson JS, Grann VR, Neugut AI. Risk of perforation after colonoscopy and sigmoidoscopy: a population-based study. J Natl Cancer Inst. 2003;95:230–6.

37. Sung JJ, Chan FK, Leung WK, et al. Screening for colorectal cancer in Chinese: comparison of fecal occult blood test, flexible sigmoidoscopy, and colonoscopy. Gastroenterology. 2003;124:608–14.

38. Graser A, Stieber P, Nagel D, et al. Comparison of CT colonography, colonoscopy, sigmoidoscopy and faecal occult blood tests for the detection of advanced adenoma in an average risk population. Gut. 2009;58: 241–8.

39. Rockey DC, Koch J, Yee J, McQuaid KR, Halvorsen RA. Prospective comparison of air-contrast barium enema and colonoscopy in patients with fecal occult blood: a pilot study. Gastrointest Endosc. 2004;60: 953–8.

40. Rockey DC, Paulson E, Niedzwiecki D, et al. Analysis of air contrast barium enema, computed tomographic colonography, and colonoscopy: prospective comparison. Lancet. 2005;365:305–11.

41. Baxter NN, Goldwasser MA, Paszat LF, Saskin R, Urbach DR, Rabeneck L. Association of colonoscopy and death from colorectal cancer. Ann Intern Med. 2009;150:1–8.

42. Brenner H, Chang-Claude J, Seiler CM, Rickert A, Hoffmeister M. Protection from colorectal cancer after colonoscopy: a population-based, case-control study. Ann Intern Med. 2011;154:22–30.

43. Winawer SJ, Zauber AG, Ho MN, et al. Prevention of colorectal cancer by colonoscopic polypectomy. The National Polyp Study Workgroup [see comments]. N Engl J Med. 1993;329:1977–81.

44. Winawer SJ, Zauber AG, O'Brien MJ, et al. Randomized comparison of surveillance intervals after colonoscopic removal of newly diagnosed adenomatous polyps. The National Polyp Study Workgroup [see comments]. N Engl J Med. 1993;328: 901–6.

45. Ransohoff DF. How much does colonoscopy reduce colon cancer mortality? Ann Intern Med. 2009;150: 50–2.

46. Khiani VS, Soulos P, Gancayco J, Gross CP. Anesthesiologist involvement in screening colonoscopy: temporal trends and cost implications in the Medicare population. Clin Gastroenterol Hepatol. 2012;10(1):58–64.e1.

47. Rex DK. Reducing costs of colon polyp management. Lancet Oncol. 2009;10:1135–6.

48. Bressler B, Paszat LF, Vinden C, Li C, He J, Rabeneck L. Colonoscopic miss rates for right-sided colon cancer: a population-based analysis. Gastroenterology. 2004;127:452–6.

49. Toma J, Paszat LF, Gunraj N, Rabeneck L. Rates of new or missed colorectal cancer after barium enema and their risk factors: a population-based study. Am J Gastroenterol. 2008;103:3142–8.

50. Lieberman D. Progress and challenges in colorectal cancer screening and surveillance. Gastroenterology. 2010;138:2115–26.

51. Winawer SJ, Zauber AG, Fletcher RH, et al. Guidelines for colonoscopy surveillance after polypectomy: a consensus update by the US Multi-Society Task Force on Colorectal Cancer and the American Cancer Society. Gastroenterology. 2006;130:1872–85.

52. Imperiale TF, Sox HC. Guidelines for surveillance intervals after polypectomy: coping with the evidence. Ann Intern Med. 2008;148:477–9.
53. Laiyemo AO, Murphy G, Albert PS, et al. Postpolypectomy colonoscopy surveillance guidelines: predictive accuracy for advanced adenoma at 4 years. Ann Intern Med. 2008;148:419–26.
54. Mysliwiec PA, Brown ML, Klabunde CN, Ransohoff DF. Are physicians doing too much colonoscopy? A national survey of colorectal surveillance after polypectomy. Ann Intern Med. 2004;141:264–71.
55. Ransohoff DF, Yankaskas B, Gizlice Z, Gangarosa L. Recommendations for post-polypectomy surveillance in community practice. Dig Dis Sci. 2011;56:2623–30.
56. Lasisi F, Rex DK. Improving protection against proximal colon cancer by colonoscopy. Expert Rev Gastroenterol Hepatol. 2011;5:745–54.
57. Rex DK, Kahi CJ, Levin B, et al. Guidelines for colonoscopy surveillance after cancer resection: a consensus update by the American Cancer Society and the US Multi-Society Task Force on Colorectal Cancer. Gastroenterology. 2006;130:1865–71.
58. Zou H, Taylor WR, Harrington JJ, et al. High detection rates of colorectal neoplasia by stool DNA testing with a novel digital melt curve assay. Gastroenterology. 2009;136:459–70.
59. Ahlquist DA, Sargent DJ, Loprinzi CL, et al. Stool DNA and occult blood testing for screen detection of colorectal neoplasia. Ann Intern Med. 2008;149:441–50, W81.
60. Imperiale TF, Ransohoff DF, Itzkowitz SH, Turnbull BA, Ross ME. Fecal DNA versus fecal occult blood for colorectal-cancer screening in an average-risk population. N Engl J Med. 2004;351:2704–14.
61. Ahlquist DA, Skoletsky JE, Boynton KA, et al. Colorectal cancer screening by detection of altered human DNA in stool: feasibility of a multitarget assay panel. Gastroenterology. 2000;119:1219–27.
62. Lind GE, Danielsen SA, Ahlquist T, et al. Identification of an epigenetic biomarker panel with high sensitivity and specificity for colorectal cancer and adenomas. Mol Cancer. 2011;10:85.
63. Schoofs N, Deviere J, Van Gossum A. PillCam colon capsule endoscopy compared with colonoscopy for colorectal tumor diagnosis: a prospective pilot study. Endoscopy. 2006;38:971–7.
64. Eliakim R, Yassin K, Niv Y, et al. Prospective multicenter performance evaluation of the second-generation colon capsule compared with colonoscopy. Endoscopy. 2009;41:1026–31.
65. Van Gossum A, Munoz-Navas M, Fernandez-Urien I, et al. Capsule endoscopy versus colonoscopy for the detection of polyps and cancer. N Engl J Med. 2009;361:264–70.
66. Sieg A, Friedrich K, Sieg U. Is PillCam COLON capsule endoscopy ready for colorectal cancer screening? A prospective feasibility study in a community gastroenterology practice. Am J Gastroenterol. 2009;104:848–54.
67. Sacher-Huvelin S, Coron E, Gaudric M, et al. Colon capsule endoscopy vs. colonoscopy in patients at average or increased risk of colorectal cancer. Aliment Pharmacol Ther. 2010;32:1145–53.
68. Rokkas T, Papaxoinis K, Triantafyllou K, Ladas SD. A meta-analysis evaluating the accuracy of colon capsule endoscopy in detecting colon polyps. Gastrointest Endosc. 2010;71:792–8.
69. Spada C, Hassan C, Marmo R, et al. Meta-analysis shows colon capsule endoscopy is effective in detecting colorectal polyps. Clin Gastroenterol Hepatol. 2010;8:516–22.
70. Bunger S, Haug U, Kelly FM, et al. Toward standardized high-throughput serum diagnostics: multiplex-protein array identifies IL-8 and VEGF as serum markers for colon cancer. J Biomol Screen. 2011;16:1018–26.
71. Ward DG, Suggett N, Cheng Y, et al. Identification of serum biomarkers for colon cancer by proteomic analysis. Br J Cancer. 2006;94:1898–905.
72. Walgenbach-Brunagel G, Burger B, Leman ES, et al. The use of a colon cancer associated nuclear antigen CCSA-2 for the blood based detection of colon cancer. J Cell Biochem. 2008;104:286–94.
73. Ran Y, Hu H, Zhou Z, et al. Profiling tumor-associated autoantibodies for the detection of colon cancer. Clin Cancer Res. 2008;14:2696–700.

CTC Background and Development

3

Darren Boone, Stuart A. Taylor, and Steve Halligan

Introduction

Computed tomography (CT) following laxative cleansing and gaseous insufflation was first described for imaging the colorectum in the mid-1980s [1]. However, the technique did not gain widespread recognition until 1994 when advances in computer technology enabled Vining et al. [2] to demonstrate the feasibility of using volumetric CT data to generate a three-dimensional, endoluminal reconstruction—"virtual colonoscopy". Since then, research relating to CT colonography (CTC) has continued apace, developing its implementation, interpretation and diagnostic performance. Consequently, CTC has grown from a novel technique practised in a handful of specialist academic centres to one that has widely surpassed the barium enema as the preferred colorectal imaging modality in radiological departments. This chapter charts the evolution of CTC over the last 17 years, focusing in particular on research that has shaped current practice.

D. Boone, M.B.B.S. • S.A. Taylor, M.B.B.S., M.D. (✉)
S. Halligan, M.B.B.S., M.D.
Centre for Medical Imaging, University College Hospital, London, UK
e-mail: csytaylor@yahoo.co.uk

The Fall of Double-Contrast Barium Enema

For many years, the double-contrast barium enema (DCBE) was the preferred radiologic investigation for suspected colorectal cancer (CRC) or adenomatous polyps (Fig. 3.1). Comparative studies showed reasonable diagnostic accuracy compared to the gold standard, optical colonoscopy (OC), with a sensitivity for detecting cancer or large polyps in excess of 80% [3, 4]. However, by the turn of the century, evidence was accumulating that barium enema interpretation was deteriorating [5] and that accuracy was considerably lower than previously believed [6]. The turning point came in 2000 when the National Polyp Study [7] found a sensitivity of 48% for polyps larger than 1 cm prompting an accompanying editorial to suggest that double-contrast barium enema was no longer suitable for colorectal screening [8]. Despite opposition from the radiological community [9], no hard evidence has emerged since to refute these claims.

The Rise of Multi-detector Helical CT

Around this time, while barium enema was falling out of favour, CT was enjoying a renaissance as a result of the potential offered by helical and, later, multi-detector machines. The potential to

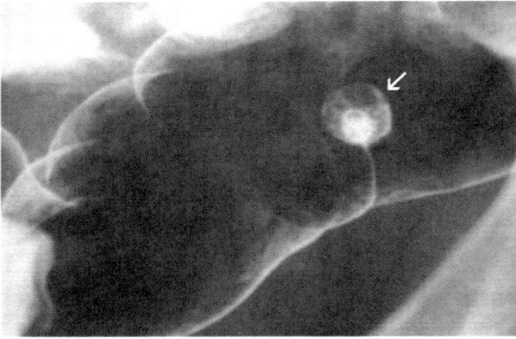

Fig. 3.1 Single oblique, magnified projection from a double-contrast barium enema examination. This optimally prepared examination demonstrates a 6-mm sigmoid polyp with a central depression (*arrow*)

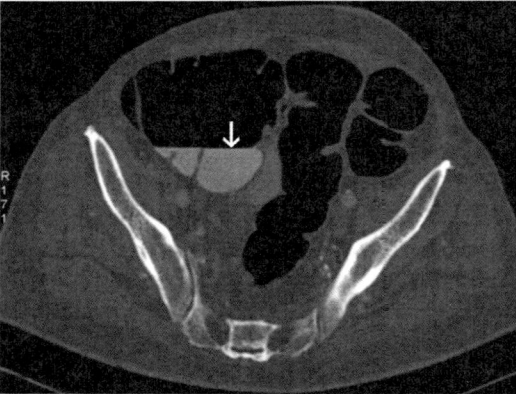

Fig. 3.2 Axial CT following full bowel catharsis, spasmolysis and carbon dioxide insufflation. Note the use of oral contrast to "tag" residual colonic content (*arrow*) and that intravenous contrast has been administered. Extensive research has taken place over recent years to optimise technical implementation

acquire volumetric data within one breath-hold stimulated research interest in abdomino-pelvic CT. For example, while seeking an alternative to barium enema in frail, elderly patients, researchers from Cambridge, UK, found CT could be used to demonstrate colorectal cancer, particularly after administering dilute oral contrast [10, 11]. Therefore, it was not long before established barium enema techniques such as bowel catharsis, spasmolysis and gaseous insufflation were applied to CT (Fig. 3.2); UK researchers named

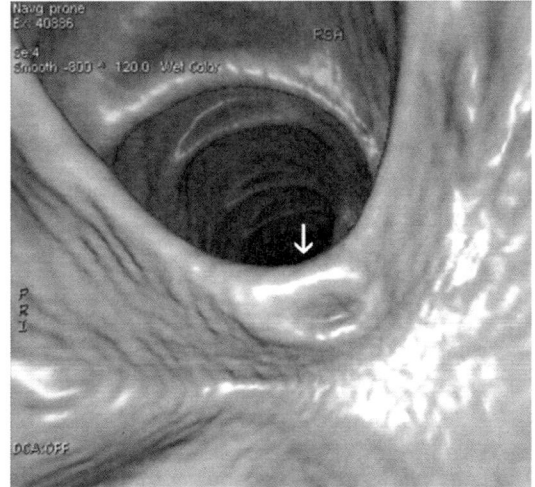

Fig. 3.3 Endoluminal CT colonography viewed from the caecum. Note the normal ileocaecal valve (*arrow*). Although "virtual colonoscopy" initially required many hours of painstaking rendering, three-dimensional representations can be obtained almost immediately on most modern workstations

the resulting procedure, "CT pneumocolon"—a term which remains in use sporadically [12]. Although related research continued in specialist academic centres, barium enema was well established in daily practice and remained the mainstay of radiologic colonic investigation for several years.

The Birth of Virtual Colonoscopy

By 1994, the radiology community eagerly awaited a technique that could exploit the latest CT technology to improve upon barium enema and provide a viable imaging alternative for colorectal screening. Thus, the scene was set for a celebrated presentation at the 23rd Annual Meeting of the Society of Gastrointestinal Radiologists where Vining et al. introduced "virtual colonoscopy" presenting an endoluminal flythrough video set to Wagner's "Flight of the Valkyries". The subsequent publication [2] is widely regarded as the earliest description of CT colonography (Fig. 3.3).

Optimising Technical Implementation

Although "virtual colonoscopy" subsequently gained international exposure, access to computer technology capable of endoluminal reconstruction was limited and, where available, processing remained time-consuming. Therefore, initial research focused on two-dimensional interpretation [12, 13] which could be carried out on a regular workstation directly after image acquisition. Moreover, it soon became apparent that technical implementation needed refinement before CTC's full potential could be realised. Consequently, research groups formed and published the initial groundwork, which is largely responsible for today's CTC implementation. For example, initial research demonstrated that performing scans with the patient prone and supine (Fig. 3.4a, b) could improve overall colonic distension [14] and that insufflation with CO_2 was superior to room air [15]. Nevertheless, research was less conclusive regarding the use of intravenous contrast [16], spasmolytics [17, 18] and bowel preparations [19]. Furthermore, early attempts at "tagging" residual stool using oral barium or iodine gave conflicting results, with some groups finding improved sensitivity with tagging [20], while others found it less helpful [21]. Moreover, these studies initiated the quest for "prepless" CTC [22] which remains a current goal for many researchers in the field.

Another concern since the outset of CTC development and implementation has been the anticipated increase in diagnostic radiation exposure compared to barium enema, a factor that continues to raise concerns today. Initial research employing phantom models [23–25] was instrumental in optimising scanning parameters. Low-dose protocols exploiting the intrinsic contrast between soft tissue and gas were introduced with promising results [26]. Nevertheless, once individual research groups had settled upon suitable preparation and scanning parameters, it was not long before researchers began to perform CTC on patients with colonoscopic abnormalities to compare appearances of various colorectal lesions [27, 28]. Having demonstrated feasibility [29], early observational studies rapidly ensued to establish the efficacy of this new technique.

Exploratory Reader Studies

Initial studies used small retrospective samples of high-risk patients undergoing colonoscopy. For example, Royster et al. [30] studied 20 high-risk patients and found all colonic masses (>2 cm) and 12 of 15 polyps (>6 mm). Similarly, Dachman et al. performed CTC in 44 high-risk patients [31] achieving a per-polyp sensitivity of 83 and 100% for two observers compared to the colonoscopic reference standard. Ferrucci's group was also instrumental in providing these initial performance

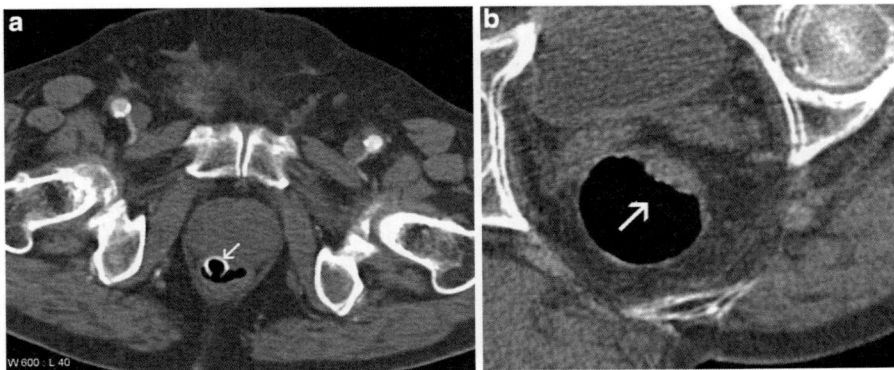

Fig. 3.4 (**a**) Supine, axial CT colonography. The lumen is collapsed around the rectal insufflation catheter (*arrow*). (**b**) The same patient was re-examined in the prone position. Note the improved rectal distension has revealed irregular mural thickening (*arrow*); colonoscopy confirmed a 35-mm flat carcinoma

data from small, high prevalence cohorts [29, 30]. However, while good sensitivity was demonstrated, a prospective trial was needed, preferably without such high disease prevalence. This was provided in 1997 by Hara et al. [32] who compared 70 patients undergoing CTC to routine abdomino-pelvic CT or colonoscopy. Two observers read the cases, and each achieved 75% sensitivity and 90% specificity for polyps 10 mm or larger. Furthermore, this was the first study to demonstrate superiority over regular CT, which obtained a sensitivity of 58% for polyps >10 mm. Interestingly, patients were scanned only in the supine position, illustrating that consensus had not been reached regarding even the most fundamental elements of CTC implementation. Indeed, it was seven years before convincing research by Yee et al. closed the debate on the value of prone and supine acquisitions [33].

New Meeting, New Name

By the late 1990s, several research groups were independently pioneering this new technique, and in October 1998, key researchers arranged the first international meeting dedicated to CTC. The International Symposium on Virtual Colonoscopy in Boston remains the premier congress for researchers in the field today [34]. It is also worthy to note that many opinion leaders in CTC research at this time were gastroenterologists. Later that year, the community settled on "CT colonography" as the accepted scientific terminology [35]. Although other descriptive terms such as "CT coloscopy", "CT pneumocolon" and "virtual endoscopy" were subsequently abandoned, "virtual colonoscopy" remains in widespread use, likely because the terminology is readily understood by the public.

International Interest

The following year, international interest was raised considerably by an article published in the New England Journal of Medicine led by Dr Helen Fenlon [36], an Irish radiologist undertaking a fellowship with Dr Joseph Ferrucci in Chicago. This prospective trial of 100 high-risk patients (49 with endoscopically proven colorectal neoplasia, 51 with negative colonoscopy) was the largest to date and utilised "state-of-the-art" technique. For example, interpretation used both 2D and 3D assessment in all patients—a factor some considered instrumental in achieving excellent performance. CTC achieved a sensitivity of 100% for cancer, 91% for polyps 10 mm or larger and 82% for polyps 6–9 mm in diameter. On a per-patient basis, a 10-mm threshold would have resulted in 96% sensitivity and 96% specificity.

Until this time, CT colonography development had been confined almost exclusively to North America. However, publication of Fenlon's work stimulated considerable worldwide interest; within a few months, the British Medical Journal commissioned a review of the technique [37]. Moreover, several other European radiologists on fellowships in the USA returned home and introduced CT colonography to their practice. Subsequently, European research groups formed and began conducting their own studies.

Early Research from Europe

European studies initially focused on the technical aspects of CTC, such as optimization of acquisition parameters [15, 25, 38, 39], bowel preparation [40–42], effect of spasmolytics and rectal catheter type [18, 43]. European researchers were also early to recognise that radiation concerns could hinder CTC uptake and investigated reduced-dose techniques [44, 45].

On the surface, repeating this groundwork may appear superfluous, yet it was necessary due to Europe's differing legislation, regulation and patient case-mix. For example, in the UK, hyoscine butylbromide is licensed for diagnostic spasmolysis, and researchers soon showed it improved distension during CTC [43]. In addition, European studies have paid particular attention to patient acceptability [46–50], particularly by reducing or avoiding cathartic bowel preparation [22, 51]. Around this time, European CTC researchers

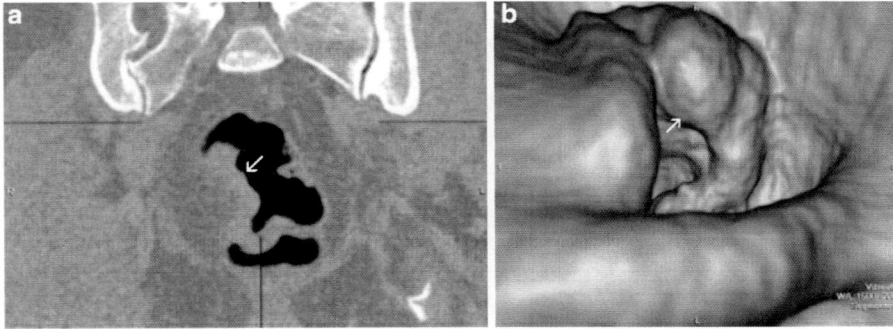

Fig. 3.5 2D coronal (**a**) and 3D endoluminal CT colonography (**b**) at the level of the mid-rectum. Although the emphasis of early research focused upon polyp detection in screening populations, CTC can be used to detect polyps or invasive cancer in symptomatic patients. Here, a large annular carcinoma (*arrow*) is clearly demonstrated

began to collaborate with their neighbours via the European Society of Gastrointestinal and Abdominal Radiology (ESGAR).

In 2003, research leads from the UK (Halligan, Taylor, Frost, Breen), Italy (Laghi), Belgium (Lefere) and the Netherlands (Stoker) established the ESGAR CTC committee and initiated training workshops. The committee has since expanded and has been instrumental in promoting pan-European academic collaboration and training. Subsequently, ESGAR has actively facilitated CTC research and has funded several multicentre studies [52–54].

Above all, the most striking international difference in CTC research has related to the patients studied; the focus in the US has traditionally been establishing a viable screening tool, while European radiologic colorectal investigations have been reserved for symptomatic patients (Fig. 3.5a, b). Inevitably, CTC research specifically investigating patients at increased colorectal cancer risk soon followed [47, 55–58]. However, European researchers also recognised that the vast majority of published studies from the USA had actually examined symptomatic patients (although the emphasis was directed towards a role for screening when data were interpreted). ESGAR funded a systematic review and meta-analysis which established CTC had a high sensitivity for diagnosis of symptomatic colorectal cancer [59] and paved the way for CTC implementation in Europe.

The First Large Multicentre Trials

While European research was gathering momentum, additional prospective trials in the USA continued to demonstrate good sensitivity for large polyp detection [60, 61]. However, 2003 saw the publication of one of the largest and most influential studies in CTC's history, Dr Perry Pickhardt's Department of Defence (DoD) trial [62]. This 3-centre prospective study of 1,233 asymptomatic, average-risk adults compared CTC against the enhanced reference standard of "unblinded colonoscopy". Most prior studies had been potentially subject to verification bias due to an imperfect gold standard (i.e. a polyp seen on CTC and not subsequently identified by colonoscopy would be considered a CTC false positive but potentially could in reality represent a colonoscopic false negative). The DoD study "unblinded" the colonoscopist to CTC findings once they had completed their segmental analysis, to allow re-evaluation of each colonic segment in the light of CTC findings. Another state-of-the-art technique was primary 3D endoluminal reading in all cases; again, most studies thus far had used 3D for problem-solving only. CTC achieved sensitivities of 94% and 89% for polyps at least 10 mm and 6 mm, respectively. Using the same thresholds, optical colonoscopy's sensitivity was 88% and 92%. However, these data were confounded by the publication of findings from the American

College of Radiology Imaging Network (ACRIN) National CT colonography trial [63] led by Dr Daniel Johnston. Johnson et al. studied 703 higher-than-average-risk and asymptomatic patients who underwent CT colonography followed by same-day colonoscopy. Results were disappointing with large intra-observer variability and sensitivities for detecting large polyps of only 34%, 32% and 73%, for three experienced readers. The following year, Cotton et al. [64] published further disappointing results in a multi-centre study which examined 615 patients undergoing CTC and same-day, unblinded colonoscopy. CTC had a sensitivity of 55% for polyps at least 10 mm in size, compared to 99% for colonoscopy. Furthermore, CTC missed two of eight cancers. Finally, in 2005, Rockey et al. [65] obtained similar results to Cotton in a prospective evaluation of high-risk patients: CTC achieved a sensitivity of only 59% for polyps of 10 mm or larger compared to 99% for colonoscopy.

The reasons for these conflicting results were debated fiercely. Overall, the success of the DoD trial was attributed to well-trained, experienced observers using primary 3D interpretation of fluid-tagged cases. In any event, these discrepant results highlighted the need for and prompted the development of clearly defined standards for both implementation and interpretation.

International Consensus on CTC Implementation

On the background of these results, discussion at the 2005 annual Boston VC symposium led to the development of the first international CTC standards document. Barish et al. [66] surveyed 31 key opinion leaders' attitudes to cathartic preparation, faecal tagging, prone and supine positioning, intravenous contrast, scanning parameters, spasmolytics, optimal reading paradigm and polyp threshold size. The results were collated, sent to respondents for approval and a consensus statement published. At around the same time, Zalis et al. published the CRADS system for CTC reporting [67], and shortly thereafter, ESGAR commissioned its own consensus statement to address issues specific to Europe [68].

It is important to note at this juncture that in 2006, the American Gastroenterological Association (AGA) Institute released a position statement [69], aimed primarily at gastroenterologists with an interest in reporting CTC. Disappointingly, the ensuing controversy provided clear evidence of an evolving "turf battle" between specialities which is beyond the scope of this chapter, but has doubtlessly shaped the direction of research and its interpretation in recent years. Therefore, it is encouraging to note that the most recent guidelines from the *International Collaboration for CT Colonography Standards* have been developed in direct collaboration between a radiologist, Dr David Burling, and the UK National Lead for Endoscopy Services, Dr Roland Valori, supported by an extensive multidisciplinary team [70].

Ongoing Research Themes

By 2005, comparative trials and meta-analyses had suggested that CTC could achieve a sensitivity approaching that of colonoscopy for large polyps, and the technique was starting to gain acceptance outside academic environments [71]. Furthermore, publication of consensus guidelines shifted the research focus away from technical implementation and towards several discrete themes: training, reading technique, computer-aided detection, patient experience and reducing bowel preparation. These topics are covered in greater detail elsewhere in this volume but major milestones are described briefly below.

Training, Validation and Audit

It is unsurprising, given limited experience, that some of the earliest CTC performance studies suggested a learning curve for this novel technique. For example, Spinzi et al. [72] studied a random selection of 96 patients having CTC followed by colonoscopy and failed to detect five out of six polyps during review of the first 25 cases, with a resulting sensitivity of just 32%. However, by the final 20 cases, a far more satisfactory sensitivity of 92% was obtained. The authors openly attributed early perceptive errors to inexperience. In 2005, an editorial by Soto et al. [73] discussed the available evidence and concluded a variable learning curve exists for all readers and that many readers may never achieve satisfactory performance regardless of training. Nevertheless, the nature of the learning curve remains elusive, as does the optimal training programme. For example, an early study of three radiologists of differing general experience revealed interesting results; performance varied considerably, and one observer actually deteriorated after training [74]. The authors extended this work to a multicentre European setting, funded by ESGAR, investigating the effect of administering a directed training schedule of 50 cases to novice readers and then comparing their performance to that of experienced observers. Again, the authors found that there was considerable variation and that competence could not be assumed after training. Moreover, the performance of some experienced readers was far from "expert" [52]. Therefore, the precise mechanism and minimal level of training required to ensure safe practice remains elusive.

Guidelines from The American College of Radiology [75], the American Gastroenterological Association Institute [76] and the International Collaboration for CT Colonography Standards [70] have all recommended individual training with exposure to a range of endoscopically validated pathology. Hands-on training workshops are now well established to meet this need; ESGAR CTC courses have trained over 1,000 radiologists worldwide [77], while in the USA, the Society of Gastrointestinal Radiologists, American Roentgen Ray Society and International Symposium on Virtual Colonoscopy all offer validated hands-on workshops. However, at present, training uptake remains worryingly low: A recent survey of European CTC workshop participants [77] showed that 69% of respondents had been interpreting CTC in daily practice despite having no previous hands-on training and limited experience.

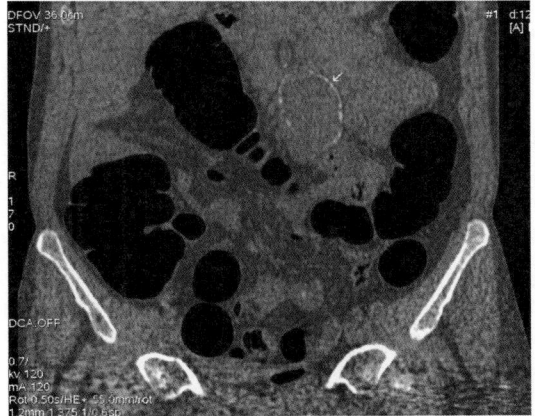

Fig. 3.6 Coronal CT colonography. Note the calcified, ectatic abdominal aorta (*arrow*) detected incidentally on this unenhanced CTC examination. The potential impact of these serendipitous extracolonic detections has become the subject of extensive debate

In any event, satisfying recommended levels of experience and training does not ensure diagnostic competence. For example, despite either completing a 1.5-day training course or reading over 500 cases, more than half of would-be observers in the ACRIN II study [78] failed to meet the basic entry requirements for the trial (90% sensitivity for polyps >1 cm over 50 cases). These data continue to raise serious concerns regarding generalisability to daily practice and reinforce the need for ongoing assessment.

Furthermore, once outside of a research environment, assessment of CTC performance becomes more challenging, not least because it is impossible in most cases to compare against a reference standard. To address this, in 2009, the American College of Radiology recommended quality metrics including complication rates, the proportion of technically inadequate studies and significant extracolonic findings (Fig. 3.6) to establish benchmarks against which departments can audit their performance [75]. Given the heterogeneous response to training, it is likely that only ongoing performance review will enable readers to ascertain their fitness to practise the technique.

Optimal Reading Method

It is difficult to speculate about what would have become of CT colonography without the advent of three-dimensional (3D) endoluminal reconstructions; "virtual colonoscopy" sparked medical and media interest in a technique that had remained quiescent for several years. However, many researchers with neither the time nor resources to generate 3D reconstructions initially capitalised on this renewed attention by performing research using a two-dimensional reading approach.

Nevertheless, computer hardware developed very rapidly, and it was not long before workstations capable of endoluminal reconstruction were readily available (albeit rather expensively), and debate surrounding the relative benefits of two and three-dimensional reading has existed ever since. The explanation for this revolves primarily around reading time: even once resource-intensive 3D reconstructions could be generated rapidly, studies soon confirmed what many researchers already suspected—primary 3D reading was considerably slower than 2D interpretation [79]. Indeed, as early as 1998, Dachman et al. had suggested using a compromise of 2D images for the primary read while reserving endoluminal views for "problem-solving" [31]; this reading paradigm remains the most widely employed to this day [77].

Nevertheless, studies by Fenlon et al. [36] and Pickhardt et al. [62] which used 3D interpretation prompted some authors to claim that primary three-dimensional interpretation was responsible for the impressive sensitivity in these trials. Furthermore, the inadequacy of 2D reading provided a convenient explanation for the poor performance achieved by Johnson et al. [63], Cotton et al. [64] and Rockey et al. [65] around the same time. In 2005, the majority of key opinion leaders were familiar with 2D interpretation and, given the considerable differences that existed between software platforms [80], the International Consensus Statement recommended 2D reading [66].

However, before long, most software platforms were considered equivalent, and by the time the ACRIN II protocol was designed, readers were encouraged to read cases using the technique with which they were most familiar. Subgroup analysis showed no significant difference in performance between reading paradigms [78], and recent consensus guidelines do not favour one method over another [70]. This debate subsequently subsided, and the matter has largely become one of personal preference [81].

Computer-Aided Detection

The time-consuming, laborious nature of interpretation, together with the well-documented problems of perceptive error, makes CTC an ideal candidate for computer-aided detection (CAD). Indeed, development and validation of CAD algorithms began in tandem with the early observer studies outlined above (Fig. 3.7). In 2000, Summers et al. reported one of the first documented CTC CAD systems by applying a prototype system developed for "virtual bronchoscopy" to artificially generated polyps in CTC data sets [82]. The following year, the same group published a preliminary validation study using 20 patients with 50 endoscopically proven polyps and achieved a sensitivity of 64% for polyps

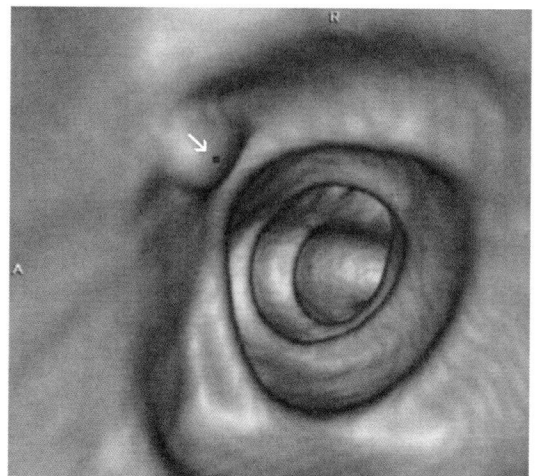

Fig. 3.7 Endoluminal CT colonography with computer-aided detection. The CAD prompt (*arrow*) correctly directs the reader to a 6-mm sessile polyp

10 mm or larger [83]. These cases were optimally prepared, but nonetheless, the sensitivity was comparable with many human readers at that time. Within months, Yoshida and Nappi validated a separate CAD system with 43 endoscopically confirmed cases and achieved comparable results [84].

By now, CAD was well established for assisting mammographic interpretation. yet research from this field suggested that unless a CAD system could achieve near-perfect sensitivity, its role would remain one of alerting the reader to potentially missed regions (i.e. "second-reader" CAD) rather than acting autonomously ("first-reader CAD"). The first study to explore potential "second-reader" interaction also came from Summers' group who applied CAD to the results of an observer study in which readers had relatively poor sensitivity (48% for polyps >10 mm). CAD detected four large polyps out of 13 which had not been reported by human readers, allowing the authors to infer that CAD could potentially increase reader sensitivity by alerting them to polyps which they had missed during their unassisted read [85].

However, despite the clinical relevance of observer studies for assessing the incremental benefit of CAD, they are time-consuming and expensive. Therefore, the algorithm's standalone performance is usually used as a surrogate to gauge its potential impact on interpretative accuracy. Consequently, several studies of unassisted CAD performance have been published in recent years, their size reflecting the ever-increasing availability of algorithms and endoscopically validated data. For example, a screening cohort of 1,186 well-characterised data sets, all of which had undergone unblinded colonoscopy, was used to test standalone CAD performance [86] and achieved a sensitivity of 89% for polyps >1 cm and, on average, 2.1 false-positive detections per patient.

Excellent standalone performance does not necessarily translate into equivalent levels of diagnostic accuracy when integrated with radiologist interpretation in clinical practice. There are likely two main reasons for this: readers may be misled by false-positive CAD prompts, reducing

their specificity, or they may incorrectly classify a true positive CAD prompt as false negative, reducing potential gains in sensitivity. Taylor et al. examined 111 polyps that had been incorrectly dismissed by radiologists in previous studies, despite appropriate CAD prompting [87], and found large polyps with atypical appearances were incorrectly disregarded. Furthermore, the optimal reading paradigm for integrating CAD into workflow is yet to be established [88].

Ultimately, the most realistic estimates of how CAD may improve clinical practice require experienced readers to interpret cases with and without CAD assistance. Recently, two groups have published multi-reader, multi-case studies [89, 90]. These are the largest CAD reader studies to date and concur that second-read CAD would be beneficial if used in clinical practice.

Patient Experience

Although early diagnosis and removal of adenomatous polyps can significantly reduce colorectal cancer mortality [91], only 50–60% of eligible patients in the USA attend colorectal screening [92]. The reasons for this are complex but inconvenience, embarrassment, discomfort and safety concerns are all likely to contribute. Given that patients may intuitively expect "virtual colonoscopy" to be less invasive than other whole-colon tests, high hopes exist that a CTC screening programme could increase compliance. Consequently, recent years have seen considerable efforts to compare patient preferences for CTC, colonoscopy and barium enema.

Early questionnaire surveys [46, 50] comparing the attitudes of patients who had undergone both CTC and colonoscopy found the majority favoured CTC. Subsequently, more elaborate studies also suggested patients would prefer subsequent investigation with CTC rather than colonoscopy [93] or barium enema [47]. However, in common with diagnostic performance studies conducted at the time, research relating to patient preference was rapidly evolving from small, high-risk cohorts to large screening populations. Therefore, in 2003, Glueker et al. published a large prospective study of asymptomatic individuals [49]; 696 patients scheduled to undergo colonoscopy and 617 patients due to have barium enema were offered additional CTC. Patients completed questionnaires exploring their attitudes to inconvenience, discomfort, preparation, willingness to repeat examinations and examination preference. Overall, patients preferred CTC to colonoscopy (72% vs. 5%) and to barium enema (97% vs. 0.4%). Moreover, regardless of the modality, the majority of patients found bowel preparation uncomfortable and inconvenient.

However, most patient preference surveys thus far had been led by a radiologist with an interest in CTC (often without gastroenterologist co-authors) which prompted some accusations of bias. Studies led by gastroenterologists found that CTC failed to offer any advantage over colonoscopy among their patient group [64]. Consequently, multidisciplinary research has been considered essential for ensuring patients' views are fairly represented and for the results to be considered unbiased. For example, in 2005, a study by van Gelder [94], working with health psychologists and gastroenterologists, obtained interesting results: while patients initially preferred CTC to colonoscopy, this was no longer the case after a 5-week interval. The authors suggested that once short-term concerns such as pain and inconvenience had subsided, long-term considerations such as test accuracy became more influential. Moreover, a recent qualitative study has suggested that patients may be willing to trade considerable discomfort for very modest increases in sensitivity [95], yet no preference survey to date has provided patients with any diagnostic performance information.

In any event, the rationale for comparing CTC to colonoscopy is questionable; patients with positive or equivocal findings will continue to need therapeutic colonoscopy regardless. Therefore, stimulated by the CTC cost-effectiveness debate, research focus has returned to the original question: the potential effect of CTC on screening uptake. Recently, a questionnaire survey of 250 asymptomatic, average-risk patients undergoing CTC showed that 36% would have forgone screening altogether had CTC been unavailable [96]. However, again, the result must be interpreted with caution; the respondents had made a decision to undergo CTC, and consequently, their attitudes are unlikely to reflect those of patients who choose not to attend colorectal cancer screening by any test. Despite these limitations, all the studies to date concur that CTC is generally well tolerated and that reducing the burden of bowel preparation is likely to improve patient experience.

Optimising Bowel Preparation

Although a certain degree of overlap exists with patient acceptability research, studies investigating reduced bowel preparation have a somewhat different emphasis: although reducing the laxative burden during CTC preparation may improve the experience, ensuring comparable sensitivity with full laxative preparations is the primary concern.

Initially, bowel preparation prior to CTC reflected that used for barium enema or colonoscopy. Although this varied from one institution to the next, as a general rule, laxative "wet" preparations involving four or more pints of polyethylene glycol (PEG) were favoured in the USA, while "dry" preparations based around sodium picosulfate were preferred in Europe. However, it soon became apparent that residual faecal fluid and residue represented a barrier to diagnosis, and researchers began to investigate alternative preparations. An early study confirmed picosulfate resulted in less residue than PEG [19], while others found drinking large volumes of PEG was considered by some patients worse than the resulting diarrhoea [97]. Subsequently, dryer preparations replaced PEG in many US centres.

While studies continued to compare the quality of various laxative regimens [42], a small number of researchers directed their efforts on avoiding catharsis altogether. The first study suggesting adequate performance could be achieved by a non-laxative CTC was published in 2001 [22], and since then, a limited number of studies have continued to produce impressive results [51, 98, 99]. Despite the obvious attraction of prepless CTC,

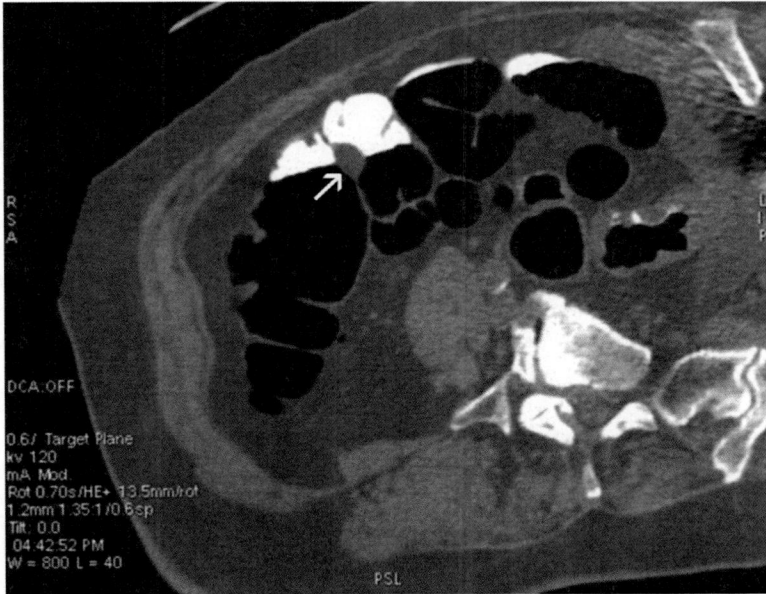

Fig. 3.8 Axial CT colonography following oral contrast. Homogenous fluid "tagging" enables confident diagnosis of a 10-mm pedunculated polyp (*arrow*) despite being partially submerged in colonic residue. Note the fat attenuation in this endoscopically proven lipoma

it remains unpopular with readers who favour a 3D approach, and despite considerable research, stool tagging often remains incomplete. Nevertheless, it is likely that early research on laxative-free preparation was responsible for the introduction of positive oral contrast faecal tagging during full-preparation CTC [100]. From experience with barium enema, colonoscopy was considered unsatisfactory in the presence of colonic barium, so to enable same-day colonoscopy, oral iodine solutions were included in the DoD [62] and ACRIN [78] study protocols. Given the performance demonstrated by these studies, full colonic cleansing coupled with iodine solutions is generally regarded as the "gold standard" [70] (Fig. 3.8). However, it is important to note that oral iodine solutions act as a strong laxative in its own right and in combination with full catharsis may give a rather harsh preparation. Nevertheless, iodine solution's laxative properties have been used to advantage by several groups for designing new regimens: These so-called "reduced preparation" techniques have proved particularly popular in Europe where

CTC is mainly used to investigate symptomatic patients [48, 101–103]. However, in common with non-laxative preparations, the main obstacle to reduced preparation is the difficulty in reading 3D endoluminal CTC in the presence of residual fluid. Therefore, the development of "digital cleansing" [20, 98] has undoubtedly made reduced preparation CTC a realistic compromise between diagnostic performance and tolerability. Recently, Nagata et al. [104] published the most convincing evidence to date that full preparation is no longer required: 101 consecutive high-risk patients scheduled to undergo CTC were alternately assigned to either full or minimal preparation. Reduced bowel preparation CTC achieved a comparable, high sensitivity for detecting polyps 6 mm or larger (88% compared to 97% for the full laxative CTC), and a questionnaire survey indicated a strong preference for the reduced preparation. However, as previously demonstrated, retaining this high sensitivity comes at a cost: the specificity was reduced from 92 to 68%. Intriguingly, the authors concluded that patients should be offered the reduced-laxative CTC if they were willing to accept the decrease in specificity—very little is known about patient attitudes to specificity, least of all how they might be weighed against side effects.

Therefore, although excellent progress has been made in terms of reducing the burden of bowel preparation, the consequences of reducing specificity may concern patients and policy makers. Therefore, research into different regimes continues apace, and the results of ongoing large prospective studies are expected in the near future.

So What Happened to the Barium Enema?

By now, the reader would be forgiven for wondering if the appetite and justification for performing barium enema had all but disappeared. However, despite comparative studies suggesting that CT colonography is superior [105], barium examinations have not been universally abandoned. Indeed, it is estimated that 3.7 million procedures were performed worldwide in 2008 (personal communication, Bracco Diagnostics Inc.). The reasons for this are beyond the scope of this chapter, but suffice it to say, barium enema has been entrenched in clinical practice worldwide for many years and remains approved (albeit no longer recommended) for colorectal screening. Furthermore, the recent landmark decision by the Centers for Medicare and Medicaid Services (CMS) to decline coverage of CT colonography for screening [106] has led some to suggest that the technique seems to be held to a higher standard than the established alternatives [107]. While it is widely accepted that randomised controlled trials (RCT) provide the "strongest" evidence, they are time-consuming and costly, and their design does not necessarily lend itself to radiologic research. Nevertheless, the UK Department of Health, via the Health Technology Assessment programme (HTA), commissioned a randomised controlled trial to determine the likely future role of CT colonography within the National Health Service

(NHS) by comparison with barium enema or optical colonoscopy. As previously stated, the emphasis of CTC research in Europe has typically involved investigation of symptomatic patients: therefore, the primary end point was detection rates for colorectal cancer or polyps ≥ 1 cm in symptomatic adults. The resulting SIGGAR trial [108], (named after the UK Special Interest Group in Gastrointestinal and Abdominal Radiology) was led by Professor Steve Halligan and Professor Wendy Atkin with the first patient randomised in April 2004 and accrual completed by November 2007. Radiologists, surgeons and gastroenterologists in 21 centres participated, registering 9,012 patients in total. The RCT comparing CTC with barium enema recruited 3,838, and the RCT comparing CTC with colonoscopy recruited 1,610 [109].

In the barium enema trial, patients aged 55 or over with symptoms suggestive of colorectal cancer who were referred by their clinician for barium enema were randomised (in a 2:1 ratio) to either barium enema (2,541) or CTC (1,280). In an intent-to-treat analysis, colorectal cancer or polyps ≥ 10 mm were diagnosed significantly more frequently in patients assigned CTC than barium enema (7.4% vs. 5.6%, $p=0.03$). Using national registry data to capture cancer miss rates (diagnosed within 2 years of randomisation), barium enema had twice the miss rate of CTC (14% vs. 7%). Additional colonic investigations occurred significantly more frequently following CTC than barium enema (23% vs. 18%), mainly due to higher polyp detection rates. One thousand three hundred and thirty-eight previously unknown extracolonic findings were reported in the 1,206 patients who underwent CTC as their randomised procedure. Eighty-six patients were referred for further tests as a result of their extracolonic findings, leading to diagnosis of a malignant tumour in 12 patients [110]. As a result of these data, the UK Department of Health has deleted barium enema from its faecal occult blood testing based national screening programme for colorectal cancer and recommends CTC in its place, and the results are expected to have worldwide impact on CTC implementation.

Table 3.1 Milestones in the history of CT colonography

1983	First report of CT imaging of the cleansed, distended colorectum [1]
1994	Vining et al. present "virtual colonoscopy" [2]
1997	First exploratory observer study of CTC performance [32]
1998	Feasibility demonstrated in patients with endoscopically proven findings [29]
1998	Boston International Symposium on Virtual Colonoscopy introduced [34]
1998	"CT colonography" becomes preferred terminology [35]
1999	Landmark study shows very favourable performance for CTC and initiates international interest [36]
2000	The National Polyp Study published; poor performance brings barium enema use into question [7]
2000	First CAD systems developed for CTC [82]
2001	Iodine tagging of liquid stool shown to benefit [20, 98]
2001	First attempts at non-laxative CTC reported [22]
2001	CAD undergoes preliminary clinical validation [83]
2003	Prospective patient attitude survey finds CTC preferable colonoscopy and to barium enema[49]
2003	ESGAR form CTC working group
2003	DoD trial published [62]
2003	ACRIN trial published [63]
2004	Comparative study shows CTC superior to barium enema [105]
2005	Meta-analysis of CTC performance for cancer detection published [59]
2005	First International CTC standards document published [66]
2007	AGA release own guidelines [76]
2007	ESGAR publish consensus statement [68]
2008	ACRIN II study published [78]
2009	CMS declines coverage of CT colonography for screening [106]
2010	Studies provide convincing evidence for "second-reader" CAD [89, 90]
2010	Preliminary results of first RCT of CTC presented (SIGGAR trial) [109]
2010	UK Department of Health discontinues barium enema in favour of CTC for CRC screening programme

ACR American College of Radiology, *ACRIN* American College of Radiology Imaging Network, *AGA* American Gastroenterological Association, *CAD* computer-aided detection, *CMS* Centers for Medicare and Medicaid Services, *CRADS* CTC reporting and data system, *CTC* computed tomographic colonography, *CRC* colorectal cancer, *DoD* Department of Defense (US), *ESGAR* European Society of Gastrointestinal and Abdominal Radiology, *RCT* randomised controlled trial, *SIGGAR* Special Interest Group in Gastrointestinal and Abdominal Radiology—now known as the British Society of Gastrointestinal and Abdominal Radiology (BSGAR)

The End of the Beginning

Advances in both CT and computer technology have allowed established techniques from barium enema to be successfully transferred to CT colonography. Since then, developments in the USA, and later worldwide, have seen the technique grow from feasibility studies in academic units to international daily practice (Table 3.1).

Recent research has established excellent comparative performance with colonoscopy and an accuracy that supersedes barium enema, but concerns remain regarding generalisability of these results to daily practice. Research continues apace to refine technical implementation, particularly reduced preparation methods which may increase adherence with screening programmes, and to ensure that readers, potentially with the assistance of CAD, achieve the same diagnostic performance as those in large multicentre trials. International training programmes have been developed to ensure the guidance laid down in international consensus proposals can be met.

Key Points

- Colorectal CT imaging following cathartic cleansing and gaseous insufflation was described in the 1980s, but the technique did not gain widespread recognition until 1994 when advances in computer technology enabled the development of "virtual colonoscopy".
- Research rapidly followed to optimise technical implementation, much of which continues to guide best practice today.
- Fenlon's landmark study in 1999, using state-of-the-art technique, demonstrated CTC's potential and precipitated international interest.
- Large prospective trials in the USA and later in Europe provided the evidence base for widespread CTC implementation.
- Simultaneously, research was accumulating that barium enema lacked sensitivity and that more sensitive colorectal imaging was necessary.
- CTC rapidly developed from a novel technique practised in a handful of specialist academic centres to one which has widely surpassed the barium enema as the preferred colorectal imaging modality.
- Having established sound performance characteristics, research focus has turned to improving patient experience, ensuring cost-effectiveness, computer-aided detection and the impact of extracolonic findings.

References

1. Coin CG, Wollett FC, Coin JT, Rowland M, DeRamos RK, Dandrea R. Computerized radiology of the colon: a potential screening technique. Comput Radiol. 1983;7(4):215–21.
2. Vining DJ, Gelfand DW, Bechtold RE, et al. Technical feasibility of colon imaging with helical CT and virtual reality. AJR Am J Roentgenol. 1994;162(S):1.
3. Steine S, Stordahl A, Lunde OC, Loken K, Laerum E. Double-contrast barium enema versus colonoscopy in the diagnosis of neoplastic disorders: aspects of decision-making in general practice. Fam Pract. 1993;10(3):288–91.
4. Rex DK, Rahmani EY, Haseman JH, Lemmel GT, Kaster S, Buckley JS. Relative sensitivity of colonos-copy and barium enema for detection of colorectal cancer in clinical practice. Gastroenterology. 1997;112(1):17–23.
5. Halligan S, Marshall M, Taylor S, et al. Observer variation in the detection of colorectal neoplasia on double-contrast barium enema: implications for colorectal cancer screening and training. Clin Radiol. 2003;58(12):948–54.
6. Glick S. Double-contrast barium enema for colorectal cancer screening: a review of the issues and a comparison with other screening alternatives. AJR Am J Roentgenol. 2000;174(6):1529–37.
7. Winawer SJ, Stewart ET, Zauber AG, et al. A comparison of colonoscopy and double-contrast barium enema for surveillance after polypectomy. National Polyp Study Work Group. N Engl J Med. 2000;342(24):1766–72.
8. Fletcher RH. The end of barium enemas? N Engl J Med. 2000;342(24):1823–4.
9. Levine MS, Glick SN, Rubesin SE, Laufer I. Double-contrast barium enema examination and colorectal cancer: a plea for radiologic screening. Radiology. 2002;222(2):313–5.
10. Fink M, Freeman AH, Dixon AK, Coni NK. Computed tomography of the colon in elderly people. BMJ. 1994;308(6935):1018.
11. Dixon AK, Freeman AH, Coni NK. CT of the colon in frail elderly patients. Semin Ultrasound CT MR. 1995;16(2):165–72.
12. Amin Z, Boulos PB, Lees WR. Technical report: spiral CT pneumocolon for suspected colonic neoplasms. Clin Radiol. 1996;51(1):56–61.
13. Harvey CJ, Renfrew I, Taylor S, Gillams AR, Lees WR. Spiral CT pneumocolon: applications, status and limitations. Eur Radiol. 2001;11(9):1612–25.
14. Chen SC, Lu DS, Hecht JR, Kadell BM. CT colonography: value of scanning in both the supine and prone positions. AJR Am J Roentgenol. 1999;172(3):595–9.
15. Rogalla P, Meiri N, Ruckert JC, Hamm B. Colonography using multislice CT. Eur J Radiol. 2000;36(2):81–5.
16. Morrin MM, Farrell RJ, Kruskal JB, Reynolds K, McGee JB, Raptopoulos V. Utility of intravenously administered contrast material at CT colonography. Radiology. 2000;217(3):765–71.
17. Yee J, Hung RK, Akerkar GA, Wall SD. The usefulness of glucagon hydrochloride for colonic distention in CT colonography. AJR Am J Roentgenol. 1999;173(1):169–72.
18. Morrin MM, Farrell RJ, Keogan MT, Kruskal JB, Yam C-S, Raptopoulos V. CT colonography: colonic distention improved by dual positioning but not intravenous glucagon. Eur Radiol. 2002;12(3):525–30.
19. Macari M, Lavelle M, Pedrosa I, et al. Effect of different bowel preparations on residual fluid at CT colonography. Radiology. 2001;218(1):274–7.
20. Zalis ME, Hahn PF. Digital subtraction bowel cleansing in CT colonography. AJR Am J Roentgenol. 2001;176(3):646–8.

21. Fletcher JG, Johnson CD, Welch TJ, et al. Optimization of CT colonography technique: prospective trial in 180 patients. Radiology. 2000;216(3):704–11.
22. Callstrom MR, Johnson CD, Fletcher JG, et al. CT colonography without cathartic preparation: feasibility study. Radiology. 2001;219(3):693–8.
23. Beaulieu CF, Napel S, Daniel BL, et al. Detection of colonic polyps in a phantom model: implications for virtual colonoscopy data acquisition. J Comput Assist Tomogr. 1998;22(4):656–63.
24. Dachman AH, Lieberman J, Osnis RB, et al. Small simulated polyps in pig colon: sensitivity of CT virtual colography. Radiology. 1997;203(2):427–30.
25. Taylor SA, Halligan S, Bartram CI, et al. Multi-detector row CT colonography: effect of collimation, pitch, and orientation on polyp detection in a human colectomy specimen. Radiology. 2003;229(1):109–18.
26. Hara AK, Johnson CD, Reed JE, et al. Reducing data size and radiation dose for CT colonography. AJR Am J Roentgenol. 1997;168(5):1181–4.
27. Fenlon HM, Clarke PD, Ferrucci JT. Virtual colonoscopy: imaging features with colonoscopic correlation. AJR Am J Roentgenol. 1998;170(5):1303–9.
28. Hara AK, Johnson CD, Reed JE. Colorectal lesions: evaluation with CT colography. Radiographics. 1997;17(5):1157–67.
29. Fenlon HM, Nunes DP, Clarke PD, Ferrucci JT. Colorectal neoplasm detection using virtual colonoscopy: a feasibility study. Gut. 1998;43(6):806–11.
30. Royster AP, Fenlon HM, Clarke PD, Nunes DP, Ferrucci JT. CT colonoscopy of colorectal neoplasms: two-dimensional and three-dimensional virtual-reality techniques with colonoscopic correlation. AJR Am J Roentgenol. 1997;169(5):1237–42.
31. Dachman AH, Kuniyoshi JK, Boyle CM, et al. CT colonography with three-dimensional problem solving for detection of colonic polyps. AJR Am J Roentgenol. 1998;171(4):989–95.
32. Hara AK, Johnson CD, Reed JE, et al. Detection of colorectal polyps with CT colography: initial assessment of sensitivity and specificity. Radiology. 1997;205(1):59–65.
33. Yee J, Kumar NN, Hung RK, Akerkar GA, Kumar PR, Wall SD. Comparison of supine and prone scanning separately and in combination at CT colonography. Radiology. 2003;226(3):653–61.
34. Fenlon HM, Ferrucci JT. First international symposium on virtual colonoscopy. AJR Am J Roentgenol. 1999;173(3):565–9.
35. Johnson CD, Hara AK, Reed JE. Virtual endoscopy: what's in a name? AJR Am J Roentgenol. 1998;171(5):1201–2.
36. Fenlon HM, Nunes DP, Schroy III PC, Barish MA, Clarke PD, Ferrucci JT. A comparison of virtual and conventional colonoscopy for the detection of colorectal polyps. N Engl J Med. 1999;341(20):1496–503.
37. Halligan S, Fenlon HM. Virtual colonoscopy. BMJ. 1999;319(7219):1249–52.
38. Laghi A, Catalano C, Panebianco V, Iannaccone R, Iori S, Passariello R. [Optimization of the technique of virtual colonoscopy using a multislice spiral computerized tomography]. Radiol Med. 2000;100(6):459–64.
39. Laghi A, Iannaccone R, Mangiapane F, Piacentini F, Iori S, Passariello R. Experimental colonic phantom for the evaluation of the optimal scanning technique for CT colonography using a multidetector spiral CT equipment. Eur Radiol. 2003;13(3):459–66.
40. Rogalla P, Meiri N. CT colonography: data acquisition and patient preparation techniques. Semin Ultrasound CT MR. 2001;22(5):405–12.
41. Robinson P, Burnett H, Nicholson DA. The use of minimal preparation computed tomography for the primary investigation of colon cancer in frail or elderly patients. Clin Radiol. 2002;57(5):389–92.
42. Taylor SA, Halligan S, Goh V, Morley S, Atkin W, Bartram CI. Optimizing bowel preparation for multidetector row CT colonography: effect of Citramag and Picolax. Clin Radiol. 2003;58(9):723–32.
43. Taylor SA, Halligan S, Goh V, et al. Optimizing colonic distention for multi-detector row CT colonography: effect of hyoscine butylbromide and rectal balloon catheter. Radiology. 2003;229(1):99–108.
44. van Gelder RE, Venema HW, Serlie IW, et al. CT colonography at different radiation dose levels: feasibility of dose reduction. Radiology. 2002;224(1):25–33.
45. Iannaccone R, Laghi A, Catalano C, et al. Detection of colorectal lesions: lower-dose multi-detector row helical CT colonography compared with conventional colonoscopy. Radiology. 2003;229(3):775–81.
46. Svensson MH, Svensson E, Lasson A, Hellstrom M. Patient acceptance of CT colonography and conventional colonoscopy: prospective comparative study in patients with or suspected of having colorectal disease. Radiology. 2002;222(2):337–45.
47. Taylor SA, Halligan S, Saunders BP, Bassett P, Vance M, Bartram CI. Acceptance by patients of multidetector CT colonography compared with barium enema examinations, flexible sigmoidoscopy, and colonoscopy. AJR Am J Roentgenol. 2003;181(4):913–21.
48. Lefere PA, Gryspeerdt SS, Dewyspelaere J, Baekelandt M, Van Holsbeeck BG. Dietary fecal tagging as a cleansing method before CT colonography: initial results polyp detection and patient acceptance. Radiology. 2002;224(2):393–403.
49. Gluecker TM, Johnson CD, Harmsen WS, et al. Colorectal cancer screening with CT colonography, colonoscopy, and double-contrast barium enema examination: prospective assessment of patient perceptions and preferences. Radiology. 2003;227(2):378–84.
50. Thomeer M, Bielen D, Vanbeckevoort D, et al. Patient acceptance for CT colonography: what is the real issue? Eur Radiol. 2002;12(6):1410–5.
51. Iannaccone R, Laghi A, Catalano C, et al. Computed tomographic colonography without cathartic preparation for the detection of colorectal polyps. Gastroenterology. 2004;127(5):1300–11.
52. European Society of Gastrointestinal and Abdominal Radiology CT Colonography Study Group

Investigators. Effect of directed training on reader performance for CT colonography: multicenter study. Radiology. 2007;242(1):152–61.

53. Burling D, Halligan S, Altman DG, et al. CT colonography interpretation times: effect of reader experience, fatigue, and scan findings in a multicentre setting. Eur Radiol. 2006;16(8):1745–9.

54. Burling D, Halligan S, Altman DG, et al. Polyp measurement and size categorisation by CT colonography: effect of observer experience in a multi-centre setting. Eur Radiol. 2006;16(8):1737–44.

55. Laghi A, Iannaccone R, Carbone I, et al. Computed tomographic colonography (virtual colonoscopy): blinded prospective comparison with conventional colonoscopy for the detection of colorectal neoplasia. Endoscopy. 2002;34(6):441–6.

56. Taylor SA, Halligan S, Vance M, Windsor A, Atkin W, Bartram CI. Use of multidetector-row computed tomographic colonography before flexible sigmoidoscopy in the investigation of rectal bleeding. Br J Surg. 2003;90(9):1163–4.

57. Van Gelder RE, Nio CY, Florie J, et al. Computed tomographic colonography compared with colonoscopy in patients at increased risk for colorectal cancer. Gastroenterology. 2004;127(1):41–8.

58. Neri E, Giusti P, Battolla L, et al. Colorectal cancer: role of CT colonography in preoperative evaluation after incomplete colonoscopy. Radiology. 2002; 223(3):615–9.

59. Halligan S, Altman DG, Taylor SA, et al. CT colonography in the detection of colorectal polyps and cancer: systematic review, meta-analysis, and proposed minimum data set for study level reporting. Radiology. 2005;237(3):893–904.

60. Yee J, Akerkar GA, Hung RK, Steinauer-Gebauer AM, Wall SD, McQuaid KR. Colorectal neoplasia: performance characteristics of CT colonography for detection in 300 patients. Radiology. 2001;219(3):685–92.

61. Macari M, Bini EJ, Xue X, et al. Colorectal neoplasms: prospective comparison of thin-section low-dose multi-detector row CT colonography and conventional colonoscopy for detection. Radiology. 2002;224(2):383–92.

62. Pickhardt PJ, Choi JR, Hwang I, et al. Computed tomographic virtual colonoscopy to screen for colorectal neoplasia in asymptomatic adults. N Engl J Med. 2003;349(23):2191–200.

63. Johnson CD, Harmsen WS, Wilson LA, et al. Prospective blinded evaluation of computed tomographic colonography for screen detection of colorectal polyps. Gastroenterology. 2003;125(2):311–9.

64. Cotton PB, Durkalski VL, Pineau BC, et al. Computed tomographic colonography (virtual colonoscopy): a multicenter comparison with standard colonoscopy for detection of colorectal neoplasia. JAMA. 2004;291(14):1713–9.

65. Rockey DC, Paulson E, Niedzwiecki D, et al. Analysis of air contrast barium enema, computed tomographic colonography, and colonoscopy:

prospective comparison. Lancet. 2005;365(9456): 305–11.

66. Barish MA, Soto JA, Ferrucci JT. Consensus on current clinical practice of virtual colonoscopy. AJR Am J Roentgenol. 2005;184(3):786–92.

67. Zalis ME, Barish MA, Choi JR, et al. CT colonography reporting and data system: a consensus proposal. Radiology. 2005;236(1):3–9.

68. Taylor SA, Laghi A, Lefere P, Halligan S, Stoker J. European Society of Gastrointestinal and Abdominal Radiology (ESGAR): consensus statement on CT colonography. Eur Radiol. 2007;17(2):575–9.

69. Position of the American Gastroenterological Association (AGA) Institute on computed tomographic colonography. Gastroenterology. 2006; 131(5):1627–8.

70. Burling D. CT colonography standards. Clin Radiol. 2010;65(6):474–80.

71. Burling D, Halligan S, Taylor SA, Usiskin S, Bartram CI. CT colonography practice in the UK: a national survey. Clin Radiol. 2004;59(1):39–43.

72. Spinzi G, Belloni G, Martegani A, Sangiovanni A, Del Favero C, Minoli G. Computed tomographic colonography and conventional colonoscopy for colon diseases: a prospective, blinded study. Am J Gastroenterol. 2001;96(2):394–400.

73. Soto JA, Barish MA, Yee J. Reader training in CT colonography: how much is enough? Radiology. 2005;237(1):26–7.

74. Taylor SA, Halligan S, Burling D, et al. CT colonography: effect of experience and training on reader performance. Eur Radiol. 2004;14(6):1025–33.

75. McFarland EG, Fletcher JG, Pickhardt P, et al. ACR Colon Cancer Committee white paper: status of CT colonography 2009. J Am Coll Radiol. 2009; 6(11):756–72.e4.

76. Rockey DC, Barish M, Brill JV, et al. Standards for gastroenterologists for performing and interpreting diagnostic computed tomographic colonography. Gastroenterology. 2007;133(3):1005–24.

77. Boone D, Halligan S, Frost R, et al. CT colonography: who attends training? A survey of participants at educational workshops. Clin Radiol. 2011; 66(6):510–6.

78. Johnson CD, Chen MH, Toledano AY, et al. Accuracy of CT colonography for detection of large adenomas and cancers. N Engl J Med. 2008;359(12):1207–17.

79. Macari M, Milano A, Lavelle M, Berman P, Megibow AJ. Comparison of time-efficient CT colonography with two- and three-dimensional colonic evaluation for detecting colorectal polyps. AJR Am J Roentgenol. 2000;174(6):1543–9.

80. Pickhardt PJ. Three-dimensional endoluminal CT colonography (virtual colonoscopy): comparison of three commercially available systems. AJR Am J Roentgenol. 2003;181(6):1599–606.

81. Lenhart DK, Babb J, Bonavita J, et al. Comparison of a unidirectional panoramic 3D endoluminal interpretation technique to traditional 2D and bidirectional

3D interpretation techniques at CT colonography: preliminary observations. Clin Radiol. 2010;65(2): 118–25.

82. Summers RM, Beaulieu CF, Pusanik LM, et al. Automated polyp detector for CT colonography: feasibility study. Radiology. 2000;216(1):284–90.

83. Summers RM, Johnson CD, Pusanik LM, Malley JD, Youssef AM, Reed JE. Automated polyp detection at CT colonography: feasibility assessment in a human population. Radiology. 2001;219(1):51–9.

84. Yoshida H, Nappi J. Three-dimensional computer-aided diagnosis scheme for detection of colonic polyps. IEEE Trans Med Imaging. 2001;20(12): 1261–74.

85. Summers RM, Jerebko AK, Franaszek M, Malley JD, Johnson CD. Colonic polyps: complementary role of computer-aided detection in CT colonography. Radiology. 2002;225(2):391–9.

86. Summers RM, Yao J, Pickhardt PJ, et al. Computed tomographic virtual colonoscopy computer-aided polyp detection in a screening population. Gastroenterology. 2005;129(6):1832–44.

87. Taylor SA, Robinson C, Boone D, Honeyfield L, Halligan S. Polyp characteristics correctly annotated by computer-aided detection software but ignored by reporting radiologists during CT colonography. Radiology. 2009;253(3):715–23.

88. Taylor SA, Halligan S, Slater A, et al. Polyp detection with CT colonography: primary 3D endoluminal analysis versus primary 2D transverse analysis with computer-assisted reader software. Radiology. 2006;239(3):759–67.

89. Dachman AH, Obuchowski NA, Hoffmeister JW, et al. Effect of computer-aided detection for CT colonography in a multireader, multicase trial. Radiology. 2010;256(3):827–35.

90. Halligan S, Mallett S, Altman DG, et al. Incremental benefit of computer-aided detection when used as a second and concurrent reader of CT colonographic data: multiobserver study. Radiology. 2011;258(2): 469–76.

91. Atkin WS, Edwards R, Kralj-Hans I, et al. Once-only flexible sigmoidoscopy screening in prevention of colorectal cancer: a multicentre randomised controlled trial. Lancet. 2010;375(9726):1624–33.

92. Seeff LC, Nadel MR, Klabunde CN, et al. Patterns and predictors of colorectal cancer test use in the adult U.S. population. Cancer. 2004;100(10): 2093–103.

93. Ristvedt SL, McFarland EG, Weinstock LB, Thyssen EP. Patient preferences for CT colonography, conventional colonoscopy, and bowel preparation. Am J Gastroenterol. 2003;98(3):578–85.

94. van Gelder RE, Birnie E, Florie J, et al. CT colonography and colonoscopy: assessment of patient preference in a 5-week follow-up study. Radiology. 2004;233(2):328–37.

95. Von Wagner C, Halligan S, Atkin WS, Lilford RJ, Morton D, Wardle J. Choosing between CT colonography and colonoscopy in the diagnostic context:

a qualitative study of influences on patient preferences. Health Expect. 2009;12(1):18–26.

96. Moawad FJ, Maydonovitch CL, Cullen PA, Barlow DS, Jenson DW, Cash BD. CT colonography may improve colorectal cancer screening compliance. AJR Am J Roentgenol. 2010;195(5):1118–23.

97. Gryspeerdt S, Lefere P, Dewyspelaere J, Baekelandt M, van Holsbeeck B. Optimisation of colon cleansing prior to computed tomographic colonography. JBR-BTR. 2002;85(6):289–96.

98. Zalis ME, Perumpillichira JJ, Magee C, Kohlberg G, Hahn PF. Tagging-based, electronically cleansed CT colonography: evaluation of patient comfort and image readability. Radiology. 2006;239(1): 149–59.

99. Bielen D, Thomeer M, Vanbeckevoort D, et al. Dry preparation for virtual CT colonography with fecal tagging using water-soluble contrast medium: initial results. Eur Radiol. 2003;13(3):453–8.

100. Thomeer M, Carbone I, Bosmans H, et al. Stool tagging applied in thin-slice multidetector computed tomography colonography. J Comput Assist Tomogr. 2003;27(2):132–9.

101. Lefere P, Gryspeerdt S, Marrannes J, Baekelandt M, Van Holsbeeck B. CT colonography after fecal tagging with a reduced cathartic cleansing and a reduced volume of barium. AJR Am J Roentgenol. 2005; 184(6):1836–42.

102. Taylor SA, Slater A, Burling DN, et al. CT colonography: optimisation, diagnostic performance and patient acceptability of reduced-laxative regimens using barium-based faecal tagging. Eur Radiol. 2008;18(1):32–42.

103. Jensch S, de Vries AH, Peringa J, et al. CT colonography with limited bowel preparation: performance characteristics in an increased-risk population. Radiology. 2008;247(1):122–32.

104. Nagata K, Okawa T, Honma A, Endo S, Kudo SE, Yoshida H. Full-laxative versus minimum-laxative fecal-tagging CT colonography using 64-detector row CT: prospective blinded comparison of diagnostic performance, tagging quality, and patient acceptance. Acad Radiol. 2009;16(7):780–9.

105. Johnson CD, MacCarty RL, Welch TJ, et al. Comparison of the relative sensitivity of CT colonography and double-contrast barium enema for screen detection of colorectal polyps. Clin Gastroenterol Hepatol. 2004;2(4):314–21.

106. Dhruva SS, Phurrough SE, Salive ME, Redberg RF. CMS's landmark decision on CT colonography – examining the relevant data. N Engl J Med. 2009;360(26):2699–701.

107. Garg S, Ahnen DJ. Is computed tomographic colonography being held to a higher standard? Ann Intern Med. 2010;152(3):178–81.

108. Halligan S, Lilford RJ, Wardle J, et al. Design of a multicentre randomized trial to evaluate CT colonography versus colonoscopy or barium enema for diagnosis of colonic cancer in older symptomatic patients: the SIGGAR study. Trials. 2007;8:32.

109. Taylor S, Halligan S, Atkin W, et al. Clinical trials and experiences: SIGGAR. Presented at the 11th international symposium on virtual colonoscopy Westin Copley Place, Boston, MA, 25–27 Oct 2010; 2010.

110. Halligan S, Waddingham J, Dadswell E, Wooldrage K, Atkin W, SIGGAR Trial Investigators. Detection of extracolonic lesions by CTC in symptomatic patients: their frequency and severity in a randomised controlled trial. Eur Radiol. 2010;20 Suppl 1:S8.

Indications and Evidence for CTC

4

Elizabeth G. McFarland

Background

The clinical indications of CTC have broadened gradually over the past decade. Several interactive influences of this trend include the impact of validation data of clinical trials, health policy decisions of colorectal screening guidelines, and insurance reimbursement rates determined by payors. After the early clinical trials of CTC in the late 1990s, clinical use of CTC was limited to a few specific diagnostic indications [1]. Since 2003 with the emergence of multiple successful large screening trials, there has been broader use of CTC in asymptomatic patients. From these validation data however, health policy agencies responded differently in 2008 for the 5-year updates of colorectal screening guidelines. Specifically, the American Cancer Society, with the multidisciplinary consensus of the American College of Radiology and the US Multi-Society Task Force of colorectal cancer (comprised of the American Gastroenterology Association, American Society of Gastroenterology, and the American College of Gastroenterology), recommended the use of CTC for the first time for

screening of average-risk patients [2]. Contrary to this, the US Preventative Task Force (USPTF) gave CTC an *indeterminate rating of effectiveness* and did not recommend CTC for screening purposes [3].

Payors have responded differently to rates of reimbursement for CTC. Similar to the American Cancer Society guidelines, both Kaiser Permanente and Blue Cross Blue Shield gave positive endorsements in their subsequent technology assessments for screening CTC in 2008. Although 47 states had Medicare coverage for specific diagnostic indication for CTC (largely after incomplete colonoscopy (OC)), the US Centers of Medicare and Medicaid (CMS), influenced by USPTF rating, passed a national noncoverage decision for screening indications in May 2009 [4]. Concerns raised during the initial CMS deliberation included radiation exposure, diagnostic performance in Medicare population, management of small polyps, and the cost burden of extracolonic findings. Despite these challenges, CTC continues to expand as a novel, minimally invasive structural imaging evaluation of the entire colon and rectum, holding the promise of improved patient compliance for colorectal screening.

The purpose of this chapter is twofold: (1) review the current diagnostic and screening indications for CTC and (2) review important validation data of the diagnostic performance of CTC.

E.G. McFarland, M.D. (✉)
Department of Radiology, SSM St. Joseph's Hospital,
St. Charles, MO, USA
e-mail: mcfarlandb123@gmail.com

Current Indications and Uses of CTC

Diagnostic CTC

Diagnostic indications for CTC are listed in Table 4.1. The most common indication is for patients who require completion of colorectal evaluation, following an incomplete OC. This has been supported since 2004 in 47 states [1]. Other diagnostic indications for CTC that are currently reimbursed variably across states include patients at risk to undergo OC (e.g., anticoagulation or anesthesia risks) and patients who require evaluation of submucosal lesions detected at OC.

Screening CTC

Based on local reimbursement issues, only a few centers have large screening programs. At the National Naval Medical Center, in Bethesda, MD, the Colon Health Initiative (CHI) was established through a congressional grant in 2004. A dedicated team of radiologists, gastroenterologists, general surgeons, nurses, technologists, and research personnel provide a multidisciplinary clinical colon health-care program with integrated clinical research for Department of Defense beneficiaries in the national capital region. President Obama underwent screening CTC at this facility in 2010. At the University of Wisconsin, several third-party payers have provided coverage for colorectal screening with CTC. Pickhardt et al. reported very positive first-year results of screening 1,100 patients in this system in 2006, with 99% insurance coverage provided [5]. In the near future, a positive national coverage decision CTC screening in Medicare patients will have a great impact on its more widespread use.

Screening indications for CTC include patients 50 years or older with average risk for colorectal cancer (Table 4.1). This includes patients with no family history or low risk based on family history. Low-risk patients include those with first-degree relatives with colon cancer after the age of 60 years or multiple second-degree relatives with

Table 4.1 Indications for CTC

Indications for diagnostic CTC[a]
1. History of incomplete OC with colorectal symptoms
2. Patients at risk to undergo OC with colorectal symptoms
3. Further evaluation of submucosal lesion(s) found at OC

Indications for screening CTC[b]
1. Average-risk[c] patients for colorectal cancer
2. Patients at moderate risk[d] for colon cancer in appropriate clinical context
3. Patients at average risk, with history of incomplete OC
4. Noncompliant patients who will not undergo OC

OC optical colonoscopy
[a]Diagnostic CTC may be done at routine radiation dose (25.0 mGy total), with and without IV contrast
[b]Screening CTC is done at low radiation dose (12.5 mGy total), without IV contrast
[c]Average-risk patients are 50 years or older with no colorectal symptoms or risk factors, with no family history or low-risk family history (first-degree family member(s) greater than 60 years of age or multiple second-degree relatives at any age with colon cancer)
[d]Moderate risk for colon cancer based on family history is first-degree family member(s) before age 60 or multiple first-degree relatives at any age with colon cancer

colon cancer at any age. CTC is typically not the first-line test for patients with moderate or high risk based on family history; however, it can be used in appropriate settings including contraindications for optical OC or previously unsuccessful OC (Table 4.2). Moderate risk is defined as first-degree relatives with colon cancer at or before the age of 60 or multiple first-degree relatives at any age. High-risk history includes patients with family history of known genetic syndromes at increased risk for colon cancer or personal history of ulcerative colitis.

Diagnostic Performance in Clinical Trials

Early Clinical Validation

In early clinical trials of CTC from 1997 to 2002, studies were predominantly validated in polyp-rich cohorts using OC as the reference standard.

Table 4.2 Relative contraindications for CTC

1. High-risk patients[a] for colon cancer, unless OC contraindicated or history of incomplete OC
2. Routine evaluation of anal disease
3. Recent colorectal surgery
4. Recent deep endoscopic biopsy or polypectomy/mucosectomy
5. Symptomatic or high-grade small bowel obstruction
6. Known bowel perforation
7. Colon-containing abdominal or pelvic hernia
8. Acute symptoms of colitis, diverticulitis, or diarrhea
9. Evaluation of pregnant woman

[a]High risk for colon cancer includes patients with inflammatory bowel disease or family history of known genetic syndromes at increased risk for colon cancer

As technical advances in CTC evolved over the years, a range of results were reported in different cohorts of patients using different techniques [6–15]. Two early landmark studies achieved the benchmark result of 90% sensitivity to detect polyps 10 mm and larger [14, 15]. The first study was performed at Boston University by Fenlon et al. [14]. In this study, 100 patients (60 men, 40 women; mean age 62 years) at high risk for colorectal neoplasia were evaluated. Selection criteria included patients 50 years or older who had a history of adenomatous polyps, positive FOBT, or strong family history of colon cancer in a first-degree relative. A total of 115 polyps and 3 cancers were found at OC, used as the reference standard. CTC had 100% (3/3) sensitivity to detect cancers, 91% (20/22) sensitivity to detect 10-mm and larger polyps, and 82% (33/40) sensitivity to detect 6–9-mm polyps. From this study, the authors concluded that CTC may have similar efficacy to OC to detect polyps 6 mm and larger in high-risk patients.

Following this study, Yee et al. reported a study with similar results in a larger cohort of 300 patients from the University of California, San Francisco Veterans Administration trial [15]. Participants in this trial were mostly male (291 male, 9 female), with 96 enrolled for screening and 204 enrolled for evaluation of colorectal symptoms. Two readers individually interpreted the CTC data using 2D primary review, with additional 3D endoscopic fly through (mean analysis times of 27–31 min), with the results given for the subsequent consensus reading. Sensitivities were 100% (8.8) to detect cancers, 90% (74/82) to detect polyps ≥10 mm, and 80% (113/141) to detect 5–9.9-mm polyps. This study helped to reinforce the feasibility of CTC as a modality to evaluate the colon in polyp-rich cohorts.

Other studies helped define the role of CTC in the setting of incomplete OC. Several early studies demonstrated the feasibility of CTC to complete the colon evaluation in same-day incomplete OC due to an obstructing cancer [16–18].

Large CTC Trials in Higher Risk Cohorts

Following the promising results of early validation trials, three larger trials demonstrated less favorable results in studies published from 2003 to 2005 [19–21] (Table 4.3). These three trials evaluated patient cohorts of 600–700 patients, who are at increased risk for colorectal cancer based on history of prior polyps, family risk, or colorectal symptoms. Specifically, Johnson et al. published a single-center trial of 703 patients with 153 lesions (≥6 mm in size) in 2003, using primarily 2D image display techniques for lesion detection [19]. Wide variability across results of three readers was reported with per-patient sensitivities to detect 5–9-mm and ≥10-mm polyps ranging from 41% to 69% and 35% to 72%, respectively. Cotton et al. published a multicenter trial of 615 patients with 173 lesions in 2004 [20]. Per-patient sensitivities to detect 6–9-mm and

Table 4.3 Large CTC trials in higher risk cohorts[a]

Trial Author, journal, year	Subjects (n)	Total lesions ≥6 mm	MDCT Scanner rows	Per-polyp sensitivity ≥6 mm	Per-polyp sensitivity ≥10 mm	Per-patient sensitivity ≥6 mm	Per-patient sensitivity ≥10 mm	Per-patient specificity ≥6 mm	Per-patient specificity ≥10 mm
Johnson et al. Gastroenterology 2003	703	153	4 row	29–57% (5–9 mm)	32–73%	41–65% (5–9 mm)	38–72%	88–95% (5–9 mm)	95–98%
Cotton et al. JAMA 2004	615	173	2–4 row	32%	52%	39%	55%	91%	96%
Rocky et al. Lancet 2005	614	234	4–8 row	49%[b]	53%[b]	51%[b]	59%[b]	89%	96%
Regge et al. JAMA 2009	937	233[c]	88% 16–64 row	76%	84%	85%	91%	88%	85%

[a]Higher risk cohorts includes patients with history of prior polyps, family risk factors, or colorectal symptoms
[b]Re-analysis of Rockey et al. data of the 152 adenomas only (excluding the 82 non-adenomatous lesions), increased sensitivity per polyp for ≥6 mm and ≥10 mm to 61% and 64% respectively and sensitivity per patient for ≥6 mm and ≥10 mm to 68% and 70%, respectively
[c]Regge et al. data only evaluates advanced adenomas and carcinomas (excludes nonadenomas and low risk adenomas)

≥10-mm polyps were 30% and 55%, respectively, using 2D for primary detection; a follow-up analysis using 3D endoscopic fly through increased results to 36% and 60%, respectively. In this study, the requirement for reader experience was set at a low standard, requiring readers to have only read ten CTC cases. The most experienced center recruited close to one-third of the patients and reported significantly higher sensitivities than the other centers, raising the concern that differences in reader experience largely affected the results. Despite low performance in sensitivity, both of these trials reported consistently high specificity results, ranging from 88 to 98% at 6-mm and 10-mm thresholds, respectively.

Rockey et al. later published the third multi-center trial in 2005, evaluating the diagnostic performance of CTC, air-contrast barium enema, and OC in 614 patients [21]. CTC was predominantly interpreted with 2D image display techniques to detect, with 3D imaging to characterize. In this trial, reader experience was more standardized; however, similar negative results were obtained. CTC results of per-patient sensitivities to detect 6–9-mm and ≥10-mm polyps were 51% and 59%, respectively, outperforming results at ACBE of 35% and 48%, respectively. Common to all three of these larger trials of patients at increased risk, results were analyzed for all histological lesions detected 6 mm and larger, including non-adenomatous and adenomatous polyps. A subsequent analysis of the Rockey trial determined that if non-adenomatous cancerous lesions were excluded ($n = 87$), analysis of the remaining adenomatous and cancerous lesions ($n = 147$) increased, the per-patient sensitivities to detect 6–9-mm and ≥10-mm polyps to 68% and 70%, respectively [22]. This methodology of selectively evaluating adenomatous or cancerous lesions would carry forward as the accepted methodology to evaluate CTC performance.

In contrast to these three less successful trials, the Italian Multicenter Polyp Accuracy Trial (IMPACT) was performed also in higher risk cohorts in 2009, encompassing a total of 21 centers [23]. A total of 937 patients were evaluated who had positive family history, prior polypectomy of polyps, or positive FOBT. In this trial, a total of 233 lesions with advanced neoplasia were evaluated, including advanced adenomas or cancer at histology (non-adenomatous and low-risk adenoma lesions were excluded). Per-patient sensitivity to detect polyps 6–9 mm and ≥10 mm was 85% and 91%, respectively. Per-polyp sensitivity decreased to 59% and 84%, respectively. Specificity remained high, ranging from 80 to 85% at 10- and 6-mm thresholds. Requirement of the radiologist experience was review of 50 or more cases under supervision by an expert. CT scanner technology used 16–64-row MDCT in 88% of cases. Radiologists used primarily 2D (74%) rather than 3D (26%) image display techniques, according to their preference. Stool tagging was used in the minority of cases (34%). The exclusion of low-risk adenomas from the analysis could be criticized. However, the large scale of this trial including 21 centers with strong results favorably supports generalizability into more diverse practice settings.

Larger Screening Trials in Asymptomatic Patients at Average Risk

At the same time as some of the early multicenter trials in patients at increased risk, a landmark successful trial was published which exploited new technological advances in the largest screening cohort of asymptomatic patients to date in 2003 [24]. Pickhardt et al. evaluated 1,233 asymptomatic patients for colorectal screening with CT colonography in a multicenter Department of Defense trial [24]. This trial introduced the novel techniques of stool tagging with electronic subtraction and 3D fly through as the primary image display technique in all studies. It also used the "enhanced" reference standard of segmental unblinding of CTC results during OC. This technique had been used in two of the large center trials [20, 21]. Namely, the colonoscopist evaluated each colonic segment initially, followed by a second look at the colonic segment if the disclosed CTC results demonstrated a significant lesion. This trial reported per-patient sensitivities to detect adenomas at size thresholds of ≥6 mm and ≥10 mm of 88.7% and 93.8%, respectively; specificities at these two-size thresholds were reported at 79.6% and 96.0%. Based on the segmental unblinding methodology, miss rates at the original OC (before CTC results were disclosed) could be evaluated. A subsequent analysis of these results demonstrated that OC missed 10% of adenomas larger than 10 mm [25]. This study clearly sets a new benchmark of improved diagnostic performance for detection of polyps 6 mm and larger in screening cohorts.

Five years later in 2008, the ACRIN 6664 trial (American College of Radiology Imaging Network) became the next largest screening trial of 2,531 asymptomatic patients at average risk [26]. This trial involved a total of 15 centers in academic and private practice settings. High standards for radiologist requirements were set either to have performed 500 or more CTC examinations or to take part in a 1.5-day training session of close to 50 cases and subsequently pass a qualifying examination of 90% detection rate of polyps 10 mm or greater. Methods included state-of-the-art techniques of low-dose (50 effective mAs) 16–64-row MDCT, 2D and 3D image display techniques, and stool tagging. The validation methodology of segmental unblinding at OC, however, was not used. Overall, the major goal of the study was met with per-patient sensitivity for ≥10-mm polyps of 90%. Per-polyp sensitivity in this size threshold decreased to 84%. More modest results were seen for detection of polyps at the lower size threshold of ≥6 mm, with per-patient and per-polyp results of 78% and 70%, respectively. Despite the use of stool tagging, specificity was slightly lower with results of 88% and 86% at 6-mm and 10-mm polyp thresholds, respectively. Although overall results were not as good as the Pickhardt et al. study in 2003, the diversity of 15 centers in both academic and private practice settings was valued as being more representative of potential results in general practice.

In Germany, the Munich trial by Graser et al. [27] was another successful screening trial of asymptomatic patients at average risk that was published in 2009, modeled very closely in methodology to the military trial by Pickhardt. A total of 307 subjects with 221 adenomas were evaluated

with CTC, flexible sigmoidoscopy (FS), fecal immunochemical stool testing (FIT), fecal occult blood testing (FOBT), and OC. Stool tagging, 3D primary review, and segmental unblinding were used. Enhanced data acquisition at 64-row MDCT (0.75-mm slice thickness at 0.5-mm reconstruction interval), using low-dose technique (30–70 mAs, mean radiation dose of 4.5 mSv), was also performed. CTC results of per-patient sensitivities to detect polyps at ≥6-mm and ≥10-mm thresholds were 91% and 92%, respectively, less than results at OC of 98% and 100%, but far improved compared to FS of 67% and 68%, FOBT of 18% and 24%, and FIT of 40% and 33%. Interestingly, similar results between CTC and OC were obtained for per-polyp sensitivity at 6–9 mm (CTC 90% and OC 93%) and ≥10 mm (CTC 94% and OC 100%). This study represents the highest sensitivity results of small polyps in the 6–9-mm range in a screening cohort using 64-row MCDT, despite the potential increase of image noise due to the low-dose technique (Table 4.4).

Factors That May Have Influenced Differences in Results Across Studies

What then could help explain some of the differences in results among these larger trials over a decade of efforts? First, diagnostic performance does differ between early assessments of detection of multiple polyps in enriched cohorts compared to the later challenges of detecting fewer polyps in a screening cohort. Analyses of studies must be distinguished between these two types of patient cohorts. Second, clearly advancements in multirow detector CT technology over time have improved spatial resolution (Figs. 4.1 and 4.2). Additionally, awareness in knowledge of the different morphologies of polyps and the subsequent efficiency of reader training have improved, as structured courses have been developed with individual reader workstation review of CTC libraries of 50–100 case reviews both in ESGAR and the USA. There continues to some debate about the impact of 3D over 2D in reader review, as discussed

Table 4.4 Large CTC screening trials in average risk cohorts[a]

Trial Author, journal, year	Subjects (n)	Total adenomas ≥6 mm	MDCT Scanner rows	Per-polyp sensitivity		Per patient sensitivity		Per patient specificity	
				≥6 mm	≥10 mm	≥6 mm	≥10 mm	≥6 mm	≥10 mm
Pickhardt et al. N Engl J Med 2003	1,233	210	4–8 row	89%	94%	89%	94%	80%	96%
Johnson, et al. N Engl J Med 2008	2,531	374	16–64 row	70%	84%	78%	90%	88%	86%
Graser et al. JAMA 2009	307	221	64 row	90% (6–9 mm)	94%	91%	92%	93%	98%

[a]Average-risk cohorts are asymptomatic patients, with no personal history of polyps, family history of colorectal neoplasia, or colorectal symptoms

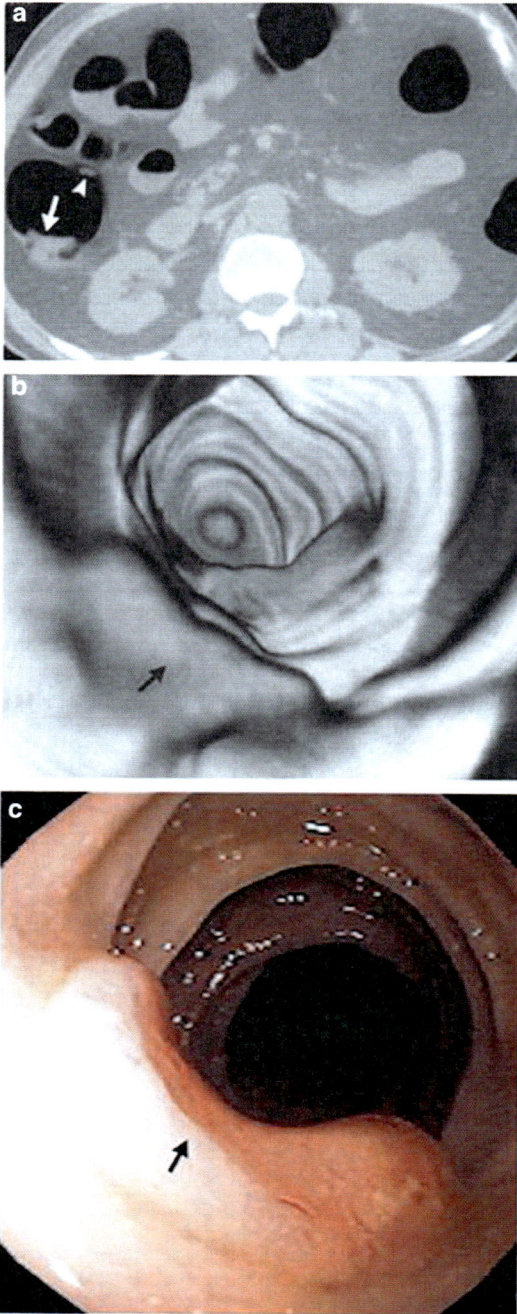

Fig. 4.1 From the Fenlon et al. trial of 1999, image quality of detection of a 2.5 cm cancer at single-row CTC at 5-mm slice thickness: (**a**) 2D axial, (**b**) 3D endoscopic view, and (**c**) optical colonoscopy image (reproduced from Fenlon HM, Nunes DP, Schroy PC, et al. A comparison of virtual and conventional colonoscopy for the detection of colorectal polyps. N Engl J Med. 341, copyright © 1999 Massachusetts Medical Society. Reprinted with permission from Massachusetts Medical Society)

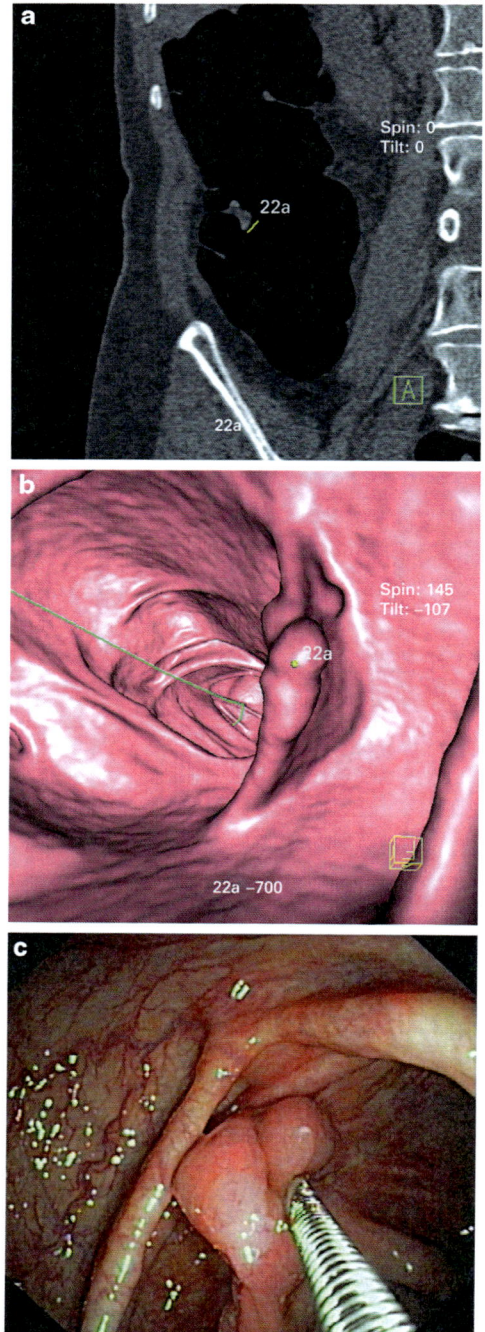

Fig. 4.2 From the Graser et al. trial of 2009, advancement of image quality of detection of a 2.2 cm sessile polyp at 64DCT at 0.75-mm slice thickness: (**a**) 2D sagittal, (**b**) 3D endoscopic, and (**c**) OC (reproduced from Graser A, Stieber P, Nagel D, et al. Comparison of CT colonography, colonoscopy, sigmoidoscopy, and fecal occult blood tests for the detection of advanced adenoma in an average-risk population. Gut. 2009;58:241–8, copyright notification year 2012, with permissions from BMJ Publishing Group Ltd.)

below. Differences may have occurred based on the analysis to evaluate all polyps in earlier studies, compared to adenomatous polyps in later studies. Finally, one less debated issue of significance is the difference in clarity of definition of polyp-size target, which Pickhardt et al. first clearly emphasized.

Among the studies of higher risk cohorts, the IMPACT trial took place 4–5 years after the first three trials of Johnson, Rockey, and Cotton. Not only were readers more familiar with the types of polyp morphologies with structured training through CTC interpretation courses, but scanner resolution with 16-DCT and 64-DCT scanners clearly improved visualization over the 2–8 row of earlier studies. Also the IMPACT trial did not include lower risk adenomas in their assessment, compared to all polyps evaluated in the first three. As discussed earlier in the reanalysis of the Rockey et al. data, sensitivity results were increased when evaluation of adenoma detection was assessed [22].

Before assessing the screening trials, there was a period of great debate during the publication of three closely spaced trials with diverging results. Namely, the screening trial of Pickhardt trial in 2003 was published at the same time as the Cotton trial and just before the Rockey trial, the latter two assessing cohorts at increased risk. The Cotton trial was largely criticized due to lack of rigorous training of radiologists at the leading edge of a new technology. However, the Rockey trial had better training and similar, if not improved, CT scanner technology, along with similar methodology of segmental unblinding of results. The enriched cohort of Rockey would have favored results over the first screening trial of Pickhardt. However, the primary technological improvements of stool tagging and 3D as a primary review were attributed to Pickhardt's success. In addition, despite having the harder task of finding fewer polyps in a screening cohort, Pickhardt also rigorously set the target size for lesion detection at 6 mm and greater, thus focusing the multi-reader task and possibly not distracting or tiring readers with the assessment of smaller polyps.

Finally, evaluation of the screening trials involves trials that are more similar in techniques. All used multirow CT scanner technology, although Pickhardt et al. had less advanced scanner technology. This likely demonstrates that good techniques in bowel preparation and insufflation clearly trump differences in 4D vs. 16–64D-scanner technique for assessment of 6-mm and larger polyps. All used stool tagging. Although ACRIN had lower specificity than Pickhardt et al. and Graser et al. despite the use of stool tagging, this might have been more influenced on the rigorous task defined by ACRIN to obtain 90% sensitivity for detection of 10-mm and larger polyps. In this context, readers did not want to miss a significant polyp, and this may have driven down specificity to some degree. All assessed adenoma detection rates. The 3D primary review in Pickhardt et al. was challenged 5 years later by equal results of 2D vs. 3D in ACRIN, with 2D being more time efficient. As readers become more familiar with image display techniques over time, 2D and 3D are both easily done, and each has advantages and disadvantages. As discussed, Pickhardt's emphasis of the target lesion size of 6 mm and larger likely focused the reader task. Finally, learning curve effects during the trials also may have been an influence. Readers who were shown the answers after cases were completed during the trial, likely benefited from awareness of case mix and improved their increased accuracy as they read additional cases [24, 27]. Lessons learned from clear definition of target lesions and feedback of results to enhance learning are key to remember as CTC clinical programs continue to expand.

Selection of Patients by CTC to Benefit from Colonoscopy

Beyond validation, Kim et al. published a study that demonstrated the efficacy of CTC to properly select patients who would benefit from therapeutic OC [28]. This was a two-pronged study comparing screening with primary CTC in 3,120 patients (with selective recommendation for polypectomy in positive patients) to screening with primary OC in 3,163 patients. In the CTC arm, patients were recommended to have a follow-up therapeutic OC based on detection of polyps 6 mm or greater in size. The two cohorts had similar demographics, other than a slightly higher proportion of individuals with a positive family history in the OC group. A total of 7.9% of patients in the CTC arm were recommended for therapeutic OC. Both groups reported a similar detection rate of advanced adenomas (3.2% in the CTC group and 3.4% in the OC group). However, the total number of polypectomies was over four times higher in the OC group compared to the CTC group (2,434 vs. 561, respectively) [28]. This study supports that using a polyp-size threshold of 6 mm or greater, CTC can efficaciously recommend therapeutic OC for removal of advanced adenomas.

Meta-analyses of CTC Diagnostic Performance

During the first decade of effort, two meta-analyses were done to review the CTC trial results [29, 30]. The most comprehensive meta-analysis of Mulhall et al. evaluated 33 studies encompassing 6,393 patients. In this analysis on a per-patient basis, CTC sensitivity and specificity for 10-mm and larger polyps was found to be 85–93% and 97%, respectively [29]. Pooled sensitivity and specificity for small polyps (6–9 mm) was 70–86% and 86–93%, respectively. Halligan et al. reported the sensitivity of CTC to detect invasive colorectal cancer was 96% [30].

In 2011, a comprehensive meta-analysis of CTC and OC for detection of colorectal cancer reviewed 49 studies evaluating 11,151 patients, spanning the years from 1994 to 2009 [31]. The sensitivity of CTC for detection of colorectal cancer was 96.1%. No cancers were missed at CTC when both cathartic and tagging agents were used in the bowel preparation. The sensitivity of OC for colorectal cancer in a subset of 25 studies of 9,223 patients was 94.7%. Thus, the high sensitivity of CTC for detection of cancer was confirmed, similar to that of OC.

CTC Performance in Other Settings

Medicare Population

A relative paucity of studies of the Medicare population partially influenced the national non-coverage decision by the CMS in 2009. Subsequent to that decision, a retrospective review was published in 2010, which evaluated 577 older patients, ranging in age from 65 to 79 years, as part of the CTC screening program at University of Wisconsin [32]. Using the polyp-size threshold of 6 mm or greater, a total of 15.3% patients were referred for therapeutic OC. This was greater than the prior published referral rate of 7.9% in average-risk patients (mean age, 57 years). Given the higher rate of neoplasia with aging, the establishment of this increased referral rate to OC was important to establish for cost considerations. For adenomas, the per-patient positivity rates at 6-mm and 10-mm polyp-size thresholds were 10.9% and 6.8%, respectively. The prevalence of advanced neoplasia was 7.6%. In addition, the effects of extracolonic findings were also evaluated, which can also add additional costs. The reported extracolonic findings led to an additional work-up rate of 7.8%. No major complications occurred in this age group. Overall, these results were favorable, suggesting that CTC could be a safe and effective screening modality in this age group.

At New York University, a retrospective evaluation of the extracolonic findings and polyp prevalence was compared between senior and non-senior patients [33]. A total of 454 patients were evaluated, with 204 non-seniors (age < 65 years) and 250 seniors (age ≥ 65 years). Among the seniors, 82 patients (33%) underwent CTC for screening indications. No significant difference in the percentage of patients with one reported clinically significant polyp (defined as ≥6 mm in size) was present, encompassing 14.2% of the non-senior and 13.2% of senior patients. The percentage of patients with at least one extracolonic finding was less in the non-senior group (55.4%) compared with the senior group (74.0%). However, most patients (92% of non-seniors and

91.8% of seniors) had extracolonic findings of low clinical significance. Subsequently, there was no statistical difference in the frequency of recommendation for additional imaging between groups (4.4% in non-seniors and 6.0% in seniors). Thus, investigators from two different demographic regions, NYU and University of Wisconsin, concurred from their colorectal screening programs that 15% or less of Medicare-aged patients would undergo therapeutic OC, using the index size threshold of 6 mm or larger for polyps detected at CTC. It is also reassuring for cost considerations that the additional imaging recommendations based on extracolonic findings were also found to be low in this population.

A reanalysis of the ACRIN data in the Medicare population of 477 patients 65 years of age and older demonstrated that the sensitivity and specificity per patient for detection of polyps 6 mm and greater was 72% and 86%, respectively, compared to 82% and 83%, respectively, for detection of polyps 10 mm and larger [34]. Per-polyp sensitivity in this age group for polyps larger than or equal to 6 mm and larger than or equal to 10 mm was 59% and 75%, respectively. Overall, the majority of these results in Medicare-aged patients did not differ significantly from patients less than 65 years of age.

Flat Lesions

Flat colorectal lesions are challenging, both at OC and CTC. Debates of both the prevalence and pathological risk have occurred. The diagnostic performance of CTC for flat lesions has varied, with recent improvements reported as technological improvements with 3D software and CT spatial resolution have occurred. Some of this variability may be due to differences in definitions of the morphology and terminology of flat lesions.

Using the definition of "sessile" (height of lesion less than half of length), Fidler et al. reported a sensitivity to detect sessile lesions of less than 50% [35]. In a subanalysis of sessile lesions, Pickhardt et al. reported a sensitivity of 83% [36].

Other terminology for flat lesions has included a recent description by Soetikno et al. [37]. Polypoid lesions are defined as sessile or pedunculated in morphology. Non-polypoid lesions are defined as superficially elevated, flat, or depressed. In a series of OC screening of veterans, the overall prevalence of non-polypoid neoplasia was 9.4% vs. 5.8% [37]. In this report, concerns for failed detection of such lesions at CTC were raised. However, all CTC trials reported to date have not described significant trends of false negatives of flat lesions at CTC, using OC as a gold standard. In addition, this morphological type of lesion is well recognized in CTC and is a part of standardized training.

The Paris classification of flat lesions defines these lesions as being less than 3 mm in height. A subcategory is the carpet lesion or laterally spreading lesion, which spans a distance of over 3 cm. Using this terminology, Pickhardt et al. published a series evaluating 5,107 consecutive asymptomatic patients at screening CTC [38]. All lesions larger than 6 mm in size were labeled as sessile or pedunculated (combined as polypoid type) vs. flat. Lesions larger than 3 cm in length that were flat were labeled as carpet lesions. A total of 125 out of 964 polyps (13.1%) were labeled as flat in 106 adults. Flat lesions between 6 and 30 mm averaged a maximum height of 2.2 mm (≤3 mm in 86%). Further improvements in CT acquisition, computed-aided diagnosis, and 3D image display techniques should continue to improve detection of this morphological type of colorectal lesion.

Low-Dose CTC

Radiation dose imparted at CTC is a critical factor to keep efficient. Several investigators have reported successful use of low-dose CTC protocols [11, 39–41]. In 2002, a study of 105 patients was performed with the CT scan protocol of 1-mm slice thickness and low dose of 50 effective mAs [11]. The total effective dose to the patients for both supine and prone imaging of the abdomen and pelvis was 5.0 mSv for men and 7.8 mSv for women, which is comparable to dose ranges of barium enema. Excellent sensitivity of 90% for 1-cm polyps was achieved. In 2003, further dose reduction was achieved in a cohort of 158 patients predominantly at increased risk of colorectal neoplasia, using 10 effective mAs and a slightly thicker slice thickness of 2.5 mm [39]. This protocol resulted in total effective doses to the patients of 1.8 mSv in men and 2.4 mSv in women. In this study, there was 100% sensitivity for all 22 cancers, 100% sensitivity for the thirteen 10-mm and larger polyps, and 83% sensitivity for the 6–9-mm (20/24) polyps. Further decreases in radiation dose have been achieved with advances in automatic tube current exposure and dose modulation techniques [42], which differentially change the delivered dose over the anatomy scanned in real time (e.g., more dose given to penetrate the bony pelvis and less dose given over the soft tissues of the abdomen). With these new dose reduction techniques, the effective dose from CTC becomes close to, or less than, yearly background radiation. These low-dose radiation techniques have now become standard of care for screening CTC in both research and clinical practice.

Recent reports have discussed the controversy of low radiation dose exposure [43]. Brenner et al. recently addressed the issue of radiation dose screening with CTC and concluded that the benefit-risk ratio was high and that radiation-induced cancer risks were very low [43]. Brenner concluded that potential lifetime cancer risk for one CTC exam at age 50 was 0.14% (0.07% if 70), which could be reduced by factors of five or ten with optimized low-dose protocols. Potential limitations of these estimates of cancer risk include use of the linear non threshold model from whole body exposure of A bomb survivors of all ages, compared to the more limited abdominal-pelvic exposure of CTC in patients 50 years and older. Recently, the American College of Radiology created a Blue Ribbon Panel on Radiation Dose in Medicine and published recommendations and quality initiatives for the safe use of ionizing radiation, including CT, in clinical practice [44]. In addition, quality metrics for CTC developed by the ACR include the documentation of low-dose CT protocols for screening cohorts.

Summary

CTC continues to rapidly evolve with technological improvements in bowel preparation, low-dose CT acquisition, and novel 3D display techniques. Although diverse results were initially obtained in the first decade during rapid improvement in the technology, more consistent results of diagnostic performance have now been realized in larger screening cohorts. These validation data will continue to drive implementation and reimbursement, likely promoting further expansion of utilization of CTC in clinical practice.

References

1. Knechtges PM, McFarland BG, Keysor KJ, Duszak Jr R, Barish MA, Carlos RC. National and local trends in CT colonography reimbursement: past, present, and future. J Am Coll Radiol. 2007;4:776–99.
2. Levin B, Lieberman DA, McFarland B, Smith RA, Brooks D, Andrews KS, et al. Screening and surveillance for the early detection of colorectal cancer and adenomatous polyps 2008: a joint guideline from the American Cancer Society, the US Multi-society task force on colorectal cancer, and the American College of Radiology. CA Cancer J Clin. 2008;58:130–60.
3. Whitlock EP, Lin JS, Liles E, Beil TL, Fu R. Screening for colorectal cancer: a targeted, updated systematic review for the U.S. Preventative Services Task Force. Ann Intern Med. 2008;149:638–58.
4. Dhruva SS, Phurrough SE, Salive MR, Redberg RF. CMS' landmark decision on CT colonography: examining the relevant data. N Engl J Med. 2009;360: 2699–701.
5. Pickhardt PJ, Taylor AJ, Kim DH, Reichelderfer M, Gopal DV, Pfau PR. Screening for colorectal neoplasia with CT colonography: initial experience from the first year of coverage by third-party payers. Radiology. 2006;241:417–25.
6. Hara AK, Johnson CD, Reed JE, Ahlquist DA, Nelson H, Maccarty RL, et al. Detection of colorectal polyps with CT colonography: initial assessment of sensitivity and specificity. Radiology. 1997;205:59–65.
7. Dachman AH, Kuniyoshi JK, Boyle CM, et al. CT colonography with three-dimensional problem solving for detection of colonic polyps. AJR Am J Roentgenol. 1998;171:989–95.
8. Fletcher JG, Johnson CD, Welch TJ, MacCarty RL, Ahlquist DA, Reed JE, Harmsen WS, Wilson LA. Optimization of CT colonography technique: prospective trial in 180 patients. Radiology. 2000;216: 704–11.

9. Spinzi G, Belloni G, Martegani A, Sangiovanni A, Del Favero C, Minoli G. Computed tomographic colonography and conventional colonoscopy for colon diseases: a prospective, blinded study. Am J Gastroenterol. 2001;96:394–400.

10. Hara A, Johnson C, MacCarty R, Welch T, McCollough C, Harmsen W. CT colonography: single- versus multidetector row imaging. Radiology. 2001;219:461–5.

11. Macari M, Bini EJ, Xue X, Milano A, Katz S, Resnick D, Chandarana H, Klingenbeck K, Krinsky G, Marshall CH, Megibow AJ. Prospective comparison of thin-section low-dose multislice CT colonography to conventional colonoscopy in detecting colorectal polyps and cancers. Radiology. 2002;224:383–92.

12. McFarland EG, Pilgram TK, Brink JA, McDermott RA, Santillan CV, Brady PW, et al. Multi-observer diagnostic performance of CT colonography: factors influencing diagnostic-accuracy assessment. Radiology. 2002;225:380–90.

13. Laghi A, Iannaccone R, Carbone I, et al. Detection of colorectal lesions with virtual computed tomographic colonography. Am J Surg. 2002;183:124–31.

14. Fenlon HM, Nunes DP, Schroy III PC, Barish MA, Clarke PD, Ferrucci JT. A comparison of virtual and conventional colonoscopy for the detection of colorectal polyps. N Engl J Med. 1999;341:1540–2.

15. Yee J, Akerkar GA, Hung RK, Steinauer-Gebauer AM, Wall SD, McQuaid KR. Colorectal neoplasia: performance characteristics of CT colonography for detection in 300 patients. Radiology. 2001;219:685–92.

16. Fenlon HM, McAneny DB, Nunes DP, Clarke PD, Ferrucci JT. Occlusive colon carcinoma: virtual colonoscopy in the preoperative evaluation of the proximal colon. Radiology. 1999;210:423–8.

17. Copel L, Sosna J, Kruskal JB, Raptopoulos V, Farrell RJ, Morrin MM. CT colonography in 546 patients with incomplete colonoscopy. Radiology. 2007;244:471–8.

18. Neri E, Giusti P, Battolla L, et al. Colorectal cancer: role of CT colonography in preoperative evaluation after incomplete colonoscopy. Radiology. 2002;223:615–9.

19. Johnson CD, Harmsen WS, Wilson LA, Maccarty RL, Welch TJ, Ilstrup DM, et al. Prospective blinded evaluation of computed tomographic colonography for screen detection of colorectal polyps. Gastroenterology. 2003;125:311–9.

20. Cotton PB, Durkalski VL, Pineau BC, et al. Computed tomographic colonography (virtual colonoscopy): a multicenter comparison with standard colonoscopy for detection of colorectal neoplasia. JAMA. 2004;291:1713–9.

21. Rockey DC, Paulson E, Niedzwiecki D, et al. Analysis of air contrast barium enema, computed tomographic colonography, and colonoscopy: prospective comparison. Lancet. 2005;365:305–11.

22. Doshi T, Rusinak D, Halvorsen RA, Rockey DC, Suzuki K, Dachman A. CT colonography: false-negative interpretations. Radiology. 2007;244:165–73.

23. Regge D, Laudi C, Galatola G, Della Monica P, Bonelli L, Angelelli G, et al. Diagnostic accuracy of computed tomographic colonography for the detection of advanced neoplasia in individuals at increased risk of colorectal cancer. JAMA. 2009;301:2453–61.

24. Pickhardt PJ, Choi JR, Hwang I, et al. CT virtual colonoscopy to screen for colorectal neoplasia in asymptomatic adults. N Engl J Med. 2003;349:2191–200.

25. Pickhardt PJ, Nugent PA, Mysliwiec PA, Choi JR, Schindler WR. Location of adenomas missed by optical colonoscopy. Ann Intern Med. 2004;141:352–9.

26. Johnson CD, Chen MH, Toledano AY, et al. Accuracy of CT colonography for detection of large adenomas and cancers. N Eng J Med. 2008;359:1207–17.

27. Graser A, Stieber P, Nagel D, et al. Comparison of CT colonography, colonoscopy, sigmoidoscopy, and fecal occult blood tests for the detection of advanced adenoma in an average risk population. Gut. 2009;58:241–8.

28. Kim DH, Pickhardt PJ, Taylor AJ, et al. CT colonography versus colonoscopy for the detection of advanced neoplasia. N Engl J Med. 2007;357:1403–12.

29. Mulhall BP, Veerappan GR, Jackson JL. Meta-analysis: computed tomographic colonography. Ann Intern Med. 2005;142:635–50.

30. Halligan S, Altman DG, Taylor SA, et al. CT colonography in the detection of colorectal polyps and cancer: systematic review, meta-analysis, and proposed minimum data set for study level reporting. Radiology. 2005;237:893–904.

31. Pickhardt P, Hassan C, Halligan S, Marmo R. Colorectal cancer: CT colonography and colonoscopy for detection- systematic review and meta-analysis. Radiology. 2011;259:393–405.

32. Kim DH, Pickhardt PP, Hanson ME, Hinshaw JL. CT colonography: performance and program outcome measures in an older screening population. Radiology. 2010;254:493–500.

33. Macari M, Nevsky G, Bonavita J, Kim DC, Megibow AJ, Babb JS. CT colonography in senior vs nonsenior patients: extracolonic findings, recommendations for additional imaging and polyp prevalence. Radiology. 2011;259:767–74.

34. Johnson CD, et al. The National CT Colonography Trial: assessment of accuracy in participants 65 years of age or older. Radiology. 2012;263:401–8.

35. Fidler J, Johnson C, MacCarty R, Welch T, Hara A, Harmsen W. Detection of flat lesions in the colon with CT colonography. Abdom Imaging. 2002;27:292–300.

36. Pickhardt PJ, Nugent PA, Choi JR, Schindler WR. Flat colorectal lesions in asymptomatic adults: implications for screening with CT virtual colonoscopy. AJR Am J Roentgenol. 2004;183:1343–7.

37. Soetikno RM, Kaltenbach T, Rouse RV, et al. Prevalence of nonpolypoid (flat and depressed) colorectal neoplasms in asymptomatic and symptomatic adults. JAMA. 2008;299:1027–35.

38. Pickhardt PJ, Kim DH, Robbins JB. Flat (nonpolypoid) colorectal lesions identified at CT colonography in a U.S screening population. Acad Radiol. 2010;17:784–90.

39. Iannaccone R, Laghi A, Catalano C, et al. Detection of colorectal lesions: lower-dose multi-detector row

helical CT colonography compared with conventional colonoscopy. Radiology. 2003;229:775–81.

40. Van Gelder RE, Venema HW, Florie J, et al. CT colonography: feasibility of substantial dose reduction- comparison of medium to low doses in identical patients. Radiology. 2004;232:611–20.

41. Cohnen M, Vogt C, Beck A, et al. Feasibility of MDCT colonography in ultra-low-dose technique in the detection of colorectal lesions: comparison with high-resolution video colonoscopy. AJR Am J Roentgenol. 2004;183:1355–9.

42. Kalra MK, Maher MM, Toth TL, Kamath RS, Halpern EF, Saini S. Comparison of z-axis automatic tube current modulation technique with fixed tube current CT scanning of abdomen and pelvis. Radiology. 2004; 232:347–53.

43. Brenner DJ, Georgsson MA. Mass screening with CT colonography: should the radiation exposure be of concern? Gastroenterology. 2005;129:328–37.

44. Amis Jr ES, Butler PF, Applegate KE, et al. American College of Radiology white paper on radiation dose in medicine. J Am Coll Radiol. 2007;4:272–84.

Performance and Interpretation of CTC

5

Peter D. Poullos and Christopher F. Beaulieu

Introduction

It has been almost 30 years since Coin proposed that computed tomography (CT) scanning had the potential to be used as a screening tool for the detection of colonic polyps [1]. Yet it was not until 1994 that Vining and coworkers were able to employ the new technology of spiral/helical CT and modern computer graphics, catalyzing extensive research and clinical efforts that molded the field that we now call CT colonography (CTC) or "virtual colonoscopy." [2] Owing to these efforts, reasonable consensus now exists on the optimal means by which to prepare the patient, acquire the CT data, and interpret the resulting images, though some healthy debates do persist. The goal of this chapter is to describe these technical factors in CTC and to give the reader a perspective on current techniques and alternatives. We review the best evidence for current practices and recommendations. With this information, we hope the reader will have a thorough understanding of what is required to set up a high-quality clinical operation for performance of CTC.

Bowel Preparation

Background

Technical success in CTC starts with an adequate bowel preparation. A multitude of software tools available on CTC workstations are aimed at minimizing the impact that residual fecal material makes on diagnostic performance. Yet, as any experienced interpreter of CTC will admit, a clean colon makes the job of interpretation immeasurably easier, improves confidence, and ultimately improves performance. This "low-tech" approach will produce results that no presently available computer can replicate.

Adherent stool is the most common cause of false-positives at CTC [3]. It can also lead to false-negative diagnoses, as retained liquid and stool can obscure lesions, especially small ones. Interpretation times are prolonged when a large number of potential lesions must be interrogated and documented [4]. If CTC patients are to be offered same-day optical colonoscopy (OC) for a positive finding, they will have to have completed a full bowel preparation [5]. At this time, CTC bowel cleansing regimens are quite similar to those used at OC.

Diet

Solid food and fiber restriction are as essential as laxatives to an effective bowel preparation regimen.

5

P.D. Poullos, M.D. (✉) • C.F. Beaulieu, M.D., Ph.D.
Department of Radiology, Stanford University Medical Center, Stanford, CA, USA
e-mail: ppoullos@stanford.edu

Dietary fiber is resistant to enzymatic hydrolysis and to bacterial breakdown [6, 7], and whole seeds and grains can mimic polyps [8]. A low-fiber diet has been proven to improve fecal tagging at CTC [8]. We prescribe a diet free of seeds and nuts for 7 days and a clear liquid diet the entire day before the CTC. Patients are told not to eat or drink anything from midnight until the time of their examination.

Pharmacologic Cathartics

The optimal laxative preparation for CTC has been examined extensively and has been the subject of much debate. Many agents and combinations of agents have been tested, with the goals of balancing strength and safety, with emphasis placed on patient comfort and tolerance [9]. For purposes of discussion, available laxatives have been distinguished as "dry preps" (sodium phosphate and magnesium citrate) and "wet preps" (polyethylene glycol).

The distinction between dry and wet preps is their mechanism of catharsis. Sodium phosphate and magnesium citrate preparations are low-volume, hyperosmotic formulations that induce osmotic catharsis by drawing water into the colonic lumen from the intravascular compartment. Polyethylene glycol (PEG) is a high-volume, iso-osmotic, nonabsorbable preparation that causes a washout lavage. It does not cause significant fluid shifts from the intracellular to the extracellular space. These three agents were used in the American College of Radiology Imaging Network (ACRIN) trial [10], of which a recently performed retrospective analysis demonstrated that the sensitivity and specificity for detecting colon polyps ≥ 6 mm and ≥ 1 cm did not significantly differ between bowel preparations [5]. Nevertheless, it is pertinent to review their differences.

Sodium Phosphate

Oral sodium phosphate (OSP) products include the prescription Visicol and OsmoPrep [11]. Fleets Phospho-soda® was an over-the-counter sodium phosphate preparation offered without prescription. However, it was recalled in 2009 over concerns phosphate-induced nephropathy, as discussed below [12]. Onset to catharsis was approximately 1 h. Four 10-mg bisacodyl tablets were also typically taken orally in the evening after the sodium phosphate was finished. In 2007, Kim found that a single dose (45 mL) was just as effective as a double dose (90 mL) [13]. Sodium phosphate also comes in pill form, which can be taken with any clear liquid, bypassing the problem of its considerably salty taste [14].

There have been many studies over the years comparing the efficacy of sodium phosphate to PEG. 45 mL of sodium phosphate has been reported in some studies to be superior to PEG in the amount of residual fluid, efficacy of cleansing, patient preference, and compliance [15–19]. Some studies have demonstrated that PEG is better than sodium phosphate [20]. However, in two meta-analyses, the larger of which analyzed 24 studies, there was no significant difference in quality of bowel preparation between sodium phosphate and PEG [16, 21].

More recently, retrospective analysis of the ACRIN trial data showed that sodium phosphate had the best patient compliance, the least residual stool, and highest reader confidence versus PEG for examinations with polyps. It was also the most commonly prescribed cathartic [5]. However, as stated earlier, the sensitivity and specificity for polyp detection did not differ between preparations, illustrating that reader performance does not always correlate with measures of compliance, residual stool, or reader confidence [5].

The routine use of sodium phosphate has come under scrutiny due to its history of causing serious fluid and electrolyte abnormalities [22]. Patients may become dehydrated and develop hypernatremia, hypokalemia, hypophosphatemia, and hypocalcemia [23, 24]. Metabolic acidosis, tetany, and even death have been reported [25, 26]. Additionally, rare cases of acute phosphate nephropathy have been reported. Acute phosphate nephropathy, associated with renal tubular calcium-phosphate crystal deposition, may result in permanent renal insufficiency, sometimes requiring dialysis [11]. The risk of acute phosphate nephropathy appears to be related to factors such as advanced age, hypovolemia, baseline renal insufficiency, slow bowel transit time, colonic mucosal injury from colitis, or the use of nephrotoxic medications such as diuretics, angiotensin converting enzyme (ACE) inhibitors, and angiotensin receptor blockers (ARBs) [11, 12, 22]. The Food and Drug Administration (FDA) has required the manufacturer of Visicol and OsmoPrep, the two remaining prescription-only OSPs, to add a boxed warning to their labeling [11, 12]. Following that, Fleet recalled its over-the-counter sodium phosphate products.

Some CTC programs have screening questionnaires to triage at-risk patients away from sodium phosphate. However, such systems are imperfect as one study showed that as many as 2% of patients with a contraindication to sodium phosphate could not have been identified, and thus excluded, on the basis of their clinical history alone [27]. Many CTC programs have thus decided to abandon its use. If used, however, the manufacturers have advised that the dose be restricted or split and that the patient drink sufficient liquids [22].

Magnesium Citrate

Magnesium citrate is available over-the-counter in liquid form. The liquid comes in a 10-oz (296-mL) bottle, ready to drink. Like sodium phosphate, magnesium citrate is taken in the late afternoon, and bisacodyl tablets are taken the night before the exam. Time to onset of catharsis is around 1 h. Oral hydration should be maintained to prevent dehydration [12]. Magnesium citrate is preferred to sodium phosphate in patients with underlying medical conditions, given its lower sodium content, decreased incidence of electrolyte disturbances, and higher therapeutic index [9, 12, 28].

There are fewer studies in the literature comparing magnesium citrate to sodium phosphate or PEG than there are comparing the latter two with each other. In a 2005 study by Delegge et al. 506 patients undergoing optical colonoscopy (OC)

were randomized to receive either a magnesium citrate (LoSo Prep, containing magnesium citrate, bisacodyl tablets, and a bisacodyl suppository) or sodium phosphate-based prep (double dose sodium phosphate). The group that received magnesium citrate demonstrated superior colon cleansing and the frequency of reported side effects was similar for both groups (59% vs. 58% for sodium phosphate and Neutra prep/LoSo prep, respectively) [9]. A 2010 study comparing sodium phosphate and magnesium citrate showed that residual stool and fluid were comparable, but the attenuation of tagged fluid was closer to optimal with magnesium citrate, potentially increasing lesion conspicuity [29]. Interestingly, although magnesium citrate is classified as a "dry prep," analysis of the ACRIN trial data showed that magnesium citrate was associated with significantly more residual fluid compared with both PEG and sodium phosphate [5]. Our program exclusively uses magnesium citrate, given as a double dose (296 mL×2), except in those patients who require 2-day bowel prep, in whom PEG is added to the regimen.

Polyethylene Glycol

Several formulations of PEG are available by prescription, as well as over-the-counter. Bowel preparation with PEG is usually performed by drinking 4 L of the electrolyte solution, containing 236 g of PEG, on the afternoon before the CTC. Although widely used for OC preparation, PEG has increasingly fallen out of favor for use in CTC. PEG preparation frequently leaves liquid in the colon, which is suctioned at OC without difficulty, but potentially obscures lesions at CTC [17]. It also has the poorest compliance of the preparations, due to its taste and consistency, as well as the daunting volume. At one experienced center, PEG accounts for less than 1% of CTC preparations [30].

Side effects with PEG are not as alarming as with sodium phosphate, since PEG has the benefit of not causing significant fluid shifts and it is safer for those susceptible to such effects [31]. However, it too can potentially lead to electrolyte disturbances, albeit to a lesser extent. Reported adverse events attributable to oral PEG generally reflect sodium imbalance, gastrointestinal injury caused by vomiting, allergic reactions, and aspiration [22]. Interestingly, three meta-analyses showed that there were no significant differences in adverse events between sodium phosphate and PEG, suggesting that, although the adverse events may be different, PEG may not be any safer [16, 18, 21].

As discussed above, trials examining the relative efficacies of sodium phosphate versus PEG have yielded varying results. A study performed on a population with a high-residue diet showed better colonic cleansing and shorter CTC interpretation times with a PEG-based preparation compared to the sodium phosphate-based preparation [20]. However, most studies have shown that sodium phosphate is superior to PEG in residual fluid, cleansing, patient preference, and compliance [15–19]. Yet, two meta-analyses, the larger of which analyzed 24 studies, found no significant difference in quality of bowel preparation between sodium phosphate and PEG [16, 21]. More recently, retrospective analysis of the ACRIN trial data showed that the sensitivity and specificity for polyp detection did not differ between preparations [5].

The majority of patients experience inconvenience and discomfort, no matter what type of bowel preparation is used [32, 33]. Reduced, limited cathartic, or noncathartic CTC with fecal tagging has the potential to do away with the most burdensome part of the examination.

Special Considerations

For those patients referred to CTC with history of poor bowel preparation, diabetes, or neuromuscular disorders, special attention must be paid to the type of prep prescribed. In this instance, a 2-day prep should be considered. The patient is kept on a low-fiber, clear-liquid diet for 2 days prior to the examination, instead of just the day before. Two days before the examination, the patient drinks 4 L of PEG. The following day, they undergo the standard bowel preparation

with magnesium citrate and fecal tagging agents. We do not consider diverticulosis an indication for a 2-day bowel preparation, as this has been shown not to impair good bowel cleansing [34].

Fecal and Fluid Tagging

Background

Fecal tagging is the norm in CTC [32, 33, 35]. High-density oral contrast agents are typically ingested the day before the examination. Any residual feces and fluid mix with the contrast media so that they become homogeneously high in attenuation and are therefore easily differentiated from soft tissue density polyps or masses (Figs. 5.1 and 5.2) [36]. Tagging is thought to help improve the performance of CTC for polyp detection [37, 38]. The optimal tagging density in phantom studies has been shown to be 700 Hounsfield units and greater [39]. Higher attenuation may result in more artifacts and can decrease lesion conspicuity (Fig. 5.3) [29]. Fecal tagging underpins the ability to perform CTC without (or with less) bowel preparation, so-called "reduced cathartic" or "noncathartic" bowel preparation, discussed below. Many different contrast agents and combinations of agents have been used for fecal tagging [33, 40–45]. There are two main classes tagging agents: barium-based and iodine-based (both ionic and nonionic).

Barium

Also used in standard abdominal CT scanning, barium formulations are generally safe and are familiar to radiologists. Various densities of barium-based agents (e.g., Tagitol V 40% W/V; E-Z CAT 2% W/V.; Bracco Diagnostics) have been advocated [33]. Tagging protocols utilizing barium alone have been found to be effective [38, 46, 47]. Lower concentrations of barium, when used alone, may not have high enough attenuation to be helpful. In general barium agents are given in combination with iodinated contrast.

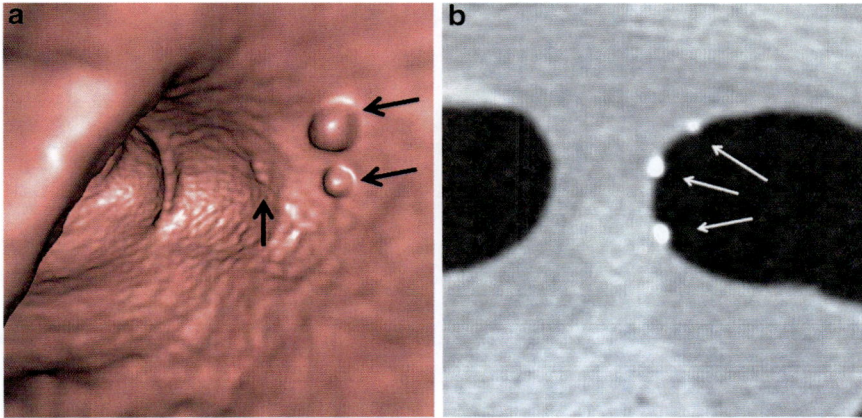

Fig. 5.1 A cluster of densely tagged stool can have the appearance of small polyps. (**a**) 3D endoluminal image of the colon demonstrates a cluster of small polypoid lesions (*arrows*). (**b**) 2D axial image demonstrates that these polypoid lesions correspond to foci of densely tagged stool (*arrows*), and can thus be disregarded

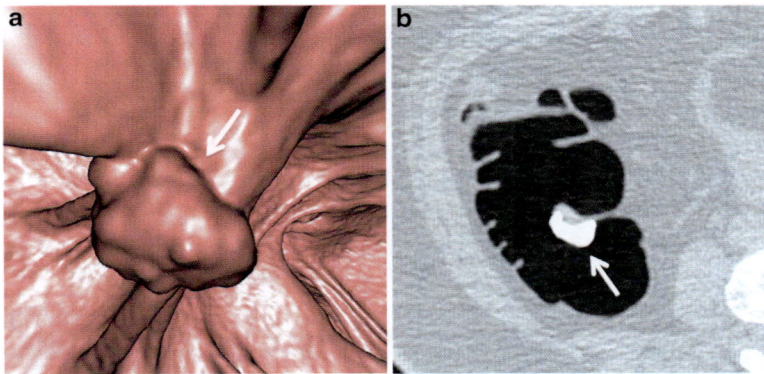

Fig. 5.2 Adherence stool on the ileocecal valve can imitate a mass lesion. (**a**) 3D endoluminal image of the ileocecal valve demonstrates an irregular, mass-like lesion (*arrow*), which appears to originate from the valve. (**b**) Corresponding 2D axial image demonstrates that the "lesion" is actually densely tagged stool (*arrow*) adherent to the valve and can thus be disregarded

Because barium preferentially tags solid stool, not liquid, it can cause inhomogeneous tagging if used alone [37]. Higher concentrations of barium have been described to leave flocculation or a "sticky coat" on the colonic wall, interfering with visualization of the colonic wall and complicating interpretation (Fig. 5.4) [48]. This problem can be solved by giving lower concentrations of barium earlier in the day, before the last dose of cathartic [48]. High-density barium, particularly if heterogeneous, causes problems for electronic cleansing software, discussed below [49]. As a side effect, barium can cause obstipation or even impaction [50]. Interestingly, there is evidence that barium selectively adheres to villous adenomas, a potentially beneficial property [51].

Iodinated Agents

As with barium, iodine-based high-osmolarity oral contrast agents are generally safe and familiar. Iodinated agents are hypertonic, can cause fluid shifts into the bowel lumen, and thus have an additional cathartic effect [52, 53]. Because they act to soften the stool, they mix homogeneously

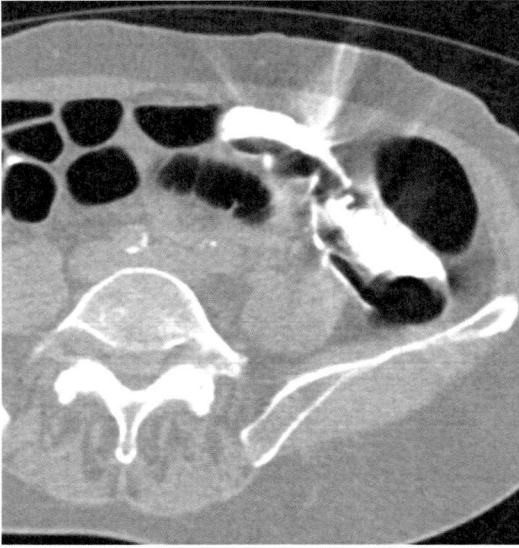

Fig. 5.3 Fecal tagging material is too dense, complicating interpretation. 2D axial image from CTC demonstrates extremely dense tagging material in the sigmoid colon. Streak artifact renders the bowel in the left lower quadrant difficult, if not impossible, to interpret

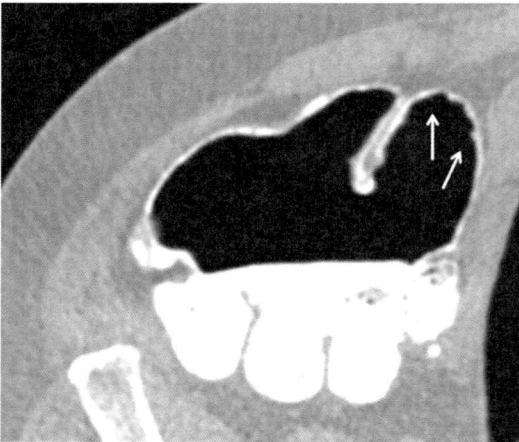

Fig. 5.4 Adherent barium can cause the appearance of a "sticky coat." 2D axial image of the right colon demonstrates circumferential, nodular high-density coating on the colonic mucosal surface, most obvious anteromedially (*arrows*). The patient ingested 40% barium as part of the fecal tagging component of their bowel preparation. Lower concentration barium has been shown to decrease this problem of the "sticky coat" [48]

with colonic contents, which results in more uniform attenuation, improving the ease of interpretation [33, 52, 53]. Iodinated contrast alone may also be used to tag residual material in the

colon [40, 41, 53] but in general are used in combination with barium. There are two varieties of iodinated contrast agents, ionic and nonionic.

Ionic Iodinated Agents

The most commonly used agent in the United States is sodium diatrizoate (Gastrografin, Bayer Shering Pharma, Berlin) also commonly used as oral contrast in standard CT examinations [40, 41]. Ionic iodinated contrast is water soluble, a property that lends itself to homogeneous tagging [30]. Although less costly than nonionic agents [33], the taste is unpleasant, especially in large amounts [54]. Despite a generally good safety profile, it can induce diarrhea and dehydration. Rare anaphylactoid reactions have been reported [55]. Sodium diatrizoate is contraindicated in those with iodine allergies, in which case barium alone is substituted. Doses as low as 20 mL have been shown to be adequate for tagging purposes [33], although up to 60 mL is commonly used.

Nonionic Iodinated Agents

As with their ionic cousins, nonionic agents are also water soluble [30]. Nonionic agents (i.e., iopromide, iohexol) have a lower risk for causing diarrhea and dehydration. Unlike sodium diatrizoate, nonionic agents are nearly tasteless and have good patient acceptance [33, 56]. Nonionic agents are less commonly used because they are more expensive than both barium and ionic iodinated contrast [33].

Combined Tagging

Barium and iodine-based tagging agents are commonly used in combination, opacifying residual solids with barium and fluid with iodine. The multicenter ACRIN National CT Colonography Trial successfully used combined tagging [10]. A total volume of 40 mL of 40% weight/volume barium (Tagitol V) was administered orally the day before the CT scan in three divided doses. A total volume of 60 mL of iodinated contrast material (Gastrografin 37% organically bound iodine) was administered in three aliquots of 20 mL starting the evening before the CT scan.

Following the lead of a large-volume CTC program and after noting that the more dense barium was causing any "sticky coat" to form, our own clinical CTC program has migrated away from using 40% barium. We now exclusively use a combined regimen with 2.1% barium and 37% Gastrografin with excellent results. Although there is no consensus regimen, the European Society of Gastrointestinal and Abdominal Radiology suggests that the choice of tagging agent should be based on local experience, taking into account any history of allergy [35]. A recently described artifact termed the "dense waterfall" is sometimes seen with CTC using fecal tagging. This artifact is caused by gravitational flow of tagged fluid between two colonic levels and appears as arciform streak artifact. It is caused by erroneous image reconstruction brought about by misregistration of moving fluid and is important because it can imitate or obscure pathology [57].

Translucency Rendering

Translucency rendering, or the "translucency view," is a specialized viewing mode in some commercial workstations that may help differentiate high-attenuation tagged stool from the soft tissue density of a true polyp (Fig. 5.5) [12, 58]. This mode is typically activated with the push of a button. The tool, when superimposed on an endoluminal lesion during 3D analysis, assigns different specific color patterns to the lesion based on its attenuation values. In general, densely tagged stool appears white. Polyps have a color signature with a red core and gradual stepwise shift to green, light blue, and dark blue hues more peripherally. Fat density lesions such as the ileocecal valve (Fig. 5.6), lipomas, and impacted diverticula are also well analyzed [59]. In a recent study of 350 patients with 482 colonoscopically verified polyps and 50 pseudopolyps, the overall average sensitivity for polyp characterization by translucency rendering was 96.6%

and average overall specificity for pseudopolyp characterization was 91.3% [59].

Reduced, Limited Catharsis, and Noncathartic CTC

Other than improving diagnostic performance, one of the reasons for developing fecal tagging regimens was the desire to improve the patient experience and compliance by decreasing or eliminating the most unpleasant aspect of CTC, the need for a full bowel preparation [60]. This would be of particular benefit to those with limited mobility, the brittle elderly, or those who have a blunted response to laxatives [33]. Additionally, it is thought that by removing the hurdle of a full preparation, patients would undergo screening with CTC more frequently [52, 61].

These types of bowel preparation are termed nonconventional and include reduced catharsis, limited catharsis, or noncathartic preparations. "Reduced catharsis" refers to the use of purgative medications in approximately half of the dose used for conventional preparation. "Limited catharsis" refers to the use of laxatives (senna, bisacodyl, lactulose) to achieve a relatively mild catharsis. "Noncathartic" or "laxative free" refers to a preparation without any purgative or laxative. All of these nonconventional bowel preparations are dependent on excellent fecal tagging [62].

Although patient acceptance is higher with lower doses of iodine and tagging agents, it has been recommended that doses of 50 mL meglumine ioxithalamate be used for optimal tagging quality in noncathartic CTC [63]. It is especially important with noncathartic preparations that good homogeneity and high tagging density be achieved. Low-density tagging increases the difficulty of polyp detection, increases false-positives, and decreases diagnostic accuracy [53].

The literature regarding the diagnostic performance of nonconventional CTC is mixed, with some studies showing favorable [37, 41, 52, 64] and others unfavorable [65–67] results. In general, although results are promising, further study is necessary because study design is inconsistent and data are limited. A systematic review of nine

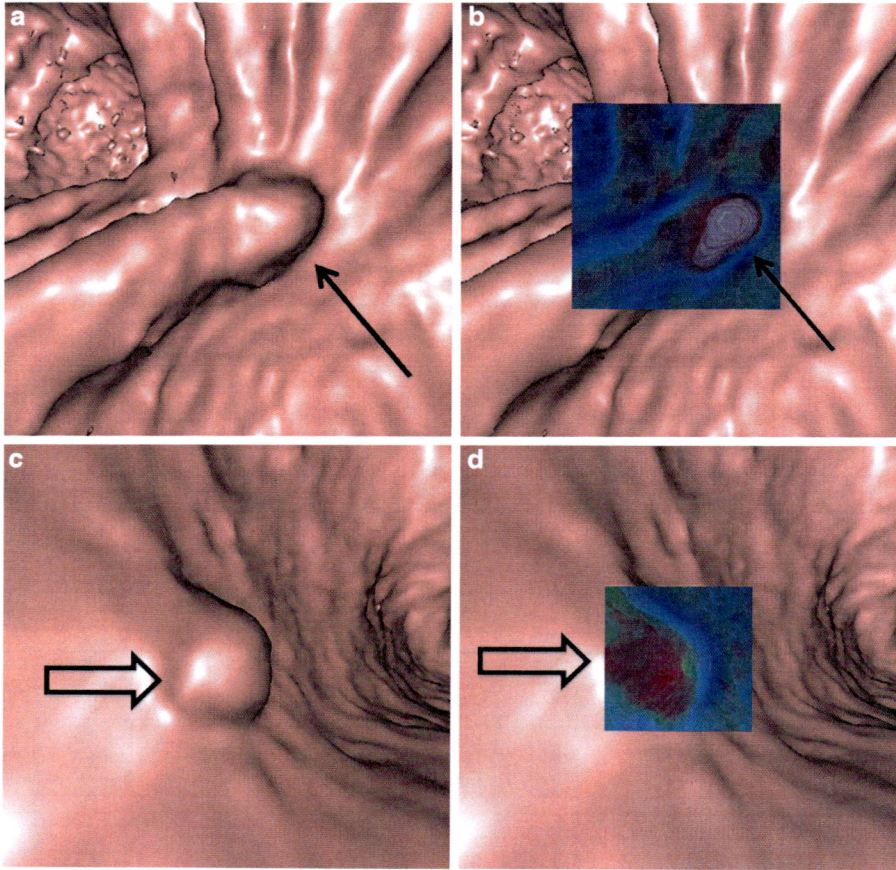

Fig. 5.5 Translucency rendering can be used to differentiate soft tissue polyps from adherent stool. (**a**) 3D endoluminal image shows a 7-mm sessile polypoid lesion on a haustral fold. (**b**) Translucency rendering applied to 3D image in "**a**" shows completely white interior, indicative of contrast material tagging. This appearance excludes a true polyp, so it is not necessary to perform 2D correlation. (**c**) 3D endoluminal image shows 1-cm sessile polyp. (**d**) Translucency rendering applied to 3D image in **c** shows typical color pattern of a soft tissue polyp, consisting of *red core* and gradual uniform shift to *green, light blue*, and *dark blue* hues more peripherally

prospective studies of CTC with nonconventional bowel preparation was recently published [62]. In six studies, detection of polyps 10 mm or larger was good [38, 41, 47, 52, 67, 68], with both per-polyp and per-patient sensitivities ranging from 82% [67] to 100% [38, 41, 68]. In the two studies in which electronic cleansing was used, per-patient sensitivity for polyps 10 mm and larger was 100% [68] and 96% [52]. In three studies [64–66], performance was relatively poor for polyps larger than 10 mm, with the per-polyp sensitivity ranging from 0% [65] to 63.3% [66] and per-patient sensitivity ranging from 0% [65] to 75.3% [64]. It should be noted that two of the poor-performing studies [64, 66] used what would be considered suboptimal doses of contrast in one [64] and iodine only in the other [66].

Sensitivity and specificity of smaller lesions is worse. In a 2008 study by Jensch et al., CTC with fecal tagging without stool subtraction and a bisacodyl-only prep was compared with colonoscopy [67]. Sensitivity for lesions 6 mm and greater was 76%. However, despite homogeneous fecal tagging, there were a large number of false-positive findings (specificity 79%) when 6 mm was used as a size threshold. In a 2009 study by Nagata, minimum laxative CTC with fecal tagging demonstrated equally high sensitivity to full

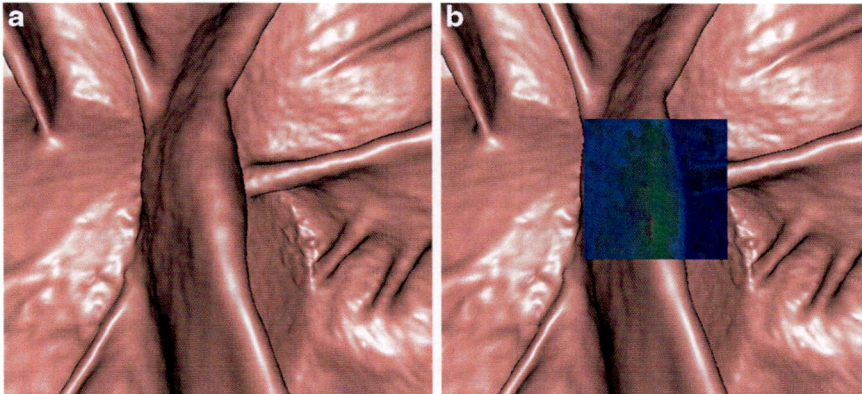

Fig. 5.6 Translucency rendering demonstrates the internal composition of the ileocecal valve. (**a**) 3D endoluminal image of the ileocecal valve demonstrates normal valve morphology with a flat, slit-like opening. (**b**) Translucency rendering applied to the 3D image in "a" shows assignment of *green* and *blue shades* to the valve, indicative of fat content

laxative examination [33]. However, the full laxative fecal-tagged CTC yielded a higher specificity. He concluded that it might be desirable to offer patients the option of the full prep for highest accuracy and the ability to perform a same-day colonoscopy, or a minimum laxative CTC for those who are willing to accept an increased risk of false-positives and attendant unnecessary colonoscopy, which not only is inconvenient but also increases risk and costs.

A problem with nonconventional preps is the difficulty of performing a primary 3D interpretation without the ability to perform electronic cleansing. Residual stool and artifacts render the 3D virtual colonoscopic view uninterpretable, as the colonic mucosa is essentially "buried." A large number of filling defects have to be addressed one by one (Fig. 5.7), an "insurmountable task." [52] Even with stool subtraction, optimal fecal tagging would be needed to make 3D interpretation possible [45]. Without the benefit of stool subtraction, a primary 2D method with 3D problem solving must be employed. Primary 2D approaches permit the reader to rapidly examine the internal density of filling defects and decide if they are soft tissue polyps or if they actually contain air or tagging agent consistent with stool [52]. In general, interpretation of noncathartic CTC is a tedious task.

Electronic Subtraction of Tagged Material

"Electronic subtraction," also called "electronic cleansing," refers to post-processing of CTC data to remove interfering high-density tagged liquid and stool, so that theoretically one is left with only the colonic mucosa and any soft tissue abnormalities to interrogate (Fig. 5.8) [49]. Electronic subtraction improves visualization whether the prep is a full prep with fecal tagging or a less rigorous limited or noncathartic one. A number of commercial platforms now feature electronic cleansing algorithms [69].

Presently, cleansing algorithms performed by post-processing software are threshold based, and artifacts often arise that complicate image interpretation. The technique is challenging from a programming aspect, mostly because of the heterogeneity of fecal tagging (Fig. 5.9), variable colonic transit times, and normal desiccation of stool as it progresses through the colon. Additionally, interfaces of air, tissue, and stool are prone to partial volume artifacts [52]. "Oversubtraction," where areas of normal tissue or polyps are subtracted along with the stool, can be a problem and must be avoided. New techniques are being developed to improve electronic cleansing. Spectral electronic cleansing,

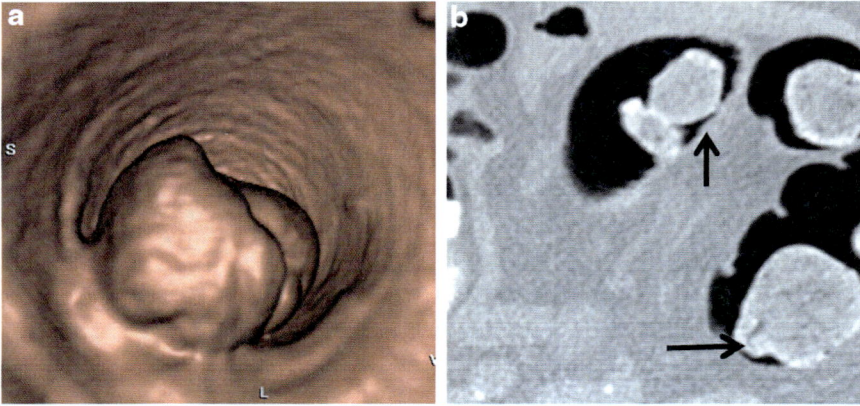

Fig. 5.7 Residual stool can imitate a mass lesion. (**a**) 3D endoluminal image of the sigmoid colon demonstrates an intraluminal lesion, which could represent a large polyp or mass. (**b**) 2D axial image shows multiple stool balls (*arrows*) in this patient who had a very poor bowel preparation. The lesion in question corresponded to one of these stool balls

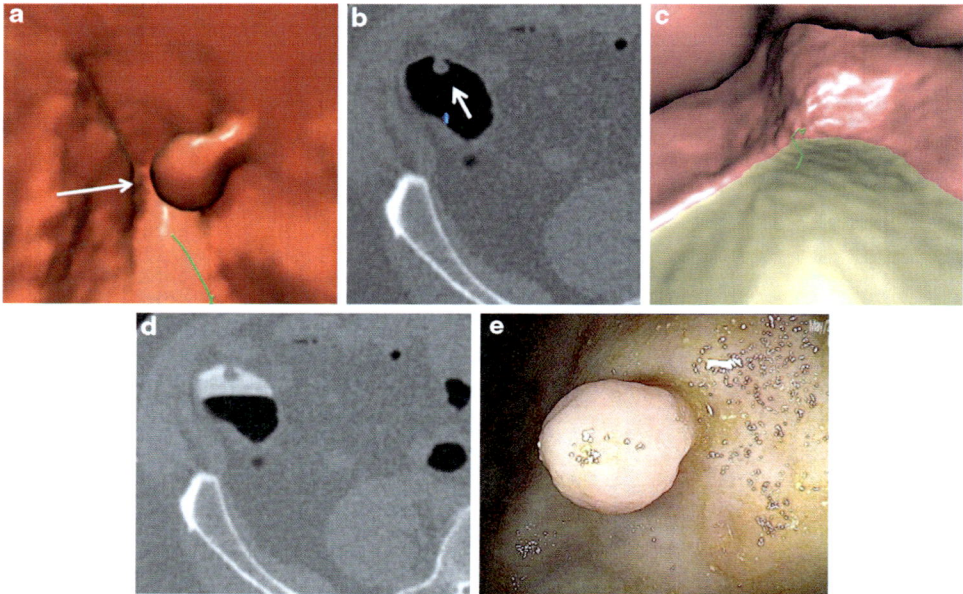

Fig. 5.8 Electronic stool subtraction can be useful to detect lesions submerged in liquid. (**a**) 3D endoluminal image of the base of the cecum demonstrates a 1-cm pedunculated lesion (*arrow*). Electronic stool subtraction was applied to this image. (**b**) Prone 2D axial view of the lesion in **a** (*arrow*) demonstrates that it is soft tissue density, concerning for a polyp. (**c**) Prone 3D endoluminal image generated on a different workstation without stool subtraction using discriminate differential color coding, shows only tagged fluid (assigned a *golden color*) within the lumen. The lesion is submerged under the liquid and is not visible. (**d**) Corresponding prone 2D axial image without stool subtraction applied shows the lesion (*arrow*) is submerged under the tagged fluid. The lesion is still easily appreciable on the 2D view but impossible to see on the unsubtracted 3D endoluminal image. (**e**) Photograph from the optical colonoscopy shows that the cecal lesion has a polypoid morphology, but on close inspection its surface was not characteristic of an adenomatous polyp. The patient had a remote history of appendectomy, and this lesion represents an inverted appendiceal stump, a potential pitfall [183]

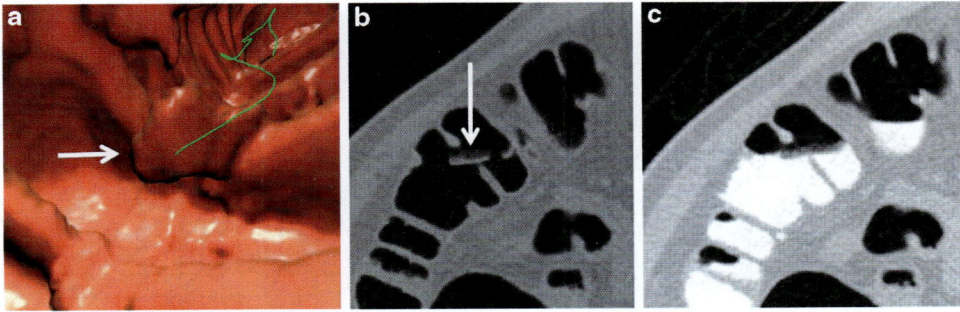

Fig. 5.9 Electronic stool subtraction artifacts can create pseudo-lesions. (**a**) 3D endoluminal image of the transverse colon demonstrates an irregular polypoid protrusion (*arrow*). (**b**) Supine 2D axial image through the area of interest in **a**, using electronic stool subtraction, demonstrates a heterogeneous, linear, soft tissue density (*arrow*). (**c**) Corresponding 2D axial image without stool subtraction applied demonstrates a thin layer of poorly tagged fecal material (*white*) floating on top of radiodense contrast. This material did not meet minimum Hounsfield units to be recognized and subtracted by the computer software and thus remained within the colonic lumen after the higher density liquid was subtracted, creating a distracting pseudo-lesion

based on dual-energy CT, may decrease the number of artifacts and improve image quality. In a 2008 study of a group of patients drawn from the Walter Reed Army Medical Center database, Serlie found that electronic cleansing shortened interpretation time, lowered assessment effort, and had a positive effect on observer confidence [70]. Although stool subtraction has been shown to improve the sensitivity of CTC, studies have also shown that specificity can decrease, especially for the detection of moderate sized polyps [52].

Discriminative Color Coding

An additional technique taking advantage of fecal tagging is discriminative color coding. This is a color enhancement technique available on some workstations that can be used during primary 3D interpretation. When activated, computer software color codes high-attenuation material on the 3D images so that residual liquid and adherent tagged stool can be easily discriminated from soft tissue density polyps, decreasing the need for 2D correlations (Figs. 5.8 and 5.15). This technique has been shown to shorten interpretation times when compared with a standard primary 3D interpretation approach [71].

Performance of CT Colonography

Patient Arrival

Examinations are scheduled first thing in the morning. After checking in to the radiology department, the patient is escorted to a dressing room and instructed to change into a gown. The technologist speaks with the patient and explains what to expect in the CT suite. The nurse requests that the patient attempts to evacuate one last time and inquires about the compliance with the preparation as well as the appearance of the stool. If the patient has not completed the preparation as instructed or continues to have semisolid stools, rather than rescheduling the CTC, more cathartic agents may be administered in the department, schedule permitting. Routine administration of a self-administered phosphate enema before the examination is not indicated, having been shown in a study of noncathartic CTC to not decrease residual stool, to increase retained fluid, and to reduce diagnostic confidence [72].

Insufflation

Ample colonic distention is of fundamental importance for CTC. Collapsed segments can

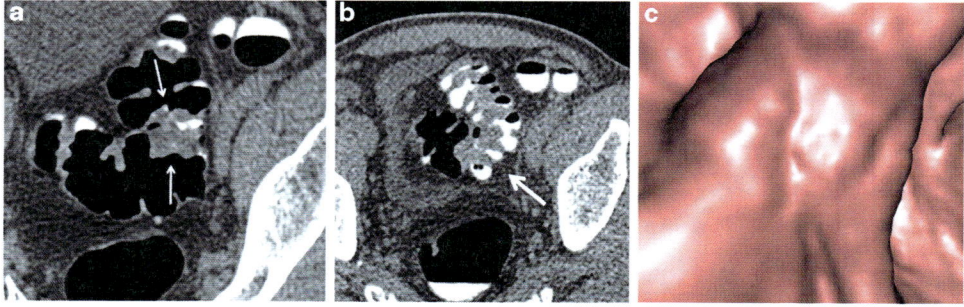

Fig. 5.10 Poor distention of the colon can simulate mass lesions. (**a**) Prone 2D axial image of the sigmoid colon shows a possible mass lesion (between *arrows*) in the sigmoid. This could also represent a pseudo-mass due to under distention. (**b**) Corresponding supine axial 2D image of the sigmoid colon (*arrow*) shows that this area remains poorly distended, limiting evaluation. (**c**) Prone 3D endoluminal view of the area in question demonstrates a possible mass versus a poorly distended complex fold. A decision was made to perform same-day sigmoidoscopy. No mass was found. This was a pseudo-lesion from underdistention, a common cause of false-positives

obscure or mimic pathology (Fig. 5.10), reducing sensitivity and specificity. With inadequate colonic distention, diagnostic confidence can be diminished and interpretation times prolonged [3, 73]. Insufflation can be achieved by administration of either room air or carbon dioxide (CO_2), via a manual pump or electronic insufflator. The most basic technique is room air insufflation using a handheld plastic bulb [74]. This method can even be performed by patients themselves [45]. Of the possible combinations, electronic insufflation of CO_2 is highly favored for reasons given below.

Burling demonstrated that automated CO_2 insufflation significantly improved colonic distention compared to manual carbon dioxide insufflation, particularly the left colon in the supine position and the transverse colon when both supine and prone scans were combined [74]. Slow, continuous, low-pressure administration of CO_2 can only be achieved with the electronic insufflator. This helps alleviate colonic spasm, especially in segments with diverticular disease [30]. CO_2 has superior lipid solubility and higher partial pressure gradient than room air and is thus more rapidly absorbed from the colon into the blood stream and exhaled with respiration [75]. Post-procedural gaseous discomfort is less than with room air [12, 76], and

patients often feel back to normal by the time they get off the CT table.

Electronic CO_2 insufflation also improves the safety of the examination. The perforation risk with electronic CO_2 insufflation is negligible in the screening population. Close to all of the reported perforations from CTC have involved staff-controlled manual insufflation of room air [77]. In two large series, the risk of colonic perforation at CTC was approximately 0.06% [78, 79]. In a review of 11,870 CTCs, seven perforations occurred, all of which involved manual insufflation of room air [79]. Risk factors for perforation include advanced age, recent colonoscopy, diverticular disease, recent colonic biopsy (Fig. 5.11), inguinal hernia, and obstructive carcinoma [78, 79].

In patients who have undergone incomplete OC and are referred for same-day CTC, it is important to inquire whether a biopsy or polypectomy was performed. Patients who have undergone deep cold forceps biopsy, hot snare polypectomy, or endoscopic mucosal resection should wait at least 1 week before undergoing CTC. In patients who have had an incomplete OC, even if they have not undergone shallow cold forceps biopsy, we obtain CT images of the abdomen and pelvis before insufflation of intra-rectal air. This is done as a safety precaution, to exclude the possibility of perforation.

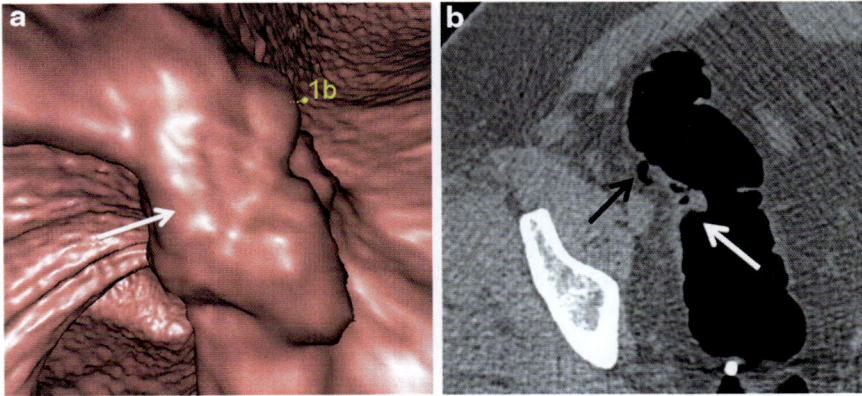

Fig. 5.11 Deep biopsy or polypectomy is a risk factor for perforation during CT colonography. (**a**) 3D endoluminal view of the sigmoid colon demonstrates a large, irregular, nearly obstructing mass lesion. This lesion had undergone biopsy earlier in the day, and the scan was ordered to clear the proximal colon of synchronous lesions. (**b**) Corresponding 2D axial supine image demonstrates the mass (*white arrow*) along the right wall of the sigmoid colon. Foci of gas can be seen in the lesion post biopsy. Additionally, there is extracolonic gas (*black arrow*). Because a scan was not performed before CO_2 insufflation, it is unknown whether this small perforation was due to the biopsy or CO_2 insufflation. The patient was asymptomatic

Patient Positioning

Insufflation techniques vary between centers [12, 30], but it is agreed that both supine and prone images are necessary. The rationale of dual positioning is to redistribute residual fluid, as well as to help redistribute air. A segment of colon may distend well on one view, but not another (Fig. 5.12) [80]. Polyp detection sensitivity has been shown to improve when both supine and prone acquisitions are performed [73, 80].

The exam is often started with the patient in the right side down decubitus position in order to facilitate rectosigmoid and descending colon distention. At our institution, with the patient on their right side on the CT table, a radiology tech or nurse inserts a thin, flexible rectal catheter. This is connected to the electronic CO_2 insufflator (PROTOCO₂L, Bracco). For comfort, we avoid using larger catheters, such as those used at barium enema, unless the patient needs help retaining the CO_2. A target pressure of 25 mmHg is programmed, and the CO_2 is administered, titrating to pressure and patient comfort. It is important to acquire the CT images during active replacement of CO_2 at equilibrium pressures [30]. Because of differences in colonic anatomy, patient tolerance,

small bowel reflux, and anal incontinence, the total volume of gas delivery can vary widely and thus has little significance [74]. Anywhere from 3 to 10 L may be needed for sufficient distention [12, 30]. Patient cooperation with gas retention is essential.

After insufflation of approximately 1.5 L, insufflation is continued in the supine position until the patient reports fullness in the right side of the abdomen, usually indicating cecal distention. One must always be aware of patient comfort, as well as the displayed pressure reading. When ready for scan acquisition, the patient exhales and then holds their breath, elevating the diaphragm, expanding the abdominal cavity, and allowing more room for the splenic flexure and transverse colon [30]. A CT scout image is used to assess colonic distention (Fig. 5.13). If distention is adequate, a supine CT scan is performed.

Unfortunately, the scout is at times unreliable for evaluation of distention. For this reason, technologists or research assistants are sometimes trained to assess the adequacy of distention by reviewing the CT images on the scanner console. This allows for problem solving in real time and reduces the need for callbacks. At our institution the interpreting radiologist or the body-imaging

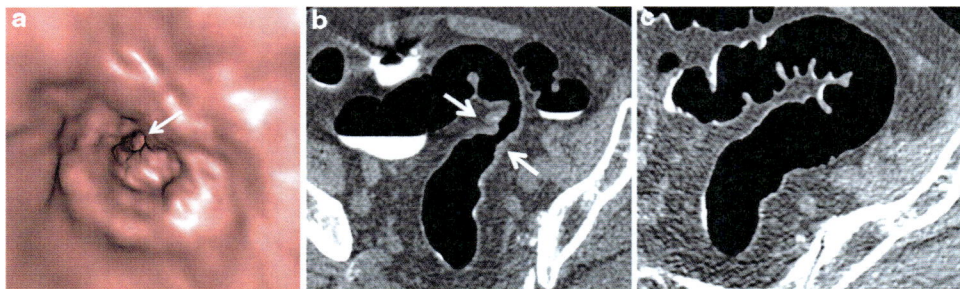

Fig. 5.12 Dual positioning may eliminate pseudo-lesions. (a) 3D endoluminal view of the sigmoid colon demonstrates apparent severe narrowing with only a pinpoint lumen (*arrow*) visible. (b) Corresponding supine 2D axial image demonstrates apparent wall thickening and luminal narrowing at the area in question (between *arrows*). This is concerning for an apple-core lesion. (c) 2D axial image obtained in the right lateral decubitus position demonstrates better sigmoid distention, without evidence of a mass lesion. This demonstrates the value of dual positioning

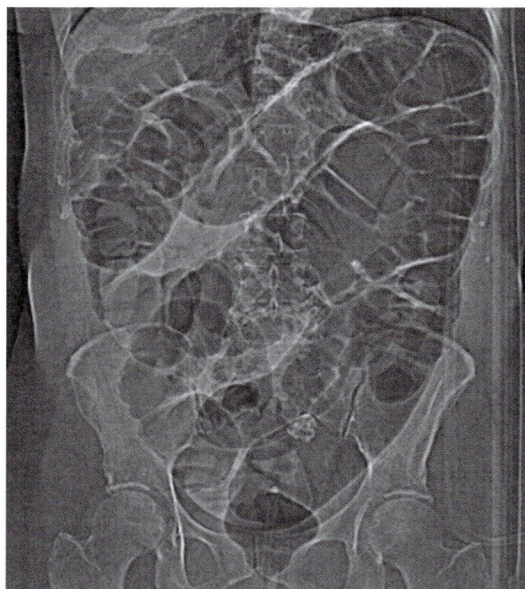

Fig. 5.13 The scout image is used to check for adequate distention before scanning. Supine scout view of CTC during CO_2 insufflation shows good distention of the entire colon, without significant small bowel reflux

fellow are involved with scan acquisition from start to finish. However, in a busy CT practice, assigning quality assurance responsibility to the CT technologist is an important goal that necessitates continued training and feedback [81]. After supine acquisition, the patient is turned prone. Elevating the torso and hips with pillows can be helpful, especially in overweight patients.

External abdominal compression in the prone position can cause poor colonic distention, especially in the transverse colon [12, 82]. Once prone, the scout is repeated. Equilibrium CO_2 pressures are maintained at 25 mmHg. At that point, axial prone images are obtained.

If, after acquisition of prone and supine data sets, a portion of the colon is not visualized well on either position, a decision can be made to obtain a third set of images, most commonly a right lateral decubitus (Fig. 5.14). To limit radiation exposure and improve efficiency, programs should limit a third series as much as possible without sacrificing diagnostic performance [81]. Most commonly, the sigmoid and/or the descending colon is the offending segment [30], and the patient in that instance would be placed in the right lateral decubitus position to facilitate distention of the nondependent sigmoid colon. As expected, the rate of obtaining a right lateral decubitus series in a diagnostic cohort is higher than that of a screening, likely because many of the reasons for failed OC (diverticulosis, redundancy, tortuosity, and obstructing masses) can lead to challenges with luminal distention at CTC [81]. Advanced diverticular disease of the sigmoid colon is a recognized cause of luminal nondistention [83]. At times, because of circular muscular hypertrophy and poor distensibility [84], the sigmoid will not be well visualized in any position. In these instances, a decision to perform unsedated flexible sigmoidoscopy may be

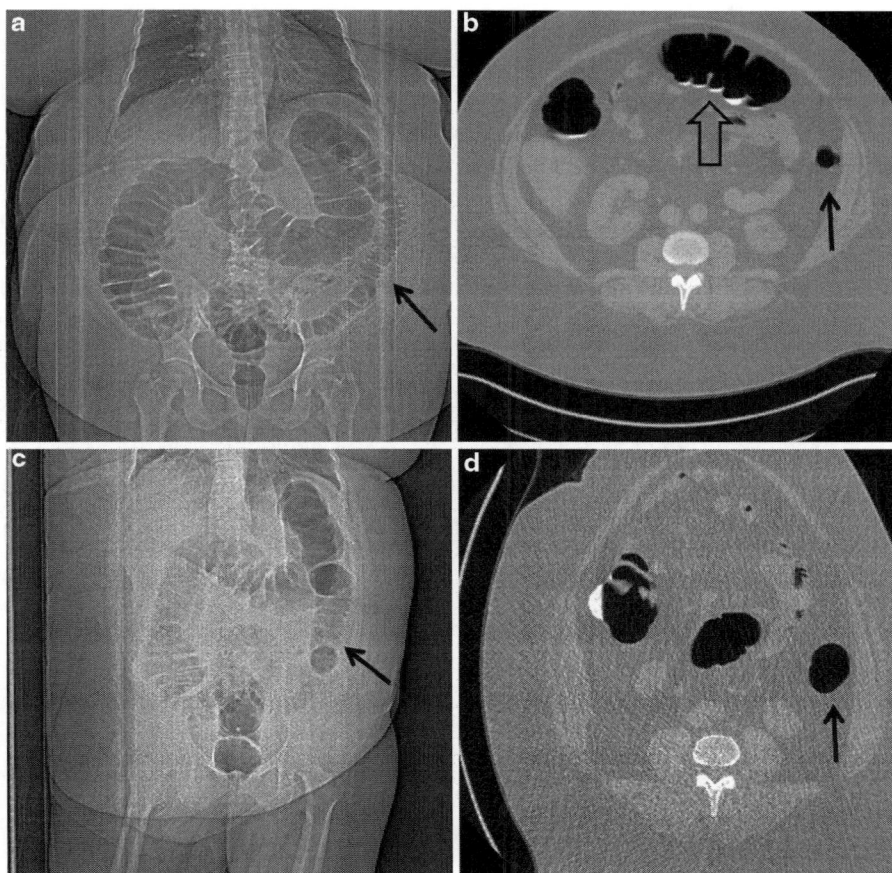

Fig. 5.14 Right lateral decubitus views may be useful when a particular segment is collapsed on both supine and prone images. (**a**) Scout supine image of the abdomen demonstrates that the descending colon (*arrow*) is suboptimally distended. (**b**) Supine 2D axial image shows that, compared with the transverse colon (*open arrow*), the descending colon (*arrow*) is suboptimally distended. Prone positioning (not shown) did not improve distention. (**c**) Scout image in the right lateral decubitus (*right-side-down*) position demonstrates somewhat improved distention of the descending colon (*arrow*). (**d**) Right lateral decubitus 2D axial images confirm better distention of the descending colon (*arrow*)

considered [83]. An additional consideration in positioning relates to patients with limited mobility, in whom supine and right lateral decubitus may be sufficient, obviating the difficult task of turning these patients prone.

Spasmolytics

Spasmolytic agents such as glucagon have been investigated with the goals of lessening patient discomfort and reducing peristalsis and resultant motion artifact. Part of the rationale for using glucagon arises from its role as an antiperistaltic in barium enema studies [85]. A placebo-controlled study of glucagon in double-contrast barium enemas demonstrated that glucagon lessened patient discomfort. However, the onset of maximum effect was after 8 min post administration [86]. Given that image acquisition with multidetector row CT (MDCT) is so fast, if given glucagon immediately before the exam, patients will have already completed the CTC before glucagon achieves its maximum effect [87]. The alternative, waiting for glucagon to take effect, increases total duration of the examination [76] and decreases efficiency. Glucagon is also costly (wholesale cost is US$48–66 per 1-mg vial). It requires an IV or intramuscular injection, increasing discomfort [87]. It also carries a risk of side effects, such as nausea and vomiting [76].

Most importantly, studies of glucagon in CTC have shown no objective beneficial effects. In a blinded, non-randomized study of 60 patients undergoing CTC, the 33 patients who received glucagon did not show any difference in segmental or overall colonic distention [88]. Morrin studied 74 patients who were administered glucagon before CTC and found that distention scores for the glucagon and non-glucagon patients were similar [87]. Its lack of proven effectiveness in CTC is not surprising physiologically, given that the colon is recognized as the least responsive part of the bowel to the antiperistaltic effects [89].

Though not available in the USA, the spasmolytic Buscopan is available in Europe and has been suggested to be more effective than glucagon as an antiperistaltic agent [90]. However, despite improved colonic distension in certain segments, Buscopan did not necessarily translate into improved polyp detection, and thus it is not routinely used in CTC. Based on the literature, there does not appear to be justification for routine use of spasmolytics in CTC. At the same time, a small percentage of patients may have cramping and pain that significantly limits tolerance of bowel insufflation, and in these selected cases, administration of glucagon may be worthwhile [12].

CT Data Acquisition

Since the introduction of spiral or helical CT in the early 1990s, CT scanning has sped up by a factor of at least 500, such that the CT acquisition portion of the exam is not at all rate limiting. Modern scanners can acquire the CT data in 10–15 s, which is well within the breath holding capability of almost all patients. There remain, however, important considerations related to slice thickness, reconstruction interval, and radiation dose that we elaborate further here.

Imaging Parameters

Careful setting of the scan parameters is needed to balance image quality (spatial and contrast resolution, and slice thickness) and radiation dose. Now, with MDCT, data can be acquired much faster, even with thinner slices. In a 2005 meta-analysis, seven studies that used multidetector scanners had higher sensitivity than nine studies in which a single-detector scanner was used (95% versus 82%) [91]. The entire abdomen and pelvis can be now scanned within a single breath hold, which decreases both respiratory and peristalsis motion artifacts.

Initial work with single-detector CTC usually used 3–5-mm-thick sections with a high degree of image overlap for data acquisition [92–94]. However, we now realize that the acquisition of thin sections is essential for the performance of CTC because they decrease partial volume averaging and improve quality of the multiplanar reconstruction (MPR) and endoluminal reformats [12, 95]. Moreover, thinner slices improve sensitivity for polyps and improve specificity, as shown in a 2005 meta-analysis [91]. The same meta-analysis evaluated data from 19 studies and suggested that every 1-mm increase in collimation width decreases sensitivity by 4.9% [91]. There is a trade-off, of course, between slice thickness and radiation dose.

As with any type of CT exam, each time the slice thickness is reduced by half, the radiation dose must be doubled to maintain image noise constant [96]. Increasing collimation or decreasing tube current (mAs) or voltage (kVp) will decrease radiation dose but at the expense of increased noise. Because image noise increases as dose is decreased, image noise can, at a certain point, degrade image quality and may decrease diagnostic performance, especially for smaller polyps [97]. It may be more difficult to differentiate stool from polyps because the attenuation of polyps becomes more heterogeneous as noise increases.

Another advantage of MDCT is that images can be reconstructed at thicknesses larger than the collimator width, for example at 2.5 or 5 mm thickness, if desired by the radiologist.

This enables efficient interpretation of extracolonic structures [12]. The ACRIN Trial sites used a minimal detector collimation of 0.5–1.0 mm, a slice thickness of 1–1.25 mm, and a reconstruction index of 0.8 mm [10]. The 2009 ACR practice guidelines for CTC recommend that CTC be performed using an MDCT with ≥4 detector rows, a slice thickness of ≤3 mm, and a reconstruction interval of ≤2 mm [98]. We review our extracolonic structures using 5-mm slices.

Radiation Dose

Every effort should be made to maintain radiation exposure *as low as reasonably achievable (ALARA)*, especially for screening examinations, where the benefit/risk ratio must be favorable [99]. As CTC becomes increasingly employed for colon cancer screening, we must consider any possible radiation risk to the population of these potential millions of scans [99]. Concern over radiation exposure, real or imaginary, was one of the reasons given why Medicare declined reimbursement of screening CTC in 2009.

Fortunately, because of the large difference in the attenuation between bowel wall and intraluminal air, as well as the lack of need for detailed evaluation of extracolonic structures, there is potential for dose reduction. The dose/noise trade-off can be heavily weighted toward low-dose, higher-noise images, while still maintaining sensitivity and specificity, at least for polyps > 10 mm in diameter [93, 99–101]. Brenner, in a widely cited study, estimated the combined prone and supine radiation dose for CTC at around 13 mSv [102]. However, this study used data from older generation 8 and 16 row machines. In comparison, the ACRIN trial used newer MDCT scanners with low-dose technique and was able to limit dose to approximately 5 mSv per exam [10]. This is very close to the 4.5-mSv annual background exposure at high altitude [4]. Additionally, a 2008 study by Liedenbaum surveyed CTC providers about their equipment and dose parameters. He found that 62% of his questionnaire respondents were using 64 row scanners and 50%

used dose modulation. The average dose of his respondents was 5.7 mSv [103].

Ultralow-dose scans have been shown to be able to deliver an effective radiation dose of 1.8 mSv for males and 2.4 mSv for females while preserving excellent sensitivity (100% for polyps greater than 10 mm and 100% for cancers) [104]. In a 2004 feasibility study, van Gelder studied 15 patients with doses ranging from 0.05 to 12 mSv. Overall sensitivity for polyps 5 mm or larger decreased at lower doses but was 74% or higher down to 1.6 mAs (0.2 mSv) [97]. Noise-related artifacts affect image quality for 3D more than 2D [97], a potential concern for primary 3D readers. However, a recent study of low-dose CTC showed that, although cobblestone artifacts and irregularly delineated folds were significantly higher with low dose compared with standard dose, most of the artifacts were mild and no significant difference in sensitivity was found between dose levels for polyps greater than or equal to 6 mm in diameter [105].

Despite these encouraging performance data, the use of ultralow-dose scans has yet to catch on, possibly because radiologists are unwilling to sacrifice image quality and further compromise evaluation of extracolonic organs [106]. New techniques, such as adaptive statistical iterative reconstruction (ASIR) and prior image constrained compressed sensing algorithm (PICCS), have the potential to improve image quality at lower radiation doses. A 2010 study demonstrated that the standard radiation dose for CTC could be reduced 50% when ASIR was used, without significantly affecting image quality [107]. As expected, image quality scores were best in thin patients, with worse image quality and noise in larger patients. PICCS, when applied to standard FBP with low-dose multidetector CT images, results in considerable noise reduction and improved image quality [108]. Further dose reductions can be achieved with automatic tube current modulation, a standard technique on newer scanners that adjusts tube current, and thus the radiation dose, to the patient's body density in order to decrease variation in image quality. This enables a significant decrease in radiation exposure without decrease in image quality in CTC [109]. It has been shown that an additional dose reduction of 20% can be accomplished with attenuation-based tube current modulation [105].

The 2009 ACR practice guidelines for CTC specify that the recommended dose level for screening CTC should be ≤50% of the CT dose index by volume (CTDI) for routine CT of the abdomen and pelvis, which is set at an upper limit of 25 mGy [110]. Thus, for CTC, a CTDI of 6.25 mGy per position or 12.5 mGy for the entire examination is the upper limit [111].

Interpretation

Background

Depending on scan parameters, a CTC study can contain between 600 and 2,000 images. An ever-growing number of techniques for 2D and 3D reconstructions provide even more images for review. Also, advanced adenomas are relatively uncommon in a screening population, with an incidence of approximately 4% [10]. Therefore, the expectation is that the bulk of CTC studies will be "negative." This "needle in a haystack" issue, as well as the fact that CTC is difficult and time intensive, can make interpretation intimidating. It is also an issue that considerably motivates research into how to most accurately and efficiently interpret CTC, which is the focus of this section.

Training

Before interpretation can begin, one must undergo training. It is well documented that the detection of carcinoma and polyps improves with practice [112–115]. Data from the ACRIN trial shows that the odds of identifying patients with disease increase 1.5-fold for every 50-case increase in reader experience or formal training [113]. Although CTC interpretation can be challenging, even well-trained nonphysicians can achieve respectable performance [112, 116]. Multiple professional organizations, including

the American College of Radiology (ACR), the American Gastroenterological Association (AGA) Institute, and the International Collaboration for CT Colonography Standards recommend dedicated training for CTC [111, 117, 118]. The only consistently recommended format for training is the educational workshop, where attendees receive face-to-face, hands-on training using colonoscopically proven cases [119]. Despite these recommendations, many interpreters of CTC do not meet minimum recommended standards. According to a recent survey of attendees at a CTC training workshop, only 24% of those already interpreting CTC had interpreted more than 50 cases [119]. Interestingly, despite evidence that non-radiologists desire to interpret CTC [120], the great majority (97%) of those attending the workshop were radiologists [119].

Training should encompass anatomy, colorectal cancer pathogenesis, examination technique, and pitfalls. It should also include appropriateness criteria, risks and benefits, problem solving (e.g., the use of IV contrast and decubitus imaging), technologist training, facility requirements, quality control, documentation [111], and standardized reporting of intra- and extracolonic findings (C-RADS/E-RADS) [113, 121]. Although training methods may vary, a minimum of 50–75 OC-validated CTC practice cases should be reviewed [122]. That said, even this may be insufficient, as a recent study demonstrated that it required on average 164 CTC studies for novices to achieve performance equal to that of experienced interpreters [122].

Clearly, one of the major goals of training is to reduce errors. Therefore, it is necessary to be cognizant of the types of errors that degrade performance. Liedenbaum describes three types of errors: errors of search (the radiologist's gaze completely misses the abnormality), errors of detection (the eyes of the radiologist pass over the abnormality, but not long enough for it to be recognized), and errors of decision (the abnormality is not correctly characterized) [122]. One can conclude that to reduce errors, competent, trained readers must read CTC with concentration, at a reasonable speed.

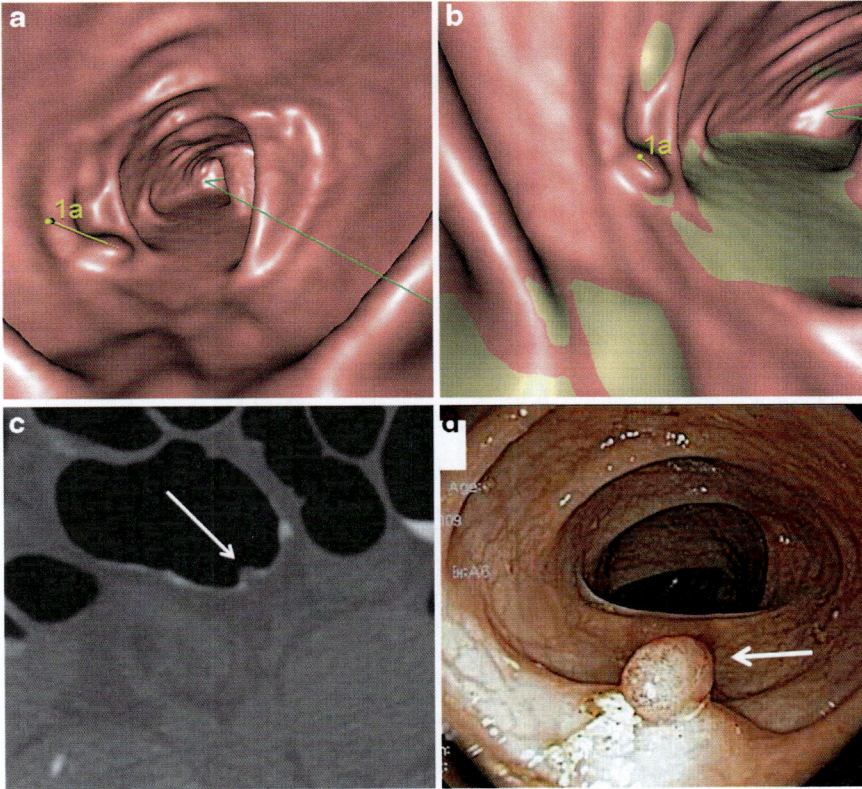

Fig. 5.15 Polyps are usually soft tissue attenuation and round in shape. (**a**) 3D endoluminal view of the sigmoid colon shows a polypoid filling defect (labeled 1a). (**b**) Application of discriminative color coding shows that high-density tagged fluid and stool is labeled a *golden color*. The lesion is not color-coded, indicating that it is soft tissue density. (**c**) Supine 2D axial image demonstrates that the lesion is indeed soft tissue, suspicious for a polyp (*arrow*). (**d**) Photograph from optical colonoscopy demonstrates snare retrieval of the polyp (*arrow*) found on CTC

Polyp Identification

The goal of CTC is to identify adenomatous polyps before they have time to turn into cancer. Polyps may develop anywhere along the mucosal lining, including on haustral folds or the ileocecal valve. The typical polyp on CTC is homogeneous soft tissue in attenuation and ovoid or round in shape (Fig. 5.15). Lesions may be sessile, pedunculated (Fig. 5.16), or flat (Fig. 5.17). Sessile lesions should not change position with respect to the colonic wall between supine and prone repositioning. In contrast, residual stool, the main source of false-positives, is often heterogeneous in attenuation and may contain air (Figs. 5.18 and 5.19). Stool can be irregular in shape and tends to change position between supine and prone scans (Fig. 5.20).

Interpretive pitfalls are abundant, a point that underscores the importance of systematic training and experience. Stool may at times be homogeneous in density. Pedunculated polyps may trap air and appear heterogeneous in attenuation [12]. Pedunculated polyps may be mistaken for pseudo-lesions (false-positives) when, because they are on a stalk, they move between supine and prone data sets. Additionally, colonic rotation may cause interpretive confusion. The ascending colon may have a deficient mesocolon [123] and may rotate from supine to prone positions, resulting in a change in the radial polyp position of as much as 79°, causing it to

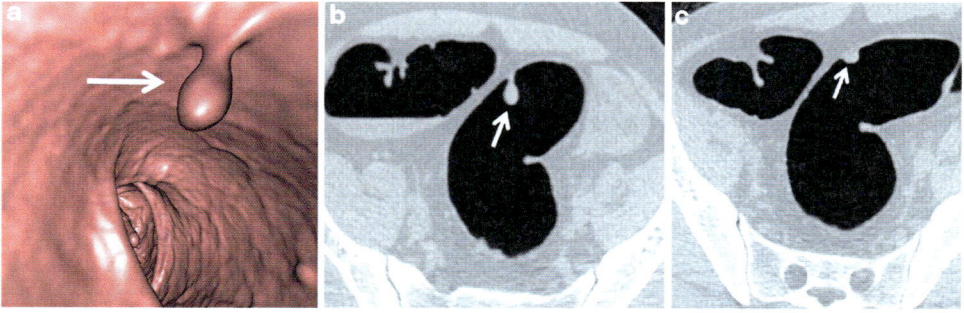

Fig. 5.16 Pedunculated polyps can change their appearance with dual positioning. (**a**) Supine 3D endoluminal view of the sigmoid colon demonstrates a 1-cm pedunculated polyp dangling into the colonic lumen (*arrow*). (**b**) Corresponding 2D supine axial image demonstrates the same polyp (*arrow*). (**c**) 2D prone axial image demonstrates that the polyp (*arrow*) has assumed a different configuration because it is now lying dependently along the anterior colonic wall. The stalk is no longer evident

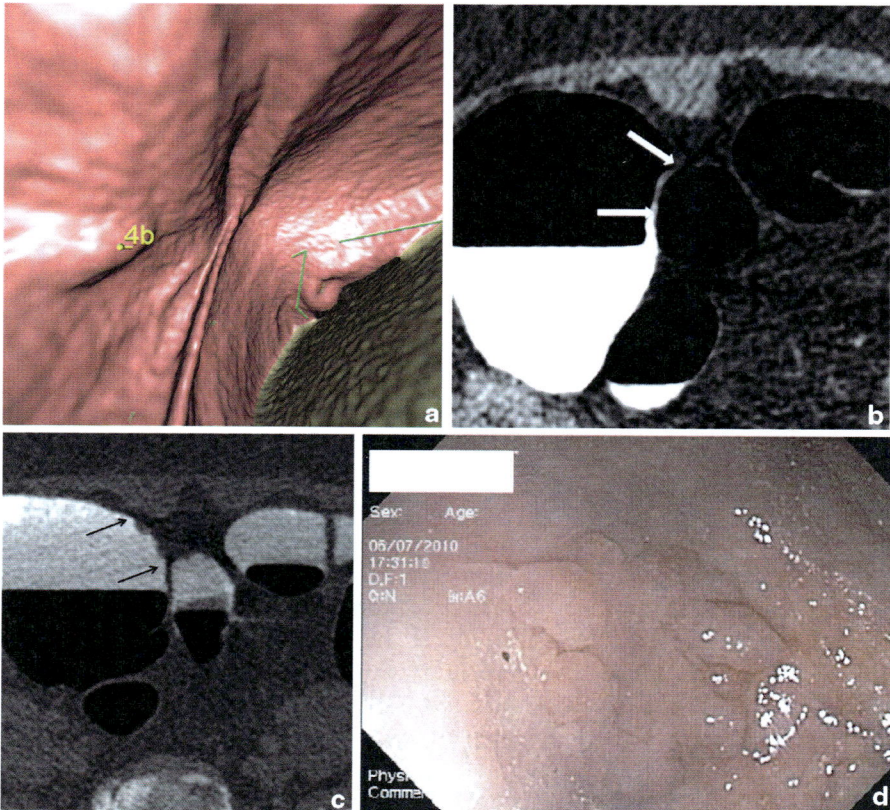

Fig. 5.17 Flat lesions can be difficult to visualize. (**a**) 3D endoluminal view of the cecum demonstrates a contour abnormality (labeled 4b) along the medial wall. This image is taken from the base of the cecum-looking Retrograde. The ileocecal valve is seen in the background (between *green lines*). The tagged fluid in the cecum is color-coded *gold*. (**b**) Corresponding supine 2D axial view of the cecum demonstrates a subtle sessile lesion arising from the medial wall (between *white arrows*). (**c**) Corresponding prone 2D axial view of the cecum demonstrates the sessile lesion (between *black arrows*) is entirely submerged by contrast, thus masking it on the 3D endoluminal reformats (not shown). (**d**) Photograph from optical colonoscopy shows a 3-cm lobulated flat lesion within the cecum. Biopsies were performed, and histology was consistent with tubular adenoma

falsely appear mobile [124]. Characteristics of difficult-to-detect polyps include flat morphology, undulating surface contour, visibility on only one view, location on a fold, or morphology that imitates a bulbous fold (Fig. 5.21) [113, 125]. On 2D images, thickened or complex folds, real or artifactual, may also be mistaken for polyps or masses (Fig. 5.22).

While the debate about the relevance of flat, superficially elevated, or "non-polypoid" lesions [126, 127] is beyond the scope of this chapter, awareness of their presence and appearance is important. These lesions are defined as having a height less than or equal to 3 mm [126]. While less conspicuous than polypoid lesions, they are still detectable with meticulous technique. Of note, this 3-mm definition does not include "carpet lesions."

Differential Diagnosis

Differential diagnosis of mucosal lesions includes not only neoplastic entities such as adenomas (tubular, tubulovillous, or villous in histology) and adenocarcinoma (Fig. 5.23), but also nonneoplastic lesion such as hyperplastic, juvenile, inflammatory, or hamartomatous polyps. These are impossible to distinguish on CTC, although it is postulated that hamartomatous polyps are flatter because they are soft and compress easily with insufflation [128]. Submucosal lesion such as lipomas, carcinoids, gastrointestinal stromal tumors, and hematogenous metastases can also imitate polyps (Fig. 5.24). Extrinsic lesions, such as impression from extracolonic structures (Fig. 5.25), appendiceal lesions (Fig. 5.26), and intussusception can also cause interpretive difficulties. Diverticula, especially when impacted,

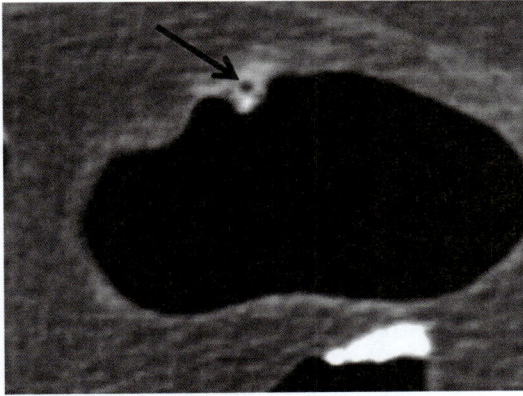

Fig. 5.18 Stool is often irregular in morphology and contains gas. Prone 2D axial image demonstrates a polypoid lesion within the colonic lumen. This can be confidently diagnosed as stool because it contains a focus of air (*arrow*) and has an irregular morphology. It is also higher attenuation than soft tissue due to fecal tagging

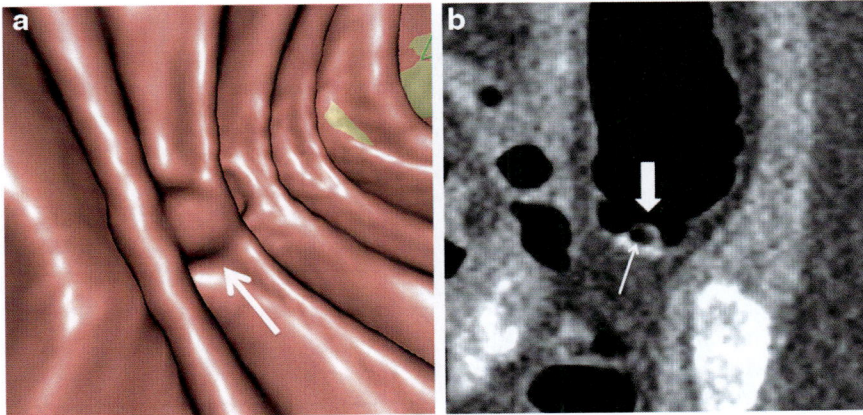

Fig. 5.19 Stool may be round in morphology. In this case, intralesional gas helps exclude a true lesion. (**a**) 3D endoluminal view of the descending colon demonstrates a polypoid lesion (*arrow*) between two haustral folds.

(**b**) 2D supine axial image demonstrates that the lesion (*larger arrow*) is heterogeneous and contains a focus of gas (*smaller arrow*), confirming that it is residual fecal material

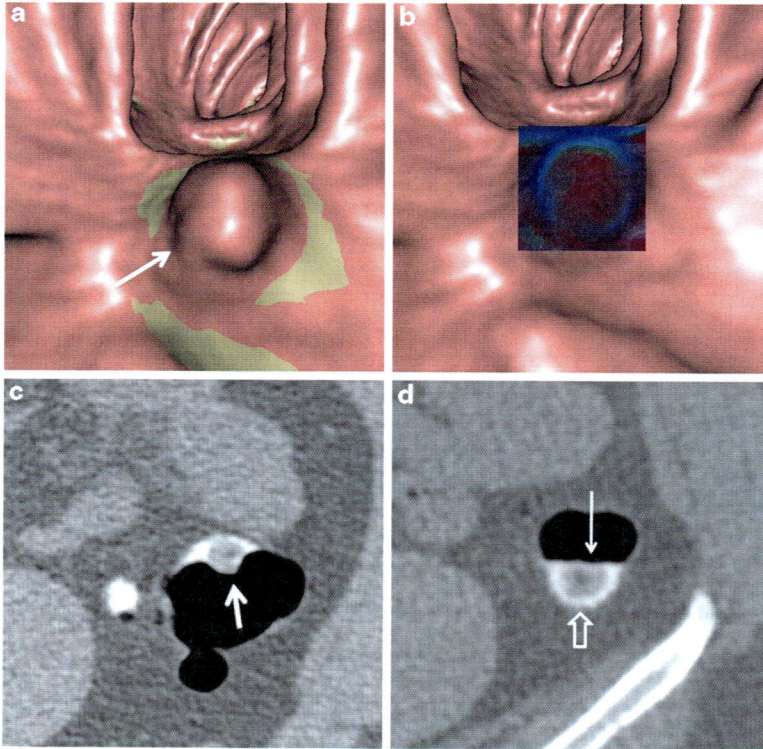

Fig. 5.20 Stool usually changes position between supine and prone scans. In this example, dual positioning was critical because the stool was homogeneous soft tissue density. (**a**) 3D endoluminal view of the left colon demonstrates a polypoid luminal protrusion. Note that the discriminative color coding (*golden colored*) did not identify the lesion as tagged stool. (**b**) Application of the translucency views demonstrates that the core of the lesion is *red*, corresponding to soft tissue density. This appearance is highly suspicious for a true polyp. (**c**) 2D axial prone view demonstrates that the lesion (*arrow*) layers dependently. (**d**) 2D supine axial image shows that the lesion again layers dependently, changing position. This lesion is consistent with residual stool. Note that high-density tagging material (*open arrow*) outlines and undercuts the lesion

can imitate disease (Fig. 5.27). Anorectal lesions such as hemorrhoids or hypertrophied anal papilla can simulate polyps or cancers.

Workstation Selection

Alongside advancements in MDCT, computer graphics technology has also evolved, such that there are now on the order of ten FDA-approved commercial workstations with CTC interpretation software. Some are thin-client web based, some are stand-alone workstations, and others are integrated into PACS. While they share many features in common, there is substantial variability in capabilities and user-friendliness. Basic features include the ability to perform MPR and 3D endoluminal reconstructions as well as length and volume measurements (Fig. 5.28). Additional features may include wide-angle or panoramic views, "virtual dissection" or "filet" views, translucency rendering, stool labeling or color coding, electronic stool subtraction, "missed region" identification, and computer-aided detection (CAD) among others. All of these features are designed to improve diagnostic performance, as well as increase reader confidence and efficiency. Because one "optimal" means of CTC interpretation does not fit all readers, there is considerable debate about the best approach to use.

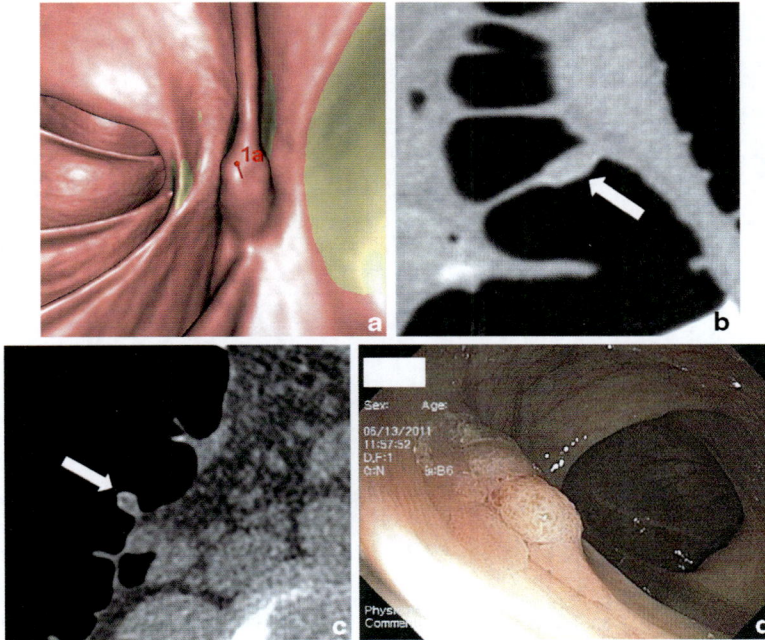

Fig. 5.21 Polyps can be mistaken for bulbous haustral folds. (**a**) 3D endoluminal view of the ascending colon demonstrates a polypoid contour abnormality of the base of a haustral fold (labeled 1a). (**b**) Corresponding supine 2D axial image demonstrates asymmetric fold thickening along the medial wall (*arrow*). (**c**) Prone axial view of the area in question demonstrates a thickened fold along the medial wall. (**d**) Photograph from optical colonoscopy shows a lobulated, sessile polyp that was subsequently removed. The lesion was a tubular adenoma

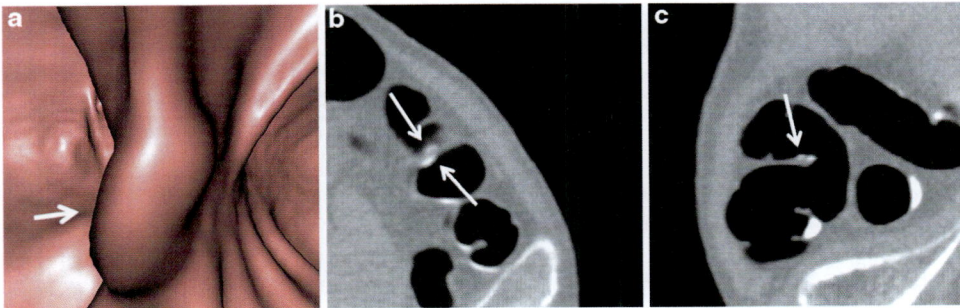

Fig. 5.22 Pseudo-fold thickening can be mistaken for a pedunculated polyp. (**a**) 3D endoluminal view of the left colon demonstrates a possible pedunculated polyp (*arrow*). (**b**) 2D axial image of the area in question demonstrates that the bulbous component of the lesion actually consists of labeled stool on both sides of a non-thickened fold (between *arrows*). (**c**) Corresponding 2D sagittal MPR confirms that the fold is not thickened and that the bulbous component is composed of tagged stool

2D Versus 3D Interpretation

Without a doubt, comprehensive assessment of CTC data requires interrogation of both 2D and 3D views. That said, upon opening a case at the workstation, one can choose to begin the primary search for polyps with either 2D or 3D projections. The 2D data set is the standard grayscale display, optimized for polyp detection by employing high contrast window settings (width = 1,400,

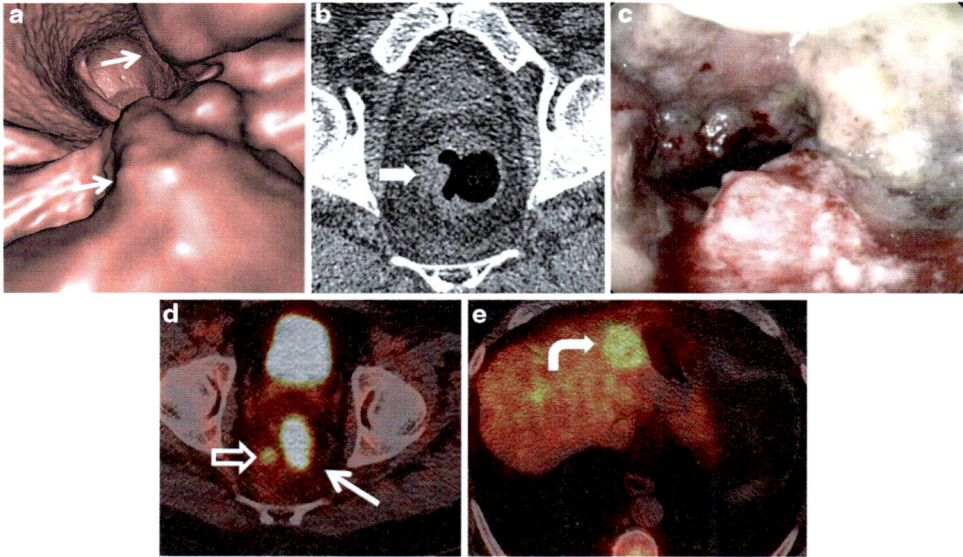

Fig. 5.23 The differential diagnosis of mucosal lesions includes adenocarcinoma. (**a**) 3D endoluminal view of the rectum demonstrates a large, irregular, nearly circumferential mass lesion (*arrows*) in the low rectum. (**b**) Corresponding prone 2D axial image of the lower rectum demonstrates the mucosal mass lesion (*arrow*) extending from approximately the 4:00 to the 2:00 position. (**c**) Photograph from optical colonoscopy demonstrates a friable, ulcerated, annular mass in the low rectum. Pathology was consistent with adenocarcinoma. (**d**) Single axial image from staging PET/CT demonstrates the hypermetabolic primary mass (*arrow*), as well as a hypermetabolic perirectal lymph node (*open arrow*). (**e**) The same PET/CT at the level of the liver demonstrates a hypermetabolic liver metastasis (*curved arrow*)

level = −350) [12]. Multiplanar reformats such as coronal and sagittal views fall under the umbrella of 2D. The 3D data set refers to other data reconstructions, most commonly virtual endoluminal views. A "primary 2D reader" first reviews the data in the axial plane with interrogation and problem solving of suspected lesions using 3D reformations [129]. A "primary 3D reader" does the opposite, examining the colon with the 3D endoluminal view and using the 2D data to investigate suspected findings.

It has been known for some time that endoluminal viewing improves the sensitivity for polyp detection at CTC above that achievable with 2D alone [45, 130]. Before 2003, most CTC readers used a primary 2D technique, reflecting the majority opinion that this was the optimal method of data interpretation [131, 132]. This technique was also more comfortable and familiar than the endoluminal fly-throughs. As technology has improved and CTC software systems have become capable of time-efficient 3D review, attitudes have begun to change [133]. As evidence of its superiority accumulates, there has been a more recent migration toward primary 3D interpretation [134, 135].

To date, there have been five major CTC trials evaluating cohorts of patients with a low prevalence of disease. The Department of Defense (DOD) CTC screening trial [45] used a primary 3D approach and demonstrated that the sensitivity of CTC for clinically relevant polyps was comparable to that of OC. In contrast, three other trials restricted readers to a primary 2D approach, and results were inferior [136–138]. The most recent of the trials, the ACRIN trial, randomized readers to interpret in primary 2D or 3D. It demonstrated the there was no difference in performance between the two techniques [10]. Confounding the results, however, the majority of ACRIN sites used a cumbersome software platform, which at the time, could not really support

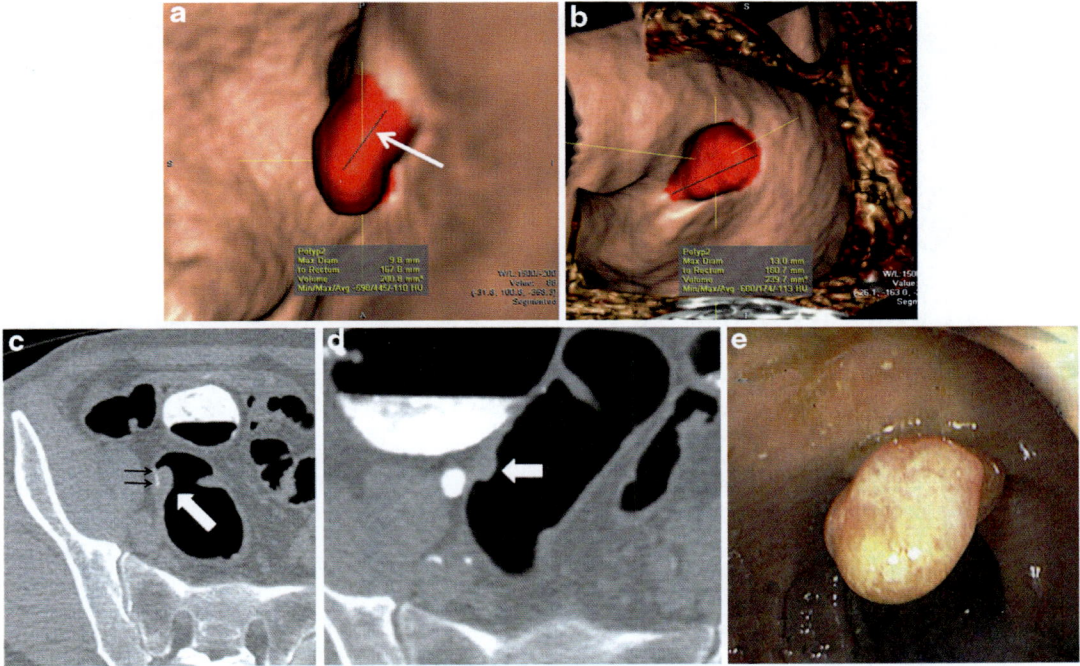

Fig. 5.28 Length and volume measurements are a basic feature of any CTC software package. (**a**) Prone 3D endoluminal view of the sigmoid colon demonstrates a pedunculated polyp. This software has an automated measurement feature. The user clicks on the suspected abnormality. The software then labels it *red*, creating a bookmark. Maximum diameter, distance to rectum, and volume measurements are displayed. Note that in this instance, the length of the automatic measurement caliper (*arrow*) has likely under-measured the polyp diameter (shown in *red*). (**b**) Supine 3D endoluminal "cube view" shows the same polyp. Its pedunculated morphology is less apparent than on the prone view. The cutaway of the cube view allows the area of interest to be rotated and viewed from different angles, removing the voxels, which interfere with the desired viewing angle. Note that in this view, the automated measurement calipers are placed more accurately. (**c**) Corresponding prone 2D axial image demonstrates a soft tissue polyp (*large white arrow*) in the sigmoid colon. Note that tagged liquid (*small black arrows*) undercuts the lesion, demonstrating its pedunculated morphology. (**d**) Corresponding supine 2D axial image demonstrates the polyp (*large white arrow*) in the sigmoid colon. Just as with the 3D endoluminal view, its pedunculated morphology is not well appreciated. (**e**) Photograph from optical colonoscopy shows a pedunculated polyp in the sigmoid colon. Pathology revealed a tubular adenoma

Referring gastroenterologists tend to appreciate 3D endoluminal views because they simulate colonoscopy.

Advantages of primary 2D interpretation include the ability to readily determine the density of filling defects. 2D evaluation is particularly helpful in cases with poor bowel preparation and adherent stool or in segments with luminal collapse [133]. The bowel wall integrity and fold contour are also more readily assessed with 2D evaluation [129, 140, 141]. An often-cited advantage of primary 2D over 3D is faster interpretation time [10, 45]. For example, the mean interpretation times in the DOD study were 6.7 min for 2D versus 19.6 min for 3D [45]. In the ACRIN trial, they were 19.4 min versus 25.3 min, respectively [10]. Longer interpretation times for 3D are due to the necessity of performing a total of four fly-throughs, two in each direction in both the supine and prone positions [142]. This is done in order to avoid "blind areas," parts of the mucosa hidden behind colonic folds or simply out of the field of view of the virtual colonoscope. It should be noted that even bidirectional review does not eliminate all blind spots, and some 3D workstations can display sequential

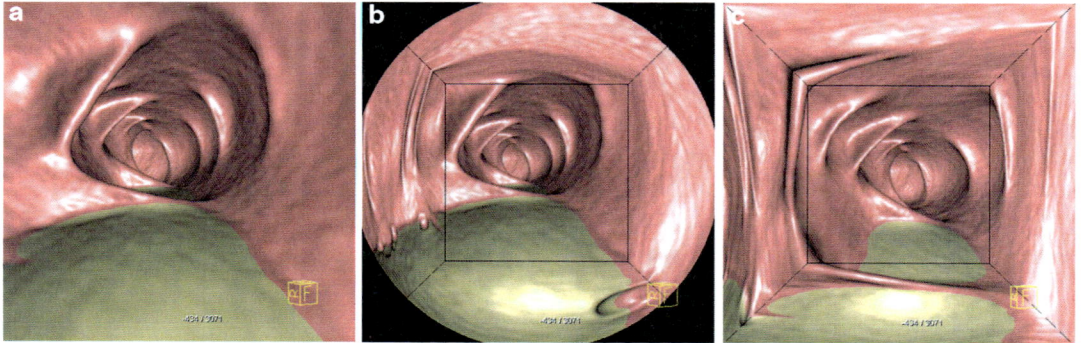

Fig. 5.29 Panoramic 3D displays widen the field of view, increasing mucosal visualization. (**a**) Standard 3D endoluminal view of the sigmoid colon demonstrates color-coded liquid layering dependently (*golden color*). (**b**) Panoramic wide-angle view of the same region demonstrates how the frontal view is mapped into a square, and the other 4 faces are mapped around it into a disk. This widens the field of view. A luminal protrusion is seen in the lower right-hand corner (*arrow*). (**c**) This panoramic view shows an even wider field of view. The filling defect is seen in the lower left-hand corner (*arrow*). Notice the distortion that thins and elongates the abnormality

blind spots until 100% of the mucosa has been displayed [143].

As both hardware and software have improved, the speed of 3D rendering has improved substantially [133]. As such, the advantage that a primary 2D viewer has in terms of speed is likely being eroded. Speed also improves with experience. At one high-volume center, interpretation times with a primary 3D approach are under 10 min for an average case [30]. Newer techniques such as panoramic views and virtual dissection were designed to reduce the need to do both antegrade and retrograde navigation, thus shortening interpretation times.

Panoramic View

Panoramic 3D display was designed to improve the visualized surface area in CTC by increasing the field of view from 90 to 120°. It is constructed by mapping the frontal view into a square, while the other four faces are mapped around it into a disk [143]. This not only widens the field of view but also essentially "stretches open" or unfolds the colon, revealing the spaces between and behind folds (Fig. 5.29). Thus, only unidirectional navigation is needed to evaluate the entire mucosa, increasing speed because theoretically

there are no unseen areas. [132, 143, 144] One criticism of this technique is mucosal distortion and its potential effect on polyp conspicuity [135]. However, this does not appear to influence performance, as shown in several studies. A 2011 retrospective study of 150 OC-validated CTC data sets was performed comparing a standard, bidirectional primary 3D approach with a unidirectional 3D panoramic view. Overall sensitivity was not significantly different, but mean interpretation times decreased from 14.6 to 7.5 min using the panoramic view [145]. These results are consistent with several other studies demonstrating improved efficiency without degraded performance. [132, 143, 144]

Virtual Dissection

The "virtual dissection" or "filet" view grew out of laboratory work demonstrating the efficacy of the panoramic view in virtual endoscopy [146]. The software was designed to allow overview of the entire colonic mucosa at once. To do this, the software "slices" along the long axis of the colonic 3D model, "fileting" it open and displaying what was once a cylindrical object as a flattened rectangular image (Fig. 5.30) [147–149]. The appearance is similar to that of a pathologic

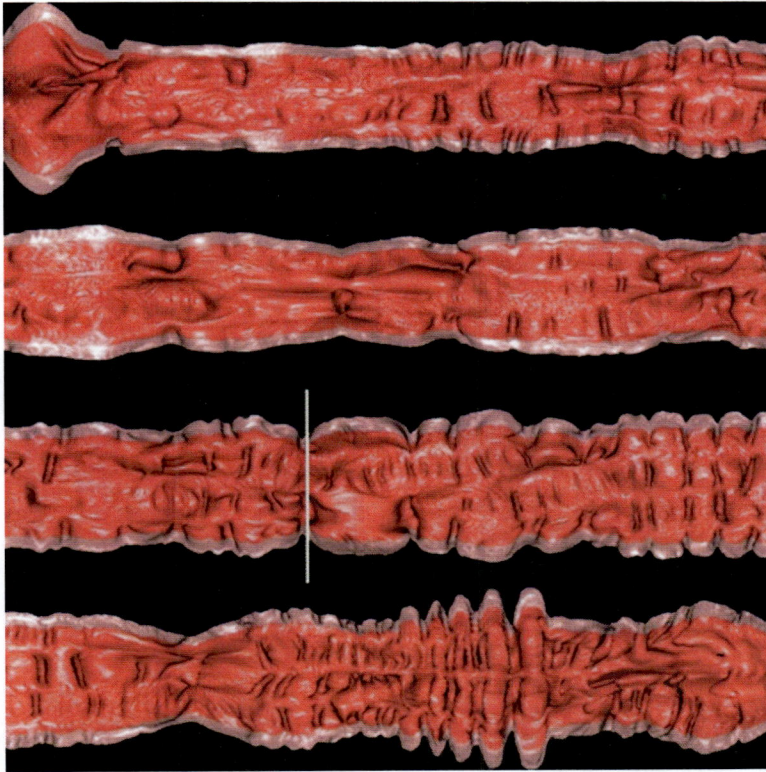

Fig. 5.30 The virtual dissection technique enables simultaneous visualization of the entire colonic mucosal surface. 3D filet view of the colon demonstrates how it is virtually straightened along the centerline and "sliced" open as if it were a pathologic specimen

specimen, thus the name "virtual dissection." The advantages of the virtual dissection view include shorter interpretation times, reduced blind spots, and elimination of the need to perform both anterograde and retrograde fly-throughs [135, 140]. The virtual dissection view has been criticized for the anatomic distortion that occurs, especially at flexures. Polyp shape and size can be misrepresented so that even some large polyps may be unrecognizable due to distortion [144]. Conversely, normal folds can take on the appearance of polyps. That said, this distortion is fairly predictable [147]. Another criticism of virtual dissection is that it must be correlated with the standard 2D and 3D views [146, 150]. However, the need for 2D problem solving is not unique to the virtual dissection view but applies to all 3D techniques [151]. An additional problem is that collapsed segments or annular masses can cause skip areas where the lesion is not displayed at all [148]. The learning curve for virtual dissection has been voiced as a concern, which could further diminish performance for this method [144].

Performance characteristics of virtual dissection are lower than those achievable with the standard 3D interpretation [140, 152, 153]. They are comparable to 2D in detection rates for both experienced [135, 140, 152] and inexperienced [154] readers. In a 2007 study, Johnson showed that interpretation times for virtual dissection were 28% faster than with the conventional 2D method (10.4 min vs. 14.5 min, respectively) [140]. Additionally, he demonstrated that double review using both conventional and virtual dissection could compensate for poorer-performing reviewers, decreasing interobserver variability,

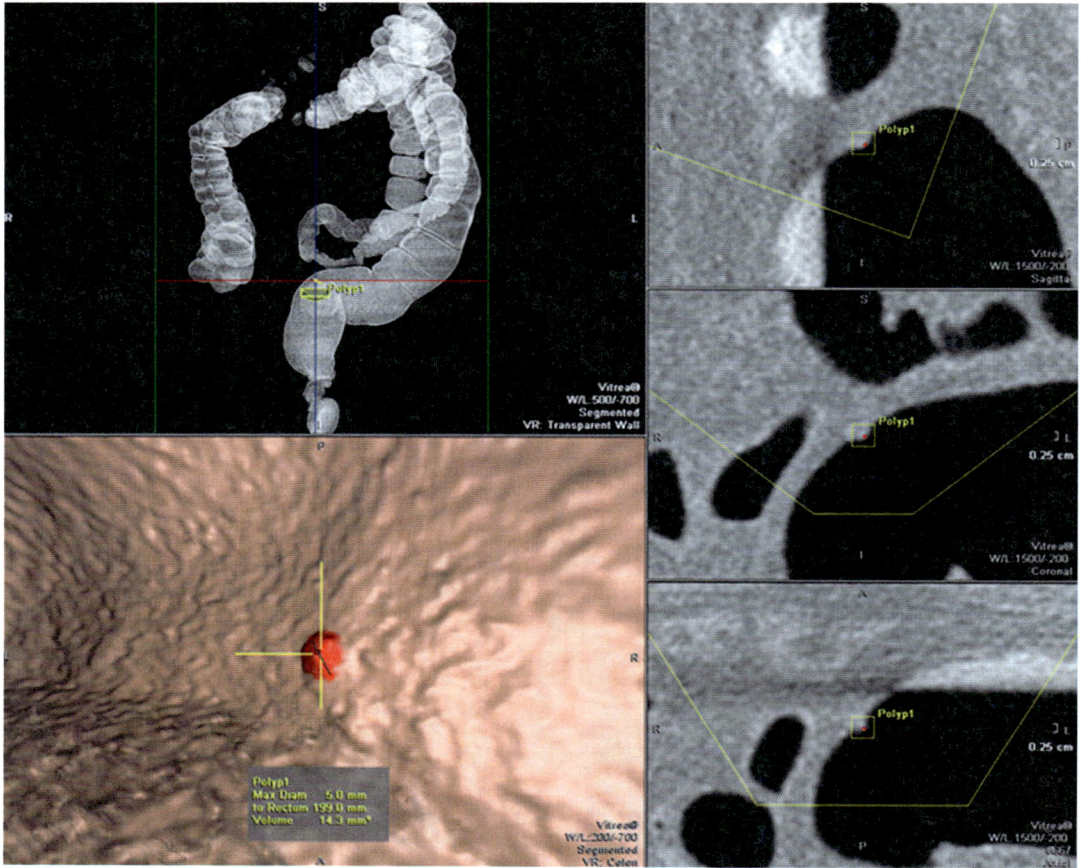

Fig. 5.31 Computer-aided detection (CAD) software can help detect and mark lesions suspicious for polyps. Screenshot from a 3D CTC workstation demonstrates a luminal protrusion detected by computer-aided detection (CAD). In the *lower left-hand corner*, the lesion is shown coded *red*, with diameter, volume, and distance from the rectum displayed. The *top left* shows a virtual barium enema view with a marker at the location of the polyp. The 3 panels on the *right* are standard 2D MPR's with the polyp marked with a *red dot*

and improving sensitivity, surpassing even the sensitivity of OC for adenomatous lesions ≥ 1 cm [140]. At this time, the filet view is not commonly used as a primary means of interpretation, but rather as a useful adjunct.

Computer-Aided Detection

Computer-aided detection refers to analysis of the 3D CTC data set by a computer software algorithm to detect and flag lesions that are likely to be polyps (Fig. 5.31). This has been proposed as a way to help readers achieve better performance.

In the majority of studies, investigators have found that CAD does improve readers' performance, particularly those with less experience [155–159]. One consistent criticism of CAD is that it typically generates a number of findings, most of which are false-positives that nevertheless have to be interrogated. This has the potential to decrease specificity, although the majority can be quickly dismissed. According to one recent study, the three most common causes of false-positive findings were the ileocecal valve (Fig. 5.32), haustral folds, and poorly tagged stool [160]. CAD can be used either concurrently with the human interpreter or used as a second reader.

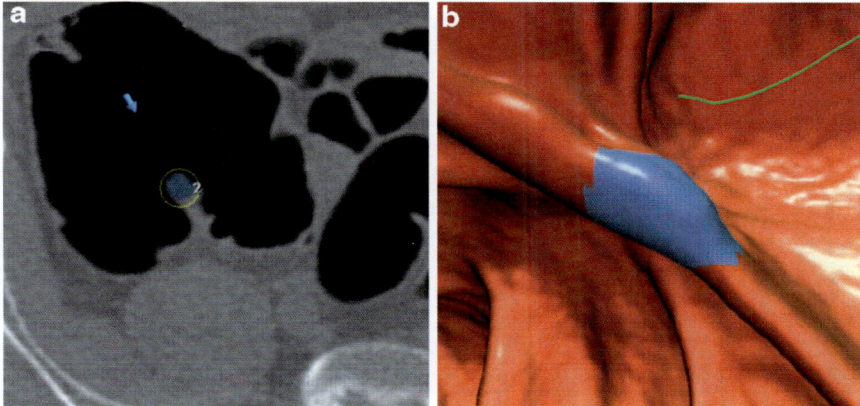

Fig. 5.32 The ileocecal valve is a common cause of false-positive findings at CTC with CAD. (**a**) Prone 2D axial image of the right colon demonstrate that CAD has marked a possible lesion (*blue color* with a *yellow circle* around it). (**b**) Corresponding 3D endoluminal view of the cecum demonstrates that the lesion marked *blue* by CAD is actually the normal ileocecal valve

A recent study by Halligan showed that second-read CAD significantly improved per-patient polyp detection without a clinically unacceptable decrease in specificity, whereas use of concurrent CAD was less effective [161].

It is remarkable that stand-alone CAD is often more sensitive than a reader assisted by CAD. This may be due to the radiologist sometimes incorrectly dismissing lesions that are correctly detected by CAD [155, 157, 162]. A study by Taylor in 2009 identified factors that lead radiologists to incorrectly dismiss lesions [163]. Interestingly, the larger the polyp and the more irregular its contour, the more likely it was to be thought to be a false-positive [163]. Thus, although CAD may generate a large number of targets and most of these may be quickly and easily dismissed, it is important to realize a potential bias against large or irregular lesions.

Measurements, Reporting, and Triage

Background

The size of an adenomatous polyp directly correlates with its cancerous potential. For this reason, accurate measurement is essential for proper patient management [164]. A difference of a millimeter can change patient disposition. As an example, a polyp ≤5 mm need not be reported under the 2009 ACR guidelines and thus a patient with such a lesion will not be offered surveillance. A consensus of three national medical societies, including the ACR, recommends immediate colonoscopy with polypectomy for both small (6–9 mm) and large (≥10 mm) polyps [165]. The C-RADS reporting system (discussed below) discriminates between small and large polyps. A CTC that depicts only one or two polyps 6–9 mm in size is reported as "C2," whereas one that demonstrates a polyp 10 mm or more in size is categorized as "C3." The recommended management in this system is surveillance or colonoscopy for C2 and colonoscopy for C3. Thus, the accuracy of polyp measurement in the 5–10 mm range is especially important [166].

Polyp Measurements

Both CTC and OC have inherent limitations in measurement capability and accuracy [167, 168]. The most accurate method of polyp measurement is debatable, as the data are mixed. Some studies demonstrate underestimation [168–172] of polyp size on CTC and others demonstrate overestimation [170, 173]. In general, polyp size measured at CTC tends to lay between measurements at OC and pathologic evaluation and may be the most accurate method compared to the in vivo size [174]. This is substantiated by a 2007 direct comparison of CTC and OC in the measurement of 86 simulated polyps in pig colonic specimens where CTC was shown to be superior in both accuracy and reliability [168].

There are several possible ways of measuring a polyp found on CTC, including the 2D axial images, 2D MPR's, "optimized" MPR's, or 3D endoluminal images, each of which has been demonstrated to give differing measurements, as does the window-level setting used to view the images [169, 175]. Additional factors affecting size include spatial resolution, partial volume averaging, motion artifacts, noise, rendering thresholds, the effects of fecal tagging agents, and unsurprisingly, observer variability [174]. This issue has been studied, and it is of practical interest to understand which methods are most effective.

A 2006 retrospective study by Yeshwant et al. [176] demonstrated that measurements from 3D images best approximate polyp size at OC. Bethea validated this in a 2009 study [166]. In his 2007 simulated polyp study, Park demonstrated that 2D measurements in an "optimized" MPR plane, an oblique plane in which the polyp has the largest diameter, were found to be the most accurate [168]. 3D measurements were the second most accurate, followed by 2D orthogonal MPR's. He concluded that the speed and ease of 3D measurements make up for any degree of the inaccuracy and are preferred over the optimized MPR method in practice [36]. It should be noted that 3D measurements in this case do not apply to nontraditional 3D techniques such as "virtual dissection," that are prone to distortion.

Many software platforms have an automated measuring tool that measures the polyp diameter and volume simply by clicking on it with the mouse (Fig. 5.33). Automated measurements tend to either overshade or under-shade the area being used for length and volume computation and no tool may be available to manually correct the errors. It has been noted that this problem is particularly exacerbated for polyps with irregular, nonspherical morphologic features. This tool should be used with caution, paying attention to the accuracy of what the software determines to be the borders of the lesion (Fig. 5.28) [166].

Polyp Location

Accurate localization of a polyp on CTC is of paramount importance so that the endoscopist can easily and efficiently find and remove the lesion at OC. Absolute distance values from the anus cannot be used to locate polyps found on CTC at OC. This is because CTC software calculates the colonic length at almost double that at OC [177]. These differences in colon length are due mostly to procedural factors that occur during OC, such as telescoping and foreshortening. Simply communicating polyp location by the colonic segment of interest is also not useful because the endoscopist is not often able to accurately determine his location during OC.

More accurate localization can be provided by computing the normalized distance along the colon centerline of a polyp found at CTC. By using this technique, the location of a polyp at OC can be predicted to within 10 cm for the majority of lesions [177]. The normalized distance at CTC is computed by dividing the distance of the polyp from the anorectal junction along the colonic centerline by the length of the entire colon. The predicted polyp location at OC is then computed by multiplying this normalized distance by the length of the entire colon at OC. For example, a polyp is identified on CTC at 50 cm from the rectum. The length of the colon is measured at 200 cm. Normalized distance is calculated as $50/200 = 0.25$. The clinician then performs OC and measures the distance from the anorectal junction to the cecum as 150 cm. Therefore, he will search for the polyp at 38 cm (0.25×150). Duncan, based on a study of 383 patients with 437 polyps, proposed standardized conversion factors for determining anus-to-polyp distance at OC from CTC measurements [178]. Conversion factors of 0.59 for right-sided or 0.78 for left-sided CTC anus-to-polyp measurements may substitute for calculating the normalized distance. He also mentioned that details about the lesions' relationship to an anatomical

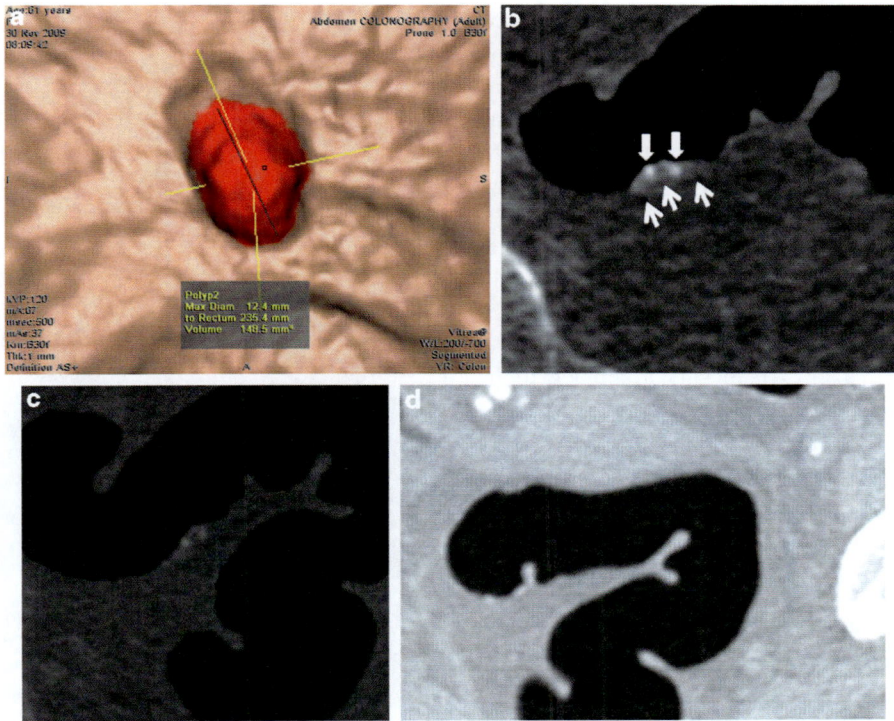

Fig. 5.33 CTC workstations have automated polyp measuring tools as a standard feature. The tools cannot help discriminate polyps from pseudo-lesions. (**a**) Prone 3D endoluminal view shows a 1.2-cm lesion in the sigmoid colon suspicious for a polyp. The lesion was slightly under-measured by the automated measurement calipers. (**b**) Corresponding prone 2D axial image shows a heterogeneous lesion arising from the posterior wall. The lesion has an irregular surface (*small arrows*) superficially coated with high-density tagging material (*larger arrows*). (**c**) Supine 2D axial image shows the lesion is nonmobile. Barium can selectively adhere to villous lesions, raising our suspicions. Because the patient was anticoagulated for severe pulmonary hypertension, rather than performing colonoscopy, the patient was followed up 1 month later. (**d**) Repeat supine 2D axial image demonstrates that the area in question is free of disease. The lesion seen on the original examination was therefore a pseudo-lesion from thickly adherent stool

reference point such as the ileocecal valve, appendiceal orifice, or a particular fold can be helpful to the endoscopist [178]. We routinely provide distance to the polyp from the anorectal junction, the colonic segment, as well as any nearby landmarks.

Systematic Reporting

A system for structured reporting of CTC studies has been proposed by a panel of experts, with the aim of replicating the benefits of the BI-RADS system used in mammography. The C-RADS system [121] captures information about preparation quality, polyp presence and size, and extracolonic findings, and places the overall study into one of five categories including recommendations for follow-up. Such a system will be very useful for large-scale research, both for epidemiological and cost-effectiveness purposes.

Same-Day Service

Same-Day OC

In a model setting, patients with positive CTC examinations would proceed directly to same day OC, thereby avoiding treatment delay and a second bowel cleansing. Arranging this workflow requires close coordination with the endoscopy department at each particular institution. Patients who undergo CTC with the option of same-day OC must adhere to guidelines intended for OC patients, who are prepared for potential polypectomy. This includes stopping anticoagulants, aspirin and NSAIDs, requiring coordination with the referring physician.

The issue of patient preparation must also be addressed by consensus. The cathartics and fecal tagging agents for CTC must be acceptable to the endoscopist for OC. Unlike residual solid material, residual fluid is not a problem at OC because it can easily be suctioned during the exam [48]. Noncathartic or limited cathartic bowel preparations are obviously not appropriate for same-day OC. If less aggressive catharsis is employed, additional bowel preparation before OC has been advocated [38].

Patients should undergo CTC in the early morning while their colon remains well prepared. For proper triage, CTC studies should be interpreted in as close to real time as possible, while the patient stays NPO and awaits results and instructions. We communicate both positive and negative findings directly to the patient. Positive cases are discussed immediately with the endoscopist, who decides together with the radiologist whether same day OC is indicated. Information such as polyp size, location, and distance from the rectum is essential. The images of the CTC should be available to the endoscopist in a format that is intuitive and informative. 3D endoluminal views as well as the "virtual barium enema" are excellent views to include (Fig. 5.34).

Some flexibility in the OC schedule is needed so that add-on patients can be accommodated when necessary. The amount of flexibility is determined by the CTC program workflow as well as the referral rate. The referral rate depends on the agreed-upon size threshold for referral. For reference, a positive CTC can be expected in approximately 13% of normal risk adults using a size threshold of 6 mm [10]. If the size threshold were 1 cm, the referral rate would of course be lower.

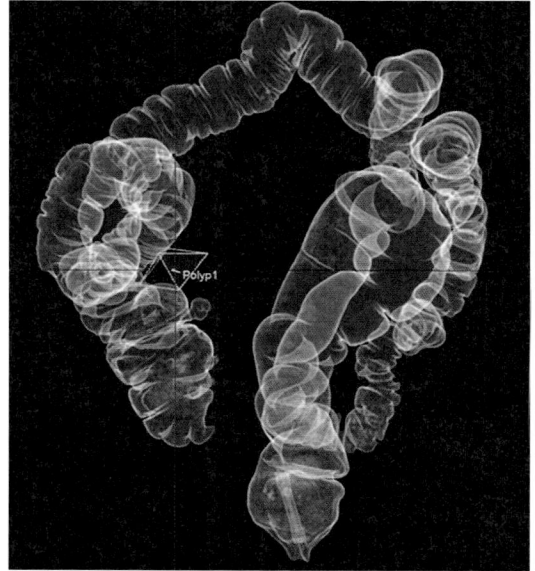

Fig. 5.34 Virtual barium enema views are easy to interpret for non-radiologists. "Virtual barium enema" 3D reconstruction of the colon demonstrates that the location of polyps can be labeled as an aid to the gastroenterologist who will be performing the subsequent colonoscopy. "Polyp 1" is seen in the ascending colon

Same-Day CTC Service

Some have postulated that if patients are offered the option of "same-day CTC," general rates of screening compliance and patient satisfaction will likely be higher [48]. Just as our endoscopy colleagues have committed to perform OC on our CTC patients with polyps, so have we agreed to perform same day CTC. We make every effort to accommodate patients who have undergone incomplete OC earlier in the day. Rates of incomplete OC range in the literature from 2 to 40%, although 5% is a commonly cited number [179]. Reasons for incomplete OC include tortuosity, redundancy, stricture, and obstructing lesions, among others. CTC is of particular use in those with obstructing neoplasms, as it can identify synchronous proximal polyps and cancers preoperatively [180, 181]. Incomplete OC is our most common indication for referral, although many are still not in the habit of referring for same-day CTC service.

In practice, the endoscopist calls us immediately after the incomplete OC. We instruct the patient, after recovery from sedation, to take 60 cc of Gastrografin 2 h before CTC. This technique has been shown to result in satisfactory opacification of the colon, especially proximal segments not seen during OC, in most patients [182]. If the OC is late in the day, the patient is administered the Gastrografin, kept on clear liquids overnight, and scanned first thing in the morning. Patients who have undergone deep biopsy or polypectomy are not candidates for same-day CTC because of the risk of perforation. Regardless of whether polypectomy was performed, we perform a thick slice low-dose scan before insufflation to check for the presence of an asymptomatic perforation.

Summary

CTC has several inherent technical components— preparation, insufflation, CT data acquisition, interpretation, and reporting—all of which must be optimized to enable a high-quality screening or diagnostic clinical practice. This field is a very good example of successful collaborative research between radiologists, basic scientists, and endoscopists. These efforts have been repeatedly validated and matured an important clinical imaging examination that, with widespread application, could significantly reduce the morbidity and mortality of a common disease.

References

1. Coin CG, Wollett FC, Coin JT, Rowland M, DeRamos RK, Dandrea R. Computerized radiology of the colon: a potential screening technique. Comput Radiol. 1983;7(4):215–21.
2. Vining DJ, Shifrin RY, Grishaw EK, Liu K, Gelfand DW. Virtual colonoscopy. Radiology. 1994;193(P): 446.
3. Fletcher JG, Johnson CD, Welch TJ, et al. Optimization of CT colonography technique: prospective trial in 180 patients. Radiology. 2000;216(3): 704–11.
4. Virtual colonoscopy workshop. San Francisco, CA; 2009.
5. Hara AK, Kuo MD, Blevins M, et al. National CT colonography trial (ACRIN 6664): comparison of three full-laxative bowel preparations in more than 2500 average-risk patients. AJR Am J Roentgenol. 2011;196(5):1076–82.
6. McRorie J, Kesler J, Bishop L, et al. Effects of wheat bran and olestra on objective measures of stool and subjective reports of GI symptoms. Am J Gastroenterol. 2000;95(5):1244–52.
7. Chen HL, Haack VS, Janecky CW, Vollendorf NW, Marlett JA. Mechanisms by which wheat bran and oat bran increase stool weight in humans. Am J Clin Nutr. 1998;68(3):711–9.
8. Liedenbaum MH, Denters MJ, de Vries AH, et al. Low-fiber diet in limited bowel preparation for CT colonography: influence on image quality and patient acceptance. AJR Am J Roentgenol. 2010;195(1): W31–7.
9. Delegge M, Kaplan R. Efficacy of bowel preparation with the use of a prepackaged, low fibre diet with a low sodium, magnesium citrate cathartic vs. a clear liquid diet with a standard sodium phosphate cathartic. Aliment Pharmacol Ther. 2005;21(12):1491–5.
10. Johnson CD, Chen M-H, Toledano AY, et al. Accuracy of CT colonography for detection of large adenomas and cancers. N Engl J Med. 2008;359(12):1207–17.
11. FDA. Oral sodium phosphate (OSP) products for bowel cleansing (marketed as Visicol and OsmoPrep, and oral sodium phosphate products available without a prescription); 2008.
12. Yee J. CT colonography: techniques and applications. Radiol Clin North Am. 2009;47(1):133–45.
13. Kim DH, Pickhardt PJ, Hinshaw JL, Taylor AJ, Mukherjee R, Pfau PR. Prospective blinded trial comparing 45-mL and 90-mL doses of oral sodium phosphate for bowel preparation before computed tomographic colonography. J Comput Assist Tomogr. 2007;31(1):53–8.
14. Aihara H, Saito S, Arakawa H, et al. Comparison of two sodium phosphate tablet-based regimens and a polyethylene glycol regimen for colon cleansing prior to colonoscopy: a randomized prospective pilot study. Int J Colorectal Dis. 2009;24(9):1023–30.
15. Berkelhammer C, Ekambaram A, Silva RG. Low-volume oral colonoscopy bowel preparation: sodium phosphate and magnesium citrate. Gastrointest Endosc. 2002;56(1):89–94.
16. Hsu C-W, Imperiale TF. Meta-analysis and cost comparison of polyethylene glycol lavage versus sodium phosphate for colonoscopy preparation. Gastrointest Endosc. 1998;48(3):276–82.
17. Macari M, Lavelle M, Pedrosa I, et al. Effect of different bowel preparations on residual fluid at CT colonography. Radiology. 2001;218(1):274–7.
18. Tan JJ, Tjandra JJ. Which is the optimal bowel preparation for colonoscopy - a meta-analysis. Colorectal Dis. 2006;8(4):247–58.
19. Vanner SJ, MacDonald PH, Paterson WG, Prentice RS, Da Costa LR, Beck IT. A randomized prospective trial comparing oral sodium phosphate with standard polyethylene glycol-based lavage solution (Golytely)

in the preparation of patients for colonoscopy. Am J Gastroenterol. 1990;85(4):422–7.

20. Kim SH, Choi BI, Han JK, et al. CT colonography in a Korean population with a high residue diet: comparison between wet and dry preparations. Clin Radiol. 2006;61(6):483–94.

21. Belsey J, Epstein O, Heresbach D. Systematic review: oral bowel preparation for colonoscopy. Aliment Pharmacol Ther. 2007;25(4):373–84.

22. Belsey J, Epstein O, Heresbach D. Systematic review: adverse event reports for oral sodium phosphate and polyethylene glycol. Aliment Pharmacol Ther. 2009;29(1):15–28.

23. Ehrenpreis ED, Nogueras JJ, Botoman VA, Bonner GF, Zaitman D, Secrest KM. Serum electrolyte abnormalities secondary to Fleet's Phospho-Soda colonoscopy prep. A review of three cases. Surg Endosc. 1996;10(10):1022–4.

24. Vukasin P, Weston LA, Beart RW. Oral Fleet phospho-soda laxative-induced hyperphosphatemia and hypocalcemic tetany in an adult: report of a case. Dis Colon Rectum. 1997;40(4):497–9.

25. Khurana A, McLean L, Atkinson S, Foulks CJ. The effect of oral sodium phosphate drug products on renal function in adults undergoing bowel endoscopy. Arch Intern Med. 2008;168(6):593–7.

26. Markowitz GS, Stokes MB, Radhakrishnan J, D'Agati VD. Acute phosphate nephropathy following oral sodium phosphate bowel purgative: an underrecognized cause of chronic renal failure. J Am Soc Nephrol. 2005;16(11):3389–96.

27. Mathus-Vliegen EM, Kemble UM. A prospective randomized blinded comparison of sodium phosphate and polyethylene glycol-electrolyte solution for safe bowel cleansing. Aliment Pharmacol Ther. 2006;23(4):543–52.

28. Wiberg JJ, Turner GG, Nuttall FQ. Effect of phosphate or magnesium cathartics on serum calcium: observations in normocalcemic patients. Arch Intern Med. 1978;138(7):1114–6.

29. Borden ZS, Pickhardt PJ, Kim DH, Lubner MG, Agriantonis DJ, Hinshaw JL. Bowel preparation for CT colonography: blinded comparison of magnesium citrate and sodium phosphate for catharsis. Radiology. 2010;254(1):138–44.

30. Pickhardt PJ. Screening CT, colonography: how I do it. AJR Am J Roentgenol. 2007;189(2):290–8.

31. Ell C, Fischbach W, Keller R, et al. A randomized, blinded, prospective trial to compare the safety and efficacy of three bowel-cleansing solutions for colonoscopy (HSG-01*). Endoscopy. 2003;35(4): 300–4.

32. Gluecker TM, Johnson CD, Harmsen WS, et al. Colorectal cancer screening with CT colonography, colonoscopy, and double-contrast barium enema examination: prospective assessment of patient perceptions and preferences. Radiology. 2003;227(2): 378–84.

33. Nagata K, Okawa T, Honma A, Endo S, Kudo S-E, Yoshida H. Full-laxative versus minimum-laxative

fecal-tagging CT colonography using 64-detector row CT: prospective blinded comparison of diagnostic performance, tagging quality, and patient acceptance. Acad Radiol. 2009;16(7):780–9.

34. Flor N, Rigamonti P, Di Leo G, et al. Technical quality of CT colonography in relation with diverticular disease. Eur J Radiol. 2012;81(3):e250–4.

35. Taylor S, Laghi A, Lefere P, Halligan S, Stoker J. European society of gastrointestinal and abdominal radiology (ESGAR): consensus statement on CT colonography. Eur Radiol. 2007;17(2):575–9.

36. Park SH, Yee J, Kim SH, Kim YH. Fundamental elements for successful performance of CT colonography (virtual colonoscopy). Korean J Radiol. 2007;8(4):264–75.

37. Lefere P, Gryspeerdt S, Marrannes J, Baekelandt M, Van Holsbeeck B. CT colonography after fecal tagging with a reduced cathartic cleansing and a reduced volume of barium. AJR Am J Roentgenol. 2005;184(6):1836–42.

38. Lefere PA, Gryspeerdt SS, Dewyspelaere J, Baekelandt M, Van Holsbeeck BG. Dietary fecal tagging as a cleansing method before CT colonography: initial results polyp detection and patient acceptance. Radiology. 2002;224(2):393–403.

39. Slater A, Taylor SA, Burling D, Gartner L, Scarth J, Halligan S. Colonic polyps: effect of attenuation of tagged fluid and viewing window on conspicuity and measurement – in vitro experiment with porcine colonic specimen. Radiology. 2006;240(1):101–9.

40. Bielen D, Thomeer M, Vanbeckevoort D, et al. Dry preparation for virtual CT colonography with fecal tagging using water-soluble contrast medium: initial results. Eur Radiol. 2003;13(3):453–8.

41. Iannaccone R, Laghi A, Catalano C, et al. Computed tomographic colonography without cathartic preparation for the detection of colorectal polyps. Gastroenterology. 2004;127(5):1300–11.

42. Jensch S, de Vries AH, Pot D, et al. Image quality and patient acceptance of four regimens with different amounts of mild laxatives for CT colonography. AJR Am J Roentgenol. 2008;191(1):158–67.

43. Lefere P, Gryspeerdt S, Baekelandt M, Van Holsbeeck B. Laxative-free CT colonography. AJR Am J Roentgenol. 2004;183(4):945–8.

44. Nagata K, Endo S, Ichikawa T, et al. Polyethylene glycol solution (PEG) plus contrast medium vs PEG alone preparation for CT colonography and conventional colonoscopy in preoperative colorectal cancer staging. Int J Colorectal Dis. 2007;22(1):69–76.

45. Pickhardt PJ, Choi JR, Hwang I, et al. Computed tomographic virtual colonoscopy to screen for colorectal neoplasia in asymptomatic adults. N Engl J Med. 2003;349(23):2191–200.

46. Gryspeerdt S, Lefere P, Herman M, et al. CT colonography with fecal tagging after incomplete colonoscopy. Eur Radiol. 2005;15(6):1192–202.

47. Taylor SA, Slater A, Burling DN, et al. CT colonography: optimisation, diagnostic performance and patient acceptability of reduced-laxative regimens

using barium-based faecal tagging. Eur Radiol. 2008;18(1):32–42.

48. Behrens C, Eddy R, Stevenson G, Audet L, Mathieson J. Bowel preparation regimen for computed tomography colonography. Can Assoc Radiol J. 2010;61(5):280–5.

49. Zalis ME, Hahn PF. Digital subtraction bowel cleansing in CT colonography. AJR Am J Roentgenol. 2001;176(3):646–8.

50. Horton KM, Fishman EK, Gayler B. The use of iohexol as oral contrast for computed tomography of the abdomen and pelvis. J Comput Assist Tomogr. 2008;32(2):207–9.

51. O'Connor SD, Summers RM. Revisiting oral barium sulfate contrast agents. Acad Radiol. 2007;14(1):72–80.

52. Johnson CD, Manduca A, Fletcher JG, et al. Noncathartic CT colonography with stool tagging: performance with and without electronic stool subtraction. AJR Am J Roentgenol. 2008;190(2):361–6.

53. Zalis ME, Perumpillichira JJ, Magee C, Kohlberg G, Hahn PF. Tagging-based, electronically cleansed CT colonography: evaluation of patient comfort and image readability. Radiology. 2006;239(1):149–59.

54. Davis GR, Santa Ana CA, Morawski SG, Fordtran JS. Inhibition of water and electrolyte absorption by polyethylene glycol (PEG). Gastroenterology. 1980;79(1):35–9.

55. Seymour CW, Pryor JP, Gupta R, Schwab CW. Anaphylactoid reaction to oral contrast for computed tomography. J Trauma. 2004;57(5):1105–7.

56. Stordahl A, Laerum F, Gjølberg T, Enge I. Water-soluble contrast media in radiography of small bowel obstruction. Acta Radiol. 1988;29(1):53–6.

57. Boyce C, Vetter J, Pickhardt P. MDCT artifact related to the intra-scan gravitational flow of opacified luminal fluid (the "Dense Waterfall" sign). Abdom Imaging. 2012;37(2):292–6.

58. Pickhardt PJ. Translucency rendering in 3D endoluminal CT colonography: a useful tool for increasing polyp specificity and decreasing interpretation time. AJR Am J Roentgenol. 2004;183(2):429–36.

59. Guerrisi A, Marin D, Laghi A, et al. Diagnostic accuracy of translucency rendering to differentiate polyps from pseudopolyps at 3D endoluminal CT colonography: a feasibility study. Radiol Med. 2010;115(5):758–70.

60. Ristvedt SL, McFarland EG, Weinstock LB, Thyssen EP. Patient preferences for CT colonography, conventional colonoscopy, and bowel preparation. Am J Gastroenterol. 2003;98(3):578–85.

61. Beebe TJ, Johnson CD, Stoner SM, Anderson KJ, Limburg PJ. Assessing attitudes toward laxative preparation in colorectal cancer screening and effects on future testing: potential receptivity to computed tomographic colonography. Mayo Clin Proc. 2007;82(6):666–71.

62. Mahgerefteh S, Fraifeld S, Blachar A, Sosna J. CT colonography with decreased purgation: balancing preparation, performance, and patient acceptance. AJR Am J Roentgenol. 2009;193(6):1531–9.

63. Liedenbaum MH, Denters MJ, Zijta FM, et al. Reducing the oral contrast dose in CT colonography: evaluation of faecal tagging quality and patient acceptance. Clin Radiol. 2011;66(1):30–7.

64. Callstrom MR, Johnson CD, Fletcher JG, et al. CT colonography without cathartic preparation: feasibility study. Radiology. 2001;219(3):693–8.

65. Dachman AH, Dawson DO, Lefere P, et al. Comparison of routine and unprepped CT colonography augmented by low fiber diet and stool tagging: a pilot study. Abdom Imaging. 2007;32(1):96–104.

66. Florie J, van Gelder RE, Schutter MP, et al. Feasibility study of computed tomography colonography using limited bowel preparation at normal and low-dose levels study. Eur Radiol. 2007;17(12):3112–22.

67. Jensch S, de Vries AH, Peringa J, et al. CT colonography with limited bowel preparation: performance characteristics in an increased-risk population. Radiology. 2008;247(1):122–32.

68. Zalis ME, Perumpillichira J, Del Frate C, Hahn PF. CT colonography: digital subtraction bowel cleansing with mucosal reconstruction initial observations. Radiology. 2003;226(3):911–7.

69. Pochaczevsky R. Digital subtraction bowel cleansing in CT colonography. AJR Am J Roentgenol. 2002;178(1):241.

70. Serlie IW, de Vries AH, van Vliet LJ, et al. Lesion conspicuity and efficiency of CT colonography with electronic cleansing based on a three-material transition model. AJR Am J Roentgenol. 2008;191(5):1493–502.

71. Park SH, Lee SS, Kim JK, et al. Volume rendering with color coding of tagged stool during endoluminal fly-through CT colonography: effect on reading efficiency. Radiology. 2008;248(3):1018–27.

72. Davis W, Nisbet P, Hare C, Cooke P, Taylor SA. Non-laxative CT colonography with barium-based faecal tagging: is additional phosphate enema beneficial and well tolerated? Br J Radiol. 2011;84(998):120–5.

73. Yee J, Kumar NN, Hung RK, Akerkar GA, Kumar PR, Wall SD. Comparison of supine and prone scanning separately and in combination at CT colonography. Radiology. 2003;226(3):653–61.

74. Burling D, Taylor SA, Halligan S, et al. Automated insufflation of carbon dioxide for MDCT colonography: distension and patient experience compared with manual insufflation. AJR Am J Roentgenol. 2006;186(1):96–103.

75. Vining DJ. Virtual colonoscopy. Semin Ultrasound CT MR. 1999;20(1):56–60.

76. Shinners TJ, Pickhardt PJ, Taylor AJ, Jones DA, Olsen CH. Patient-controlled room air insufflation versus automated carbon dioxide delivery for CT colonography. AJR Am J Roentgenol. 2006;186(6):1491–6.

77. Pickhardt PJ. Incidence of colonic perforation at CT colonography: review of existing data and

implications for screening of asymptomatic adults. Radiology. 2006;239(2):313–6.

78. Atalla MA, Rozen WM, Niewiadomski OD, Croxford MA, Cheung W, Ho YH. Risk factors for colonic perforation after screening computed tomographic colonography: a multicentre analysis and review of the literature. J Med Screen. 2010;17(2):99–102.

79. Sosna J, Blachar A, Amitai M, et al. Colonic perforation at CT colonography: assessment of risk in a multicenter large cohort. Radiology. 2006;239(2):457–63.

80. Chen SC, Lu DS, Hecht JR, Kadell BM. CT colonography: value of scanning in both the supine and prone positions. AJR Am J Roentgenol. 1999;172(3):595–9.

81. Buchach CM, Kim DH, Pickhardt PJ. Performing an additional decubitus series at CT colonography. Abdom Imaging. 2011;36(5):538–44.

82. Dachman AH. Advice for optimizing colonic distention and minimizing risk of perforation during CT colonography. Radiology. 2006;239(2):317–21.

83. Pickhardt PJ, Taylor AJ, Kim DH, Reichelderfer M, Gopal DV, Pfau PR. Screening for colorectal neoplasia with CT colonography: initial experience from the 1st year of coverage by third-party payers. Radiology. 2006;241(2):417–25.

84. Lefere P, Gryspeerdt S, Baekelandt M, Dewyspelaere J, van Holsbeeck B. Diverticular disease in CT colonography. Eur Radiol. 2003;13 Suppl 4:L62–74.

85. Skucas J. The use of antispasmodic drugs during barium enemas. AJR Am J Roentgenol. 1994;162(6):1323–5.

86. Lappas JC, Maglinte DD, Chernish SM, Hage JP, Kelvin FM. Discomfort during double-contrast barium enema examination: a placebo-controlled double-blind evaluation of the effect of glucagon and diazepam. Radiology. 1995;197(1):95–9.

87. Morrin MM, Farrell RJ, Keogan MT, Kruskal JB, Yam CS, Raptopoulos V. CT colonography: colonic distention improved by dual positioning but not intravenous glucagon. Eur Radiol. 2002;12(3):525–30.

88. Yee J, Hung RK, Akerkar GA, Wall SD. The usefulness of glucagon hydrochloride for colonic distention in CT colonography. AJR Am J Roentgenol. 1999;173(1):169–72.

89. Chernish SM, Maglinte DD. Glucagon: common untoward reactions – review and recommendations. Radiology. 1990;177(1):145–6.

90. Bruzzi JF, Moss AC, Brennan DD, MacMathuna P, Fenlon HM. Efficacy of IV buscopan as a muscle relaxant in CT colonography. Eur Radiol. 2003;13(10):2264–70.

91. Mulhall BP, Veerappan GR, Jackson JL. Meta-analysis: computed tomographic colonography. Ann Intern Med. 2005;142(8):635–50.

92. Fenlon HM, Nunes DP, Schroy 3rd PC, Barish MA, Clarke PD, Ferrucci JT. A comparison of virtual and conventional colonoscopy for the detection of colorectal polyps. N Engl J Med. 1999;341(20):1496–503 [see comments] [published erratum appears in N Engl J Med. 2000;342(7):524].

93. Hara AK, Johnson CD, Reed JE, et al. Reducing data size and radiation dose for CT colonography. AJR Am J Roentgenol. 1997;168(5):1181–4.

94. Lui YW, Macari M, Israel G, Bini EJ, Wang H, Babb J. CT colonography data interpretation: effect of different section thicknesses – preliminary observations. Radiology. 2003;229(3):791–7.

95. Macari M, Bini EJ, Xue X, et al. Colorectal neoplasms: prospective comparison of thin-section low-dose multi-detector row CT colonography and conventional colonoscopy for detection. Radiology. 2002;224(2):383–92.

96. McCollough CH. Optimization of multidetector array CT acquisition parameters for CT colonography. Abdom Imaging. 2002;27(3):253–9.

97. van Gelder RE, Venema HW, Florie J, et al. CT colonography: feasibility of substantial dose reduction – comparison of medium to very low doses in identical patients. Radiology. 2004;232(2):611–20.

98. American College of Radiology. ACR practice guideline for the performance of computed tomography (CT) colonography in adults. 2009. http://www.acr.org/~/media/A81531ACA92F45058A83B5281 E8FE826.pdf. Accessed 31 Mar 2012.

99. Hall EJ, Brenner DJ. Cancer risks from diagnostic radiology. Br J Radiol. 2008;81(965):362–78.

100. Luz O, Buchgeister M, Klabunde M, et al. Evaluation of dose exposure in 64-slice CT colonography. Eur Radiol. 2007;17(10):2616–21.

101. van Gelder RE, Venema HW, Serlie IW, et al. CT colonography at different radiation dose levels: feasibility of dose reduction. Radiology. 2002;224(1):25–33.

102. Brenner DJ, Georgsson MA. Mass screening with CT colonography: should the radiation exposure be of concern? Gastroenterology. 2005;129(1):328–37.

103. Liedenbaum MH, Venema HW, Stoker J. Radiation dose in CT colonography – trends in time and differences between daily practice and screening protocols. Eur Radiol. 2008;18(10):2222–30.

104. Iannaccone R, Laghi A, Catalano C, Mangiapane F, Piacentini F, Passariello R. Feasibility of ultra-low-dose multislice CT colonography for the detection of colorectal lesions: preliminary experience. Eur Radiol. 2003;13(6):1297–302.

105. Fisichella V, Båth M, Allansdotter Johnsson Å, et al. Evaluation of image quality and lesion perception by human readers on 3D CT colonography: comparison of standard and low radiation dose. Eur Radiol. 2009;20(3):630–9.

106. de Gonzalez AB, Kim KP, Knudsen AB, et al. Radiation-related cancer risks from CT colonography screening: a risk-benefit analysis. AJR Am J Roentgenol. 2011;196(4):816–23.

107. Flicek KT, Hara AK, Silva AC, Wu Q, Peter MB, Johnson CD. Reducing the radiation dose for CT colonography using adaptive statistical iterative

reconstruction: a pilot study. AJR Am J Roentgenol. 2010;195(1):126–31.

108. Lubner MG, Pickhardt PJ, Tang J, Chen GH. Reduced image noise at low-dose multidetector CT of the abdomen with prior image constrained compressed sensing algorithm. Radiology. 2011;260(1): 248–56.

109. Graser A, Wintersperger BJ, Suess C, Reiser MF, Becker CR. Dose reduction and image quality in MDCT colonography using tube current modulation. AJR Am J Roentgenol. 2006;187(3):695–701.

110. Amis Jr ES, Butler PF, Applegate KE, et al. American College of Radiology white paper on radiation dose in medicine. J Am Coll Radiol. 2007;4(5):272–84.

111. McFarland EG, Fletcher JG, Pickhardt P, et al. ACR Colon Cancer Committee white paper: status of CT colonography 2009. J Am Coll Radiol. 2009;6(11): 756–72.e754.

112. Dachman AH, Kelly KB, Zintsmaster MP, et al. Formative evaluation of standardized training for CT colonographic image interpretation by novice readers. Radiology. 2008;249(1):167–77.

113. Fletcher JG, Chen M-H, Herman BA, et al. Can radiologist training and testing ensure high performance in CT colonography? Lessons from the national CT colonography trial. AJR Am J Roentgenol. 2010;195(1):117–25.

114. Gluecker T, Meuwly JY, Pescatore P, et al. Effect of investigator experience in CT colonography. Eur Radiol. 2002;12(6):1405–9.

115. Taylor SA, Halligan S, Burling D, et al. CT colonography: effect of experience and training on reader performance. Eur Radiol. 2004;14(6):1025–33.

116. Jensch S, van Gelder RE, Florie J, et al. Performance of radiographers in the evaluation of CT colonographic images. AJR Am J Roentgenol. 2007;188(3):W249–55.

117. Burling D. CT colonography standards. Clin Radiol. 2010;65(6):474–80.

118. Rockey DC, Barish M, Brill JV, et al. Standards for gastroenterologists for performing and interpreting diagnostic computed tomographic colonography. Gastroenterology. 2007;133(3):1005–24.

119. Boone D, Halligan S, Frost R, et al. CT colonography: who attends training? A survey of participants at educational workshops. Clin Radiol. 2011;66(6):510–6.

120. van Dam J, Cotton P, Johnson CD, et al. AGA future trends report: CT colonography. Gastroenterology. 2004;127(3):970–84.

121. Zalis ME, Barish MA, Choi JR, et al. CT colonography reporting and data system: a consensus proposal. Radiology. 2005;236(1):3–9.

122. Liedenbaum MH, Bipat S, Bossuyt PM, et al. Evaluation of a standardized CT colonography training program for novice readers. Radiology. 2011;258(2): 477–87.

123. Saunders BP, Phillips RK, Williams CB. Intraoperative measurement of colonic anatomy and attachments with relevance to colonoscopy. Br J Surg. 1995;82(11):1491–3.

124. Kim J, Park S, Lee S, Kim A, Ha H. Ascending colon rotation following patient positional change during CT colonography: a potential pitfall in interpretation. Eur Radiol. 2011;21(2):353–9.

125. Gluecker TM, Fletcher JG, Welch TJ, et al. Characterization of lesions missed on interpretation of CT colonography using a 2D search method. AJR Am J Roentgenol. 2004;182(4):881–9.

126. Pickhardt PJ, Kim DH, Robbins JB. Flat (nonpolypoid) colorectal lesions identified at CT colonography in a U.S. screening population. Acad Radiol. 2010;17(6):784–90.

127. Soetikno R, Kaltenbach T. High-quality CT colonography can detect nonpolypoid colorectal neoplasm (NP-CRN) – science or rhetoric? Acad Radiol. 2010;17(10):1317.

128. Summers RM, Liu J, Yao J, Brown L, Choi JR, Pickhardt PJ. Automated measurement of colorectal polyp height at CT colonography: hyperplastic polyps are flatter than adenomatous polyps. AJR Am J Roentgenol. 2009;193(5):1305–10.

129. Dachman AH, Kuniyoshi JK, Boyle CM, et al. CT colonography with three-dimensional problem solving for detection of colonic polyps. AJR Am J Roentgenol. 1998;171(4):989–95.

130. Beaulieu CF, Jeffrey Jr RB, Karadi C, Paik DS, Napel S. Display modes for CT colonography. Part II. Blinded comparison of axial CT and virtual endoscopic and panoramic endoscopic volume-rendered studies. Radiology. 1999;212(1):203–12.

131. Barish MA, Soto JA, Ferrucci JT. Consensus on current clinical practice of virtual colonoscopy. AJR Am J Roentgenol. 2005;184(3):786–92.

132. Lenhart DK, Babb J, Bonavita J, et al. Comparison of a unidirectional panoramic 3D endoluminal interpretation technique to traditional 2D and bidirectional 3D interpretation techniques at CT colonography: preliminary observations. Clin Radiol. 2010;65(2):118–25.

133. Pickhardt PJ, Lee AD, Taylor AJ, et al. Primary 2D versus primary 3D polyp detection at screening CT colonography. AJR Am J Roentgenol. 2007;189(6): 1451–6.

134. An S, Lee KH, Kim YH, et al. Screening CT colonography in an asymptomatic average-risk Asian population: a 2-year experience in a single institution. AJR Am J Roentgenol. 2008;191(3): W100–6.

135. Kim SH, Lee JM, Eun HW, et al. Two- versus three-dimensional colon evaluation with recently developed virtual dissection software for CT colonography. Radiology. 2007;244(3):852–64.

136. Cotton PB, Durkalski VL, Pineau BC, et al. Computed tomographic colonography (virtual colonoscopy): a multicenter comparison with standard colonoscopy for detection of colorectal neoplasia. JAMA. 2004;291(14):1713–9.

137. Johnson CD, Harmsen WS, Wilson LA, et al. Prospective blinded evaluation of computed tomographic colonography for screen detection of

colorectal polyps. Gastroenterology. 2003;125(2): 311–9.

138. Rockey DC, Paulson E, Niedzwiecki D, et al. Analysis of air contrast barium enema, computed tomographic colonography, and colonoscopy: prospective comparison. Lancet. 2005;365(9456): 305–11.

139. Hock D, Ouhadi R, Materne R, et al. Virtual dissection CT colonography: evaluation of learning curves and reading times with and without computer-aided detection. Radiology. 2008;248(3):860–8.

140. Johnson CD, Fletcher JG, MacCarty RL, et al. Effect of slice thickness and primary 2D versus 3D virtual dissection on colorectal lesion detection at CT colonography in 452 asymptomatic adults. AJR Am J Roentgenol. 2007;189(3):672–80.

141. Macari M, Milano A, Lavelle M, Berman P, Megibow AJ. Comparison of time-efficient CT colonography with two- and three- dimensional colonic evaluation for detecting colorectal polyps. AJR Am J Roentgenol. 2000;174(6):1543–9.

142. Taylor SA, Halligan S, Slater A, et al. Polyp detection with CT colonography: primary 3D endoluminal analysis versus primary 2D transverse analysis with computer-assisted reader software. Radiology. 2006;239(3):759–67.

143. Choi JI, Kim SH, Park HS, et al. Comparison of accuracy and time-efficiency of CT colonography between conventional and panoramic 3D interpretation methods: an anthropomorphic phantom study. Eur J Radiol. 2011;80(2):e68–75.

144. Pickhardt PJ, Schumacher C, Kim DH. Polyp detection at 3-dimensional endoluminal computed tomography colonography: sensitivity of one-way fly-through at 120 degrees field-of-view angle. J Comput Assist Tomogr. 2009;33(4):631–5.

145. Mang T, Kolligs FT, Schaefer C, Reiser MF, Graser A. Comparison of diagnostic accuracy and interpretation times for a standard and an advanced 3D visualisation technique in CT colonography. Eur Radiol. 2011;21(3):653–62.

146. Paik DS, Beaulieu CF, Jeffrey Jr RB, Karadi CA, Napel S. Visualization modes for CT colonography using cylindrical and planar map projections. J Comput Assist Tomogr. 2000;24(2):179–88.

147. Johnson KT, Johnson CD, Fletcher JG, MacCarty RL, Summers RL. CT colonography using 360-degree virtual dissection: a feasibility study. AJR Am J Roentgenol. 2006;186(1):90–5.

148. Christensen KN, Fidler JL, Fletcher JG, MacCarty R, Johnson CD. Pictorial review of colonic polyp and mass distortion and recognition with the CT virtual dissection technique. Radiographics. 2010;30(5): e42.

149. Silva AC, Wellnitz CV, Hara AK. Three-dimensional virtual dissection at CT colonography: unraveling the colon to search for lesions. Radiographics. 2006;26(6):1669–86.

150. Macari M, Megibow AJ. Pitfalls of using three-dimensional CT colonography with two-dimensional imaging correlation. AJR Am J Roentgenol. 2001;176(1):137–43.

151. Rottgen R, Fischbach F, Plotkin M, et al. CT colonography using different reconstruction modi. Clin Imaging. 2005;29(3):195–9.

152. Hoppe H, Quattropani C, Spreng A, Mattich J, Netzer P, Dinkel HP. Virtual colon dissection with CT colonography compared with axial interpretation and conventional colonoscopy: preliminary results. AJR Am J Roentgenol. 2004;182(5):1151–8.

153. Juchems MS, Fleiter TR, Pauls S, Schmidt SA, Brambs HJ, Aschoff AJ. CT colonography: comparison of a colon dissection display versus 3D endoluminal view for the detection of polyps. Eur Radiol. 2006;16(1):68–72.

154. Fisichella VA, Jaderling F, Horvath S, Stotzer PO, Kilander A, Hellstrom M. Primary three-dimensional analysis with perspective-filet view versus primary two-dimensional analysis: evaluation of lesion detection by inexperienced readers at computed tomographic colonography in symptomatic patients. Acta Radiol. 2009;50(3):244–55.

155. Baker ME, Bogoni L, Obuchowski NA, et al. Computer-aided detection of colorectal polyps: can it improve sensitivity of less-experienced readers? Preliminary findings. Radiology. 2007;245(1): 140–9.

156. Dachman AH, Obuchowski NA, Hoffmeister JW, et al. Effect of computer-aided detection for CT colonography in a multireader, multicase trial. Radiology. 2010;256(3):827–35.

157. Mang T, Peloschek P, Plank C, et al. Effect of computer-aided detection as a second reader in multidetector-row CT colonography. Eur Radiol. 2007;17(10):2598–607.

158. Petrick N, Haider M, Summers RM, et al. CT colonography with computer-aided detection as a second reader: observer performance study. Radiology. 2008;246(1):148–56.

159. Taylor SA, Charman SC, Lefere P, et al. CT colonography: investigation of the optimum reader paradigm by using computer-aided detection software. Radiology. 2008;246(2):463–71.

160. Näppi J, Nagata K. Sources of false positives in computer-assisted CT colonography. Abdom Imaging. 2011;36(2):153–64.

161. Halligan S, Mallett S, Altman DG, et al. Incremental benefit of computer-aided detection when used as a second and concurrent reader of CT colonographic data: multiobserver study. Radiology. 2011;258(2): 469–76.

162. Taylor SA, Halligan S, Burling D, et al. Computer-assisted reader software versus expert reviewers for polyp detection on CT colonography. AJR Am J Roentgenol. 2006;186(3):696–702.

163. Taylor SA, Robinson C, Boone D, Honeyfield L, Halligan S. Polyp characteristics correctly annotated by computer-aided detection software but ignored by reporting radiologists during CT colonography. Radiology. 2009;253(3):715–23.

164. Dachman AH, Zalis ME. Quality and consistency in CT colonography and research reporting. Radiology. 2004;230(2):319–23.

165. Levin B, Lieberman DA, McFarland B, et al. Screening and surveillance for the early detection of colorectal cancer and adenomatous polyps, 2008: a joint guideline from the American Cancer Society, the US Multi-Society Task Force on Colorectal Cancer, and the American College of Radiology. CA Cancer J Clin. 2008;58(3):130–60.

166. Bethea E, Nwawka OK, Dachman AH. Comparison of polyp size and volume at CT colonography: implications for follow-up CT colonography. AJR Am J Roentgenol. 2009;193(6):1561–7.

167. Morales TG, Sampliner RE, Garewal HS, Fennerty MB, Aickin M. The difference in colon polyp size before and after removal. Gastrointest Endosc. 1996;43(1):25–8.

168. Park SH, Choi EK, Lee SS, et al. Polyp measurement reliability, accuracy, and discrepancy: optical colonoscopy versus CT colonography with pig colonic specimens. Radiology. 2007;244(1):157–64.

169. Burling D, Halligan S, Altman DG, et al. Polyp measurement and size categorisation by CT colonography: effect of observer experience in a multi-centre setting. Eur Radiol. 2006;16(8):1737–44.

170. de Vries A, Bipat S, Dekker E, et al. Polyp measurement based on CT colonography and colonoscopy: variability and systematic differences. Eur Radiol. 2009;20(6):1404–13.

171. Jeong JY, Kim MJ, Kim SS. Manual and automated polyp measurement: comparison of CT colonography with optical colonoscopy. Acad Radiol. 2008; 15(2):231–9.

172. Punwani S, Halligan S, Irving P, et al. Measurement of colonic polyps by radiologists and endoscopists: who is most accurate? Eur Radiol. 2008;18(5):874–81.

173. Pickhardt PJ, Lee AD, McFarland EG, Taylor AJ. Linear polyp measurement at CT colonography: in vitro and in vivo comparison of two-dimensional and three-dimensional displays. Radiology. 2005; 236(3):872–8.

174. Summers RM. Polyp size measurement at CT colonography: what do we know and what do we need to know? Radiology. 2010;255(3):707–20.

175. Halligan S, Altman DG, Taylor SA, et al. CT colonography in the detection of colorectal polyps and cancer: systematic review, meta-analysis, and proposed minimum data set for study level reporting. Radiology. 2005;237(3):893–904.

176. Yeshwant SC, Summers RM, Yao J, Brickman DS, Choi JR, Pickhardt PJ. Polyps: linear and volumetric measurement at CT colonography. Radiology. 2006;241(3):802–11.

177. Summers RM, Swift JA, Dwyer AJ, Choi JR, Pickhardt PJ. Normalized distance along the colon centerline: a method for correlating polyp location on CT colonography and optical colonoscopy. AJR Am J Roentgenol. 2009;193(5):1296–304.

178. Duncan JE, McNally MP, Sweeney WB, et al. CT colonography predictably overestimates colonic length and distance to polyps compared with optical colonoscopy. AJR Am J Roentgenol. 2009;193(5): 1291–5.

179. Church JM. Complete colonoscopy: how often? And if not, why not? Am J Gastroenterol. 1994;89(4): 556–60.

180. Fenlon HM, McAneny DB, Nunes DP, Clarke PD, Ferrucci JT. Occlusive colon carcinoma: virtual colonoscopy in the preoperative evaluation of the proximal colon. Radiology. 1999;210(2):423–8.

181. Neri E, Giusti P, Battolla L, et al. Colorectal cancer: role of CT colonography in preoperative evaluation after incomplete colonoscopy. Radiology. 2002;223(3):615–9.

182. Chang KJ, Rekhi Jr SS, Anderson SW, Soto JA. Fluid tagging for CT colonography: effectiveness of a 2-hour iodinated oral preparation after incomplete optical colonoscopy. J Comput Assist Tomogr. 2011;35(1):91–5.

183. Prout TM, Taylor AJ, Pickhardt PJ. Inverted appendiceal stumps simulating large pedunculated polyps on screening CT colonography. AJR Am J Roentgenol. 2006;186(2):535–8.

Integration of CTC into a CRC Screening Program

6

Steven Carpenter

Introduction

Screening for colorectal neoplasms has become the standard of care in advanced medical settings worldwide [1–7]. Identifying asymptomatic colorectal neoplastic lesions has been shown to reduce colorectal cancer (CRC) incidence and the overall cost of medical care. Clinicians have several alternatives at their disposal as they consider screening for their respective patient population. Many organizations have devoted considerable time weighing the evidence to establish appropriate evidence-based guidelines directing clinicians with methods to appropriately manage screening. CT colonoscopy and optical colonoscopy (OC) are viable alternatives for CRC screening. Organizations that plan to utilize both modalities must consider multiple issues to effectively integrate and ensure a high-quality screening program.

Optical Colonoscopy

Clinicians use OC as a primary means to screen the entire colon not only for cancer but also for precancerous adenomatous lesions. Most

S. Carpenter, M.D. (✉)
Mercer University School of Medicine,
Savannah Campus, Savannah, GA, USA

Department of Internal Medicine, Memorial University
Medical Center, Savannah, GA, USA
e-mail: slcarp2@gmail.com

adenomas may be removed at the time of OC. The size, location, shape, and pathologic nature of polyps may be determined during this single clinical encounter, providing the patient and clinician with valuable information to guide the future CRC screening strategy. Often, the clinician doing the endoscopic procedure has an established relationship with the patient and may provide recommendations regarding care at a subsequent clinical encounter. Established Centers of Digestive Health, worldwide, have proved to be successful in driving the CRC screening effort. Brenner et al. demonstrated a very low incidence of CRC after a negative screening OC in low-risk groups and suggested a 10-year screening interval after a negative OC [8]. Screening OC is a highly effective tool for CRC prevention.

Clearly, many patients and healthcare providers are comfortable with this protocol of patient care. However, OC has its disadvantages. The procedure requires adequate colon cleansing to allow for complete mucosal evaluation, and many patients state that the arduous task of colonic preparation is a major drawback to the entire process. In almost every case, OC requires conscious sedation of one form or another. Individual clinical evaluation of the patient's overall medical condition is required to determine candidacy for sedation. From the patient's perspective, conscious sedation provides them comfort and allays anxiety; it also requires access to reliable transportation from the medical setting. As a result, patients not only have to absent themselves from their daily responsibilities but their transporter must also take time from their routines. This is a significant issue to consider when reviewing the overall cost of the CRC screening effort. During OC and polypectomy, perforation of the colon may occur. Although this is a relatively rare complication, it can and does occur in the care of asymptomatic patients. In addition, bleeding even after the most simple of polypectomies may occur and may require hospitalization or even administration of blood products. Because of the potential for colonic perforation, post-polypectomy bleeding, and other complications, adequately trained medical personnel must carefully discuss these possibilities to obtain meaningful informed consent from all patients prior to the procedure. There is simply no substitute for an excellent patient–physician relationship.

Quality

First and foremost in managing a CRC screening program should be quality and safety [9]. Optical colonoscopy is not a perfect screening modality. There are a variety of issues that have come to the forefront in this regard. Among these are adenoma detection rates (ADR), colonoscopic withdrawal times, and preparation quality [10]. There is good evidence that quality of OC varies and that this variation has an impact on effectiveness [11–13]. Several tandem OC studies demonstrate that, for many reasons, adenomatous colon polyps may be missed during the procedure [14, 15]. Polyps may be behind folds, obscured by colonic debris, or simply not seen by the endoscopist. This issue has prompted considerable focus by gastrointestinal societies on measurement and reporting of quality parameters. Many endoscopy centers have initiated routine documentation of these important quality measures, and collectively, there is hope that these developments can improve the overall CRC screening effort. Several studies demonstrate that adequate training and experience translate into improved quality. We require additional experienced endoscopists to meet future screening needs, and quality measures are now included in gastroenterology fellowship

curricula. As the age of our patient population increases and the population grows, endoscopists and trainees need a firm grasp of advances in endoscopy (with its inherent limitations) and a fostered appreciation of their role in quality improvement during CRC screening.

Adenoma Detection Rates

Ultimately, the entire purpose of CRC screening is to prevent CRC, and this is facilitated by identification of colonic adenomas, its precursor lesion. Ideally, these polyps will be identified at an early stage when resection is relatively straightforward. The ADR has become a key measure for the relative effectiveness of OC screening [16]. Among healthy asymptomatic patients undergoing screening OC, estimates suggest adenomas should be detected in 25% or more of men and 15% or more of women 50 years of age and older. A variety of factors may influence ADR. Patient-associated variables that might affect the efficacy of OC include body mass index, medications, and comorbid illness. Various reports have documented the potential for effect of OC withdrawal time, completeness of OC (cecal intubation), adequate bowel preparation, participation of trainees in the procedure, experience, and procedural timing during the workday. Physician fatigue has received increased attention in all fields of medicine. It is not surprising that attention has been directed toward this variable. There are data that suggest the ADR may be negatively affected if the procedure is completed at the end of the endoscopist's day as opposed to the beginning. Approaching this issue may prove difficult for screening centers as they attempt to meet demand. Optimal utilization of physician and endoscopy center resources is required. Some centers have approached this issue by splitting the endoscopy workday. There is some reason to believe that endoscopists function more effectively when working in 4–5 h blocks as opposed to 8–10 blocks. Gurudu et al. [17] documented that the afternoon ADR was significantly lower than the morning ADR (21.0% vs. 26.1%; OR = 0.75; $P = 0.02$). When endoscopists were scheduled to work in half-day blocks, morning and afternoon ADR was not statistically different

(27.6% vs. 26.6%;OR = 1.05; P = 0.56). Lee et al. identified a 12.4% reduction in detected polyps when comparing morning procedures with afternoon procedures performed by the same endoscopist [18]. In fact, as each hour in the day elapsed, they reported a 4.6% reduction in polyp detection (P = 0.005).

These assertions make intuitive sense and have been documented in other manuscripts [19, 20]. Perhaps, prolonged procedure blocks create visual or mental fatigue that may adversely affect adenoma detection. Others have proposed that colonic preparation is inferior later in the day, and mucosal visualization, not fatigue, is the key variable. It is also possible that endoscopists' ADR declines if they fall behind on their schedule as the day progresses. It is imperative that endoscopists recognize the potential that fatigue and procedural timing may affect their personal ADR. Centers for digestive health must acknowledge this fact and take these data into account as patient care scheduling templates are devised.

The issue of ADR and endoscopist fatigue is a crucial consideration if one plans to integrate CTC into an existing CRC screening program [21]. The goal of CTC is to identify polyp candidates and deal with them. Patients are reluctant to take a colonic preparation to begin with and often are not interested in coming back another day for an OC requiring a second round of colonic preparation. Therefore, scheduling matrices must be established to allow for same-day OC in those patients who have identified polyp candidates by CTC. Anecdotal reports suggest that wait times for same-day OC after positive CTC may be 2 h or even longer. Many of these same-day OCs will have to be performed in the afternoon. It is undetermined whether this strategy for CRC screening is flawed due to the issue of endoscopist fatigue. Further study in this area will be required if CTC ever becomes a dominant CRC screening strategy.

Bowel Preparation

Both CTC and OC require bowel preparation to enhance visualization of colonic mucosal detail [22]. Bowel preparation may be the most despised aspect of CRC screening from the patient's perspective. Poor patient acceptance is common to both OC and CTC, and the quality of bowel preparation directly impacts the quality of both studies. In a large retrospective case study by Lebwohl et al., the adenoma miss rate for OC performed with suboptimal bowel preparation was high [23]. These authors concluded that poor bowel preparation decreases OC effectiveness and should mandate an earlier follow-up examination. Also, suboptimal bowel preparation makes OC more difficult and increases procedural time. Both the intubation and withdrawal phases are prolonged. In addition, the cecal intubation and polyp detection rates are decreased [24, 25]. Froehlich et al., in a large prospective trial, observed that small and large polyp detection rates were increased in patients with an adequate bowel preparation compared to those inadequately prepped (29% vs. 26%, P < 0.001). In this study, the cecal intubation time was significantly decreased in patients with adequate preparations (11.9 min vs. 16.1 min, P < 0.001). Careful attention to patient education regarding the preparation process will increase CRC screening center efficiency and the quality of patient care.

Polyethylene glycol electrolyte lavage solution (PEG) is widely utilized as a bowel preparative in OC (NuLYTELY, GoLYTELY, Braintree Laboratories). Patients have reported difficulty with the 4 L volume of this traditional preparation, and subsequently, 2-L preparations (HalfLytely, Braintree Laboratories) were devised using either magnesium citrate or bisacodyl tablets [26]. Later, an alternate 2-L preparation containing PEG, ascorbic acid, and sodium sulfate (MoviPrep, Salix Pharmaceuticals, Inc., Morrisville, NC) was devised. This preparation has been shown to be non-inferior to the traditional 4-L PEG preparation [27]. Previously, an oral sodium phosphate preparation (Fleet's Phospho-soda, C.B. Fleet Company, Inc., Lynchburg, VA) was widely utilized for bowel preparation. In 2008, the FDA issued a safety alert due to reports of acute phosphate nephropathy. In response, C.B. Fleet withdrew their oral sodium phosphate products intended for use as an OC preparative regimen [28, 29]. More recently, a bowel purgative regimen containing sodium sulfate 35 g, potassium sulfate 6.26 g, and magnesium sulfate 3.2 g in divided doses (total volume, 2.8 L) was devised (SuPrep, Braintree Laboratories). This split-dosed preparation favorably impacted patient acceptance [30].

Split dosing of bowel preparations has become very popular in endoscopy centers primarily due to the considerable improvement in mucosal visualization and ease of the OC associated with this administration schedule [31]. Split dosing of the bowel preparation has been recommended by the American College of Gastroenterology to improve effectiveness of bowel cleansing. Administration of one-half of the bowel preparation during the evening prior to the procedure followed by ingestion of the second half of the prep during the morning of the procedure produces considerable improvement in mucosal visualization. An interval of 6 h or less between the second dose of the preparation and OC has been shown in several studies to be superior. The duration of the interval between the completion of bowel preparation and the start of OC has been shown to impact bowel-preparation quality [32]. Bowel-preparation quality is inversely related to the time of the last preparation dose. Prior to this study, Church had concluded that small bowel contents entering the right colon after preparation completion had a deleterious effect on preparation quality, primarily in the right colon [33]. Some have proposed that this might explain the difficulty in demonstrating that OC is effective in the prevention of right-sided CRC [34]. There are a number of excellent studies that note the superiority of split-dosed colonic preparation relative to 1-day dosing regimens. Aoun et al. found that the split-dosed regimen was more likely to result in an excellent preparation rating than if the entire preparation was administered the evening before the OC (44.1% vs. 5.5%; $P<0.001$) [35]. Emerging data suggests that the improvement in bowel preparation quality with split-dosed preps results in improved detection of neoplasia [36]. Patient acceptance of the split-dosed schema is variable. If the patient is scheduled for an 8 AM procedure, it is necessary that they ingest the second dose of the bowel purgative between 12 AM and 2 AM on the day of the procedure. Nonetheless, there is some evidence that patients do prefer the divided preparation compared to the prior standard 4-L preparation, despite the potential timing inconveniences [37].

Considerable advances have been made in understanding of quality bowel preparation. CRC screening centers should maintain focus on developments in this arena. Particularly, it is important that patient education prior to the procedure remains a priority. Patient acceptance of the bowel preparation process will continue to be a barrier affecting adherence to CRC screening.

Withdrawal Time

There is considerable evidence that quality OC is directly related to the duration of the procedure [38, 39]. Polyp detection rate is directly related to mean procedural time. Many endoscopists concentrate on good technique and safety during colonoscope insertion and reserve the withdrawal period for careful mucosal visualization. The colonoscopic withdrawal time has received considerable attention in the literature. Indeed, it has been proven to be a useful and easily acquired quality measure. Barclay et al. noted that colonoscopists with mean withdrawal time of 6 min or more had higher rates of detection of any neoplasia when compared to those with mean withdrawal time of less than 6 min (28.3% vs. 11.8%, $P<0.001$) [12]. This also proved true for the detection of advanced neoplasia (6.4% vs. 2.6%, $P=0.005$).These results have been confirmed in subsequent studies. It is apparent that endoscopists do respond to monitoring and feedback. Lin et al. retrospectively reviewed 850 screening OC performed by 10 endoscopists [40]. Withdrawal times, polyp detection rates, and patient satisfaction scores were determined and then shared, confidentially, with the endoscopists. Thereafter, 541 screening OCs were prospectively evaluated measuring the same parameters. After monitoring was initiated, mean withdrawal time increased from 6.57 to 8.07 min ($P<0.0001$), and polyp detection rates improved from 33.1 to 38.1% ($P<0.05$). There was a small, statistically insignificant increase in the neoplasia detection rate from 19.6 to 22.7% ($P=0.17$). There was no change in mean patient satisfaction scores. The US Multi-Society Task Force on Colorectal Cancer recommends 6–10 min as the minimal amount of time needed for adequate inspection during the withdrawal phase.

Patient Satisfaction

It is important that all CRC screening centers make patient satisfaction a top priority [41–43]. There are many factors that influence overall patient satisfaction. Clearly, patients are concerned about their physician's technical skills and sedation adequacy. The facility's cleanliness and focus on patient privacy are also important measures impacting satisfaction. Gastrointestinal and recovery nurses play a major role in how our patients perceive the overall experience. CRC screening centers should routinely measure patient satisfaction in these, and potentially other, areas. Quality improvement initiatives need to be in place. Areas for potential improvement should be defined and then appropriate changes in process may be implemented. The latter point is the key. It does an institution little good to measure patient feedback if one is not ready and willing to act upon the information. Actually, in practice, the process of quality improvement can be quite rewarding. Once you get the team focused on quality and improvement, the entire process will self-perpetuate.

CT Colonography

CT colonography (CTC) is a promising CRC screening tool. There are several key factors that make this method of CRC screening attractive to clinicians and patients. The procedure does not require moderate conscious sedation. Therefore, patients may provide their own transportation and return to work immediately following the examination. Of course, this depends on whether the CTC has positive findings. If same-day OC is to be considered in the event of a positive CTC, then the reading of the CTC must be immediate. Thereafter, the patient may decide for intervention

on the CTC exam date. If a later date is selected, then a repeat colonic preparation will be required. As the colon is imaged digitally, the risk of procedurally related complications, such as perforation and bleeding, is vastly reduced. Improvements in CTC technology image quality and data acquisition time allow for a time-efficient examination. Patients may have their procedure completed in as little as 10 min with CTC. Importantly, CTC has resulted in increased patient awareness of the CRC screening effort. As CTC has received considerable attention in the lay press, more patients realize the value of CRC screening and may be willing to participate in the process. Anything that increases overall patient awareness and acceptance of the process of CRC screening is beneficial and improves adherence.

Despite these advantages, CTC has its own limitations. Many patients are disappointed to discover that CTC requires adequate colon preparation for optimal colonic imaging. In fact, the preparation is more complicated as contrast- and fecal-tagging agents are necessary to adequately differentiate stool from polyps. Trained medical personnel are required to describe the importance and specifics of this preparation to patients. Current screening recommendations suggest that some patients might have five or more CT examinations during their lifetime if CTC is the primary CRC screening modality. Radiation exposure remains a major concern. The singular CTC exam is not the issue. Cumulative radiation exposure, given CTC as the primary modality for CRC screening, has drawn increased scrutiny by many. Radiology societies have largely dismissed this issue [44]. The cumulative effects of medical radiation in a screening effort are poorly understood and long-term studies are needed. If a polyp is identified via CTC, most patients require OC for polyp removal. Some have suggested that small polyps may be followed with CTC at shortened screening intervals. Although some patients may be comfortable with repeated CT examinations to follow a lesion, those in primary care know other patients will have concern about the safety of this watch-and-wait approach and their cumulative radiation exposure.

Extracolonic Findings

During CTC, extracolonic information is acquired [45]. A standardized CTC reporting and data system (C-RADS) has been developed and is useful for CTC report uniformity [46]. Findings of major clinical relevance, categorized as E4 findings, arise in approximately 4–10% of CTC examinations. Examples of E4 findings include renal cell carcinoma, ovarian carcinoma, and an abdominal aortic aneurysm of worrisome size. Indeterminate extracolonic abnormalities are categorized as E3 findings in the C-RADS system and are identified in approximately 30% of examinations. Examples of E3 findings include suspicious renal and liver cysts. Findings of low clinical importance, such as simple liver and renal cysts, are placed in category E2. The frequency of E3 findings may be expected to increase, particularly if radiologists are liability averse. Furthermore, in a liability-concerned environment, some radiologists may be inclined to hedge on E2 abnormalities of low clinical importance, thereby increasing the percentage of E3 findings reported [47]. The overall cost of CRC screening would be expected to increase due to repeat radiologic (and other) tests to follow indeterminate findings. In 2009, this important cost-efficacy concern impacted the decision made by the Centers for Medicare & Medicaid Services (CMS). Individual CT reports often suggest that E3 findings be followed at the discretion of the patient and referring physician. Just as ADR and withdrawal times are important measures of quality OC, the frequencies of E2 and E3 findings are quality measures of CTC interpretation. It is important that CRC screening centers utilizing CTC as an integral component put in place a prospective measuring system to evaluate the reporting of extracolonic findings. Radiologists should receive feedback about individual reporting as compared to peers.

Experienced clinicians know that patients worry about extracolonic findings, no matter how minor. Health-related anxiety mandates time and patience when discussing even simple E2 findings with patients. In some cases, these discussions heighten the individual patient's health-care-related anxiety.

An excellent doctor–patient relationship is useful in lessening this degree of anxiety and proves invaluable in many respects. For CTC to be clinically and cost effective, it is imperative that radiologists take great care in the nature of CTC extracolonic reporting and be prudent with E2 and E3 findings. CTC findings need to be communicated in a reliable manner by the radiologist to the clinician who is primarily responsible for the patient. Likewise, primary care physicians or gastroenterologists must communicate meaningfully with patients. This seems straightforward, but in a busy clinical setting, failure to communicate is entirely possible.

Interpretation of CTC

Appropriately trained radiologists should interpret extracolonic findings identified at CTC. Although interpretation of extracolonic CT images is thoroughly covered in gastroenterology training and many practicing gastroenterologists review multiple CT images within a given workday, gastroenterologists do not have the expertise or privileges to provide an official interpretation of extracolonic CT data. In CTC centers, one prime goal is to provide the patient with the opportunity for a same-day OC. Within 20 or 30 min, a gastroenterologist or radiologist reading CTC can provide an immediate intracolonic interpretation as the patient waits. There is not a similar acute need for the extracolonic interpretation. CTC centers can send CT images digitally and thus outsource the reading of extracolonic images. Clinicians who provide CTC within their own center therefore have the opportunity to identify excellent radiologists who deliver high-quality interpretations. Small centers can even send CTC images to major university centers. Several high-quality radiologists have developed their own corporations to provide this service, allowing CRC screening centers to track the quality of extracolonic interpretations and change to an alternate vendor if necessary to ensure high-quality patient care. Extracolonic findings require careful evidence-based management. Colorectal cancer screening centered in one locale provides patients with the opportunity to review and discuss colonic and extracolonic findings with their clinician during one clinical encounter. Appropriate evidence-based management of all findings may be coordinated in this fashion.

With regard to the interpretation of colonic findings obtained during CTC, both radiologists and gastroenterologists can perform this role, provided that they commit the time to maintaining proficiency. Endoscopists have a wealth of experience with OC, and reading three-dimensional CTC flythrough images is thereby intuitive for these practitioners. Standards for gastroenterologists performing and interpreting diagnostic CTC have been established, and training programs organized by professional gastrointestinal organizations are effective in orienting endoscopists to this new technology [51]. Although courses can be helpful for introduction, there is no substitute for hands-on experience. This can be achieved via mentored leader programs. Ideally, personal hands-on experience is obtained in centers providing CTC and OC services. Gastroenterologists may interpret colonic CTC images proficiently with accuracy similar to that of radiologists [50]. Adequate training and experience is mandatory to ensure highly accurate readings. While colonoscopists may find CTC colonic interpretation intuitive, there is a learning curve to acquire proficiency with the software utilized for CTC. There are several vendors with excellent CTC software programs and platform revision is continuous. Gastroenterologists interested in CTC proficiency should select a single software and learn it well. The time commitment for CTC interpretive expertise is substantial, and maintenance of proficiency is an ongoing process.

CTC has become part of the gastrointestinal core curriculum for GI fellowship training [48, 49]. It is important that current gastroenterology fellows develop a basic familiarity with the indications, interpretation, and limitations of CTC. Coordination and cooperation with departments of radiology can provide more in-depth training, and it is reasonable to consider formal radiology rotation addition to gastroenterology fellowship curricula. Novel educational tracts within traditional gastroenterology training might be considered, with focus on technologies such as wireless capsule endoscopy and CTC. A comprehensive training curriculum would need to be established and training standards for current fellows developed.

Radiologists require a meaningful physician peer review program for accreditation. There exists no infrastructure in gastroenterology societies for this type of quality control process. Randomly selected CTC studies need to be peer reviewed on a regularly scheduled basis. Although members of one's own organization can feasibly perform this task, this method of peer review may not result in meaningful critique. Optimally, review networks would need to be organized, with reviewers able to correlate the interpretation with corresponding endoscopic and pathologic findings. Development of a national database might need to be considered. Thereby, CTC, endoscopic, and pathologic findings could be correlated and meaningfully studied. Policies and procedures must be in place to resolve discrepant peer review findings providing the means for CTC centers to achieve quality outcomes improvement [52]. Gastroenterology societies would either partner with other societies to develop appropriate peer review, quality, and safety measures or initiate the process independently. Available data confirm that gastroenterologists have the expertise to proficiently interpret CTC images, meaningfully participate in this CRC screening approach, and provide patients with CRC screening by a variety of methods within a single center.

Coordination of Care and Adherence

All members of the population should receive some form of testing to improve CRC screening outcomes. Unfortunately, this is not yet the case. There are many reasons for this lack of adherence, but some patients remain concerned about various aspects of endoscopy. CTC presents patients with an alternative, as we have no perfect CRC screening modality. Before selecting the method of CRC screening, it is desirable that each patient has an understanding of the positive and negative attributes of available methods.

This type of communication requires patience, time, and resources. A formal consultative visit can prove immensely beneficial. Primary care physicians are perfectly suited to provide this service during routine visits, but due to issues of time and complexity of primary care, a thorough review of options is not always possible. The data regarding CRC screening is far from static. Many primary care physicians are not fully versed about the sensitivity and specificity of OC and CTC in asymptomatic patients or the proper surveillance intervals for adenomas. Many patients are interested in discussing the data and options, and Centers of Digestive Health are ideally suited to provide this expertise.

Barriers that interfere with patient adherence to CRC screening must be eliminated. Patients are unlikely to accept devoting two different days to the CRC screening effort. A single center approach to CRC screening with a strong emphasis on providing the option of same day OC, should a mucosal abnormality be identified on CTC, is optimal. On occasion, OC may not provide complete colonic imaging due to technical or anatomic concerns. Immediate availability of CTC is desired from a patient convenience perspective. However, same day CTC and OC require careful schedule coordination, providing adequate time for endoscopic definitive therapy when polyps are identified on CTC. Prompt interpretation of CTC data is required to limit patient inconvenience. It is unlikely that patients will embrace an approach wherein OC follows CTC by more than 1 or 2 h. Furthermore, colonic preparation quality data suggest that if OC occurs more than 4 h after CTC, suboptimal colonic preparation can be expected. This could adversely affect the efficacy of OC. Excellent communication between the CTC interpreter and endoscopist is expected. CRC screening centers will need to prospectively follow quality parameters such false-negative and false-positive results of CTC and OC. Centers of Digestive Health may effectively follow the quality of patient care while providing comprehensive CRC screening options using the modality selected by the patient and their personal physician.

It is important that patients adhere to follow-up recommendations after a polyp is detected. Gastroenterologists are well versed in the appropriate follow-up intervals for surveillance following removal of adenomas. It is still not clear whether small polyps detected at CTC and not removed may be safely followed with serial CTC over time. This remains an area of controversy. Patients will benefit from their personal physician assisting them with this process. Follow-up of intracolonic and extracolonic abnormalities will require development of a patient health maintenance profile. A digestive center database could ensure that patients are contacted in subsequent years when due for repeat CRC screening, be it by CTC or OC. Extracolonic abnormalities will require careful attention, and this is best done between patients and their personal physicians. Worrisome E3 findings may require further diagnostic planning. E4 findings, such as hepatocellular carcinoma, cirrhosis, or large abdominal aortic aneurysms, will likely require definitive therapy. It is important that patients adhere, not only to the recommendations regarding polyp management, but also to diagnostic or therapeutic plans for extracolonic findings

Effective Integration of CTC and OC

Implementation of an efficient CRC screening program incorporating CTC requires coordination of several key processes if availability of same-day OC is to be offered. Duncan et al. recently reviewed their database of all procedures performed from 2004 to 2010 [53]. In their patient population at the National Naval Medical Center, 11% of patients required OC due to positive findings on CTC. Notably, 1,137 patients were referred for OC after CTC, but only 130 patients underwent same-day OC. The average wait time from arrival for CTC to discharge after OC was 348 min (range 178–684 min, SD 100 min, median 333 min). The process events that must occur for same-day OC after positive CTC include registration for CTC, performance of CTC, radiologist CTC interpretation time, endoscopy unit registration time, OC preparation and completion time, and discharge time following OC recovery.

There are limited data on the extent that widespread implementation of CTC might impact upon OC volume at endoscopy centers. Using mathematical modeling based on data in 2004, Hur et al. concluded that if CTC was used as the primary modality for CRC screening, one could expect a 22% decrease in OC demand. However, the polyp-size threshold utilized to define a CTC test as positive (6 or 10 mm) significantly impacts this prediction [54]. In 2008, Schwartz et al. noted that the initiation of a screening CTC program at the University of Wisconsin did not result in a decrease in total OC exams from 2004 to 2007 [55]. A mean number of 10 patients per month were sent for OC after a positive CTC. In 2010, Benson et al. published the experience from the same center in abstract form [56]. The mean per quarter total number of OC exams performed increased significantly from 1,104 in 2003 to 1,976 in 2008 ($P < 0.001$). They concluded that the initiation of a CTC screening program did not lead to a reduction in the number of OC exams performed. After the initiation of a CTC CRC screening program, OC remained the predominant screening modality. Importantly, Ladabaum et al. noted that if overall adherence to CRC guidelines is attained by a population, then overall OC volume increases, even with widespread utilization of CTC for screening [57]. An excellent working relationship between departments of radiology, general internal medicine, and gastroenterology facilitates the effort [58].

Coordination with pathology is also required for effective integration. Adenoma detection rates should be followed for both radiologists and endoscopists. A peer review process for CTC interpretation is necessary. Colonoscopic withdrawal times are yet another parameter that needs to be followed over time. The rate of E2 and E3 findings on radiologic extracolonic interpretation should be followed and compared to national database statistics. There is no need to acquire and interpret data unless one is willing to act upon the information provided. Therefore, quality improvement measures need to be in place to provide meaningful feedback to physicians as they strive to improve either their radiologic or endoscopic expertise. Following this feedback, performance measures should be continuously evaluated to ensure improvement and that the standard of care is achieved. A carefully constructed operating agreement within individual physician practices or institutional policies and procedures becomes crucial if an organization identifies and plans action regarding a physician outlier providing suboptimal patient care during the CRC screening effort.

Financial Considerations

CTC reimbursement for CRC screening remains highly variable. In May 2009, CMS published a noncoverage decision and stated, "The evidence is inadequate to conclude that CT colonography is appropriate for colorectal cancer screening" [59]. This decision had a considerable impact on the adoption of screening CTC in the United States. Still, there are a number of health plans that continue to reimburse for this procedure. There is considerable variance from state to state with regard to coverage decisions. Clinicians must contact each provider to determine the relative coverage of CTC for CRC screening. This is a cumbersome task for any organization, and the administrative complexity alone has also impacted the widespread adoption of CTC.

Over the past 7 years, there has been increased adoption of CTC by US hospitals. McHugh et al. examined American Hospital Association annual surveys and conducted interviews with several hospital representatives [60]. There was modest increase (13–17%) in the number of US hospitals offering CTC. Almost one-third of hospitals that offer CTC do not offer immediate OC after a positive CTC. Ideally, radiologists and gastroenterologists work together to schedule the follow-up OC on the same day to avoid a second colon-cleansing preparation. Lack of coordination or availability of on-site OC services, though, could increase the number of people lost to follow-up after an initial CTC screen. Lack of reimbursement for general screening and cost of implementation were major barriers that prevented hospitals not offering CTC from proceeding with implementation.

The California Technology Assessment Forum (CTAF) assesses new and emerging medical technologies. In March 2009, the CTAF concluded that CTC did not meet the technology criterion for utilization as a screening test for CRC in average-risk individuals [61]. Specifically, there were three main areas of concern. The CTAF was uncertain that there was sufficient evidence to conclude that CTC would improve net health outcomes. The main concern here was the unknown potential for harm related to radiation exposure. Secondly, the CTAF requires that new technology must be as beneficial as any established alternatives. A main additional concern here was the potential for significant adverse health outcomes related to extracolonic findings. "Many extracolonic findings require additional evaluation, but are ultimately clinically insignificant." Lastly, documented improvements in healthcare outcomes must be attainable outside of the investigational setting. Mainly due to continued concerns about long-term radiation exposure and extracolonic findings, this criterion was not achieved in the CTAF's opinion.

The Institute of Technology Assessment at the Massachusetts General Hospital evaluated the cost-effectiveness of CTC to aid CMS in their recent decision regarding CTC for the average-risk Medicare population [62]. Knudsen et al. concluded that CTC would be cost effective if the reimbursement per scan is substantially less than that for OC. However, they did note that if adherence to CRC screening was substantially improved that cost-effectiveness of CTC also improved. The undiscounted number life-years gained from CTC screening ranged from 143 to 178 per 1,000 65-year-olds. This result was slightly less than the number of life-years gained for OC every 10 years, which ranged from 152 to 185 per 1,000 65-year-olds. These findings were presented to the Medicare Evidence Development and Coverage Advisory Committee in November 2008.

Conclusion

CTC may be utilized for CRC screening, and models have been developed in which gastroenterologists and radiologists work together to implement effective CRC screening programs [63–65]. Interpretation of CTC colonic images is classically performed by radiologists, and although controversial, it has been proven that gastroenterologists may also attain competency in this area [66]. There remains continued concern about the impact of radiation exposure and identification of extracolonic findings on patient well-being and healthcare expenditure [67, 68]. Endoscopists are under increased scrutiny with regard to the overall quality of OC, and quality measures such as colonic preparation, withdrawal time, and ADR must be measured and followed over time [69]. Organizations that plan to integrate CTC and OC as options for CRC screening in their centers need to carefully measure quality parameters and make continuous quality improvement a top priority.

References

1. Rex DK, Johnson DA, Anderson JC, et al. American College of Gastroenterology guidelines for colorectal cancer screening 2009. Am J Gastroenterol. 2009;104: 739–50.
2. Levin B, Lieberman DA, McFarland B, et al. American Cancer Society Colorectal Cancer Advisory Group; US Multi-Society Task Force; American College of Radiology Colon Cancer Committee. Screening and surveillance for the early detection of colorectal cancer and adenomatous polyps, 2008: a joint guideline from the American Cancer Society, the US Multi-Society Task Force on Colorectal Cancer, and the American College of Radiology. Gastroenterology. 2008;134:1570–95.
3. Klabunde CN, Lanier D, Nadel MR, et al. Colorectal cancer screening by primary care physicians: recommendations and practices, 2006–2007. Am J Prev Med. 2009;37:8–16.
4. Rex DK, Sledge G, Harper P, et al. Colonic neoplasia in asymptomatic persons with negative fecal occult blood tests: influence of age, gender, and family history. Am J Gastroenterol. 1993;88:825–31.
5. Lynch KL, Ahnen DJ, Byers T, et al. First-degree relatives of patients with advanced colorectal adenomas have an increased prevalence of colorectal cancer. Clin Gastroenterol Hepatol. 2003;1:96–102.

6. Lieberman DA, Weiss DG, Bond JH, et al. Use of colonoscopy to screen asymptomatic adults for colorectal cancer. Veterans Affairs Cooperative Study Group 380. N Engl J Med. 2000;343:162–8.

7. Brenner H, Chang-Claude J, Seiler CM, et al. Protection from colorectal cancer after colonoscopy: a population-based, case–control study. Ann Int Med. 2011;154(1):22–30.

8. Brenner H, Haug U, Volker A, et al. Low risk of colorectal cancer and advanced adenomas more than 10 years after negative colonoscopy. Gastroenterology. 2010;138(3):87–876.

9. Baxter NN, Sutradhar R, Forbes SS, et al. Analysis of administrative data finds endoscopist quality measures associated with postcolonoscopy colorectal cancer. Gastroenterology. 2011;140:65–72.

10. Rex DK, Petrini JL, Baron TH, et al. Quality indicators for colonoscopy. Am J Gastroenterol. 2006;101:873–85.

11. Chen SC, Rex DK. Endoscopist can be more powerful than age and male gender in predicting adenoma detection at colonoscopy. Am J Gastroenterol. 2007;102:856–61.

12. Barclay RL, Vicari JJ, Doughty AS, et al. Colonoscopic withdrawal times and adenoma detection during screening colonoscopy. N Engl J Med. 2006;355:2533–41.

13. Cotton PB, Connor P, McGee D, et al. Colonoscopy: practice variation among 69 hospital-based endoscopists. Gastrointest Endosc. 2003;57:352–7.

14. Van Rijn JC, Reitsma JB, Stoker J, et al. Polyp miss rate determined by tandem colonoscopy: a systematic review. Am J Gastroenterol. 2006;101:343–50.

15. Harris JK, Froehlich F, Wietlisbach V, et al. Factors associated with the technical performance of colonoscopy: an EPAGE Study. Dig Liver Dis. 2007;39:678–89.

16. Kaminski MF, Regula J, Kraszewska E, et al. Quality indicators for colonoscopy and the risk of interval cancer. N Engl J Med. 2010;362:1795–803.

17. Gurudu SR, Ratuapli SK, Leighton JA, et al. Adenoma detection rate is not influenced by timing of colonoscopy when performed in half-day blocks. Am J Gastroenterol. 2011;106:1466–71.

18. Lee A, Iskander JM, Gupta N, et al. Queue position in the endoscopic schedule impacts effectiveness of colonoscopy. Am J Gastroenterol. 2011;106:1457–65.

19. Chan MY, Cohen H, Spiegel B. Fewer polyps detected by colonoscopy as the day progresses at a veteran's administration teaching hospital. Clin Gastroentrol Hepatol. 2009;7(11):1217–23.

20. Sanaka MR, Deepinder F, Thota PN, et al. Adenomas are detected more often in morning than in afternoon colonoscopy. Am J Gastroenterol. 2009;104:1659–64.

21. Gaba DM, Howard SK. Patient safety: fatigue among clinicians and the safety of patients. N Engl J Med. 2002;347:1249–55.

22. Summers R. The elephant in the room: bowel preparation for CT colonography. Acad Radiol. 2009;16:777–9.

23. Lebwohl B, Kastrios F, Glick M, et al. The impact of suboptimal bowel preparation on adenoma miss rates and the factors associated with early repeat colonoscopy. Gastrointest Endosc. 2011;73(6):1207–14.

24. Harewood GC, Sharma VK, de Garmo P. Impact of colonoscopy preparation quality on detection of suspected colonic neoplasia. Gastrointest Endosc. 2003;58:76–9.

25. Froehlich F, Wietlisbach V, Gonvers J-J, et al. Impact of colonic cleansing on quality and diagnostic yield of colonoscopy: the European Panel of Appropriateness of Gastrointestinal Endoscopy European multicenter study. Gastrointest Endosc. 2005;61:378–84.

26. Sharma VK, Chockalingham SK, Ugheoke EA, et al. Prospective, randomized, controlled comparison of the use of polyethylene glycol electrolyte lavage solution in four-liter versus two-liter volumes and pretreatment with either magnesium citrate or bisacodyl for colonoscopy preparation. Gastrointest Endosc. 1998;47:167–71.

27. Ell C, Fischbach W, Bronisch H-J, et al. Randomized trial of low-volume PEG solution versus standard PEG + electrolytes for bowel cleansing before colonoscopy. Am J Gastroenterol. 2008;103:883–93.

28. Desmeules S, Bergeron MJ, Isenring P. Acute phosphate nephropathy and renal failure. N Engl J Med. 2003;349:1006–7.

29. Carl DE, Sica DA. Acute phosphate nephropathy following colonoscopy preparation. Am J Med Sci. 2007;334(3):151–4.

30. Rex DK, DiPalma JA, Rodriguez R, et al. A randomized clinical study comparing reduced-volume oral sulfate solution with standard 4-liter sulfate-free electrolyte lavage solution as preparation for colonoscopy. Gastrointest Endosc. 2010;72(2):328–36.

31. Cohen LB. Split dosing of bowel preparations for colonoscopy: an analysis of its efficacy, safety, and tolerability. Gastrointest Endosc. 2010;72(2):406–12.

32. Siddiqui AA, Yang K, Spechler SJ, et al. Duration of the interval between the completion of bowel preparation and the start of colonoscopy predicts bowel-preparation quality. Gastrointest Endosc. 2009;69 Suppl 3:700–6.

33. Church JM. Effectiveness of polyethylene glycol antegrade gut lavage bowel preparation for colonoscopy – timing is the key! Dis Colon Rectum. 1998; 41:1223–5.

34. Brenner H, Chang-Claude J, Seiler CM. Protection from colorectal cancer after colonoscopy: a population-based, case-control study. Ann Int Med. 2011; 154(1):222–30.

35. Aoun E, Abdul-Baki H, Azar C, et al. A randomized single-blind trial of split-dose PEG-electrolyte solution without dietary restriction compared with whole dose PEG-electrolyte solution with dietary restriction for colonoscopy preparation. Gastrointest Endosc. 2005;62:213–8.

36. Chiu H-M, Lin J-T, Wang H-P, et al. The impact of colon preparation timing on colonoscopic detection of colorectal neoplasms – a prospective endoscopist-blinded randomized trial. Am J Gastroenterol. 2006;101:2719–25.

37. Cohen LB, Kastenberg DM, Mount DB, et al. Current issues in optimal bowel preparation: excerpts from a

roundtable discussion among colon-cleansing experts. Gastroenterol Hepatol. 2009;5 Suppl 20:1–11.

38. Corley DA, Jensen CD, Marks AR. Can we improve adenoma detection rates? A systematic review of intervention studies. Gastrointest Endosc. 2011;74(3):656–66.

39. Imperiale TF, Blowinski EA, Juliar BE, et al. Variation in polyp detection rates at screening colonoscopy. Gastrointest Endosc. 2009;69(7):1288–95.

40. Lin OS, Kozarek RA, Arai A, et al. The effect of periodic monitoring and feedback on screening colonoscopy withdrawal times, polyp detection rates, and patient satisfaction scores. Gastrointest Endosc. 2010;71(7):1253–9.

41. Cohen L, Delaney P, Boston P. Listening to the customer: implementing a patient satisfaction measurement system. Gastroenterol Nurs. 1994;17:110–5.

42. Denis B, Weiss AM, Peter A, et al. Quality assurance and gastrointestinal endoscopy: an audit of 500 colonoscopic procedures. Gastroenterol Clin Biol. 2004;28:1245–55.

43. Lin OS, Schembre DB, Ayub K, et al. Patient satisfaction scores for endoscopic procedures: impact of a survey-collection method. Gastrointest Endosc. 2007;65:775–81.

44. Brenner DJ, Hall EJ. Computed tomography – an increasing source of radiation exposure. N Engl J Med. 2007;357:2277–84.

45. Pickhardt PJ, Hanson ME, Vanness DJ, et al. Unsuspected extra-colonic findings at screening CT colonography: clinical and economic impact. Radiology. 2008;249:151–9.

46. Zalis ME, Barish MA, Choi JR, et al. CT colonography reporting and data system: a consensus proposal. Radiology. 2005;236:3–9.

47. Volk M, Ubel PA. Less is more. Arch Intern Med. 2011;171(6):487–8.

48. Wang TC, Cominelli F, Fleischer DE, et al. AGA Institute Future Trends Committee report: the future of gastroenterology training programs in the United States. Gastroenterology. 2008;135:1764–89.

49. Pickhardt P, Arluk G. Increasing exposure of gastroenterology fellows to abdominal imaging. Gastrointest Endosc. 2011;73(1):135–7.

50. Young PE, Ray QP, Hwang I, et al. Gastroenterologists' interpretation of CTC: a pilot study demonstrating feasibility and similar accuracy compared to radiologists' interpretation. Am J Gastroenterol. 2009;104:2926–31.

51. Rockey D, Barish M, Brill J, et al. CT colonography standards: standards for gastroenterologists for performing and interpreting diagnostic computed tomographic colonography. Gastroenterology. 2007;133:1005–24.

52. ACR practice guideline for the performance of computed tomography (CT) colonography in adults. http://www.acr.org/SecondaryMainMenuCategories/quality_safety/guidelines/dx/gastro/ct_colonography.aspx. Accessed 1 Oct 2011.

53. Duncan J, Ugochukwu ON, Sweeney WB, et al. Key features of an efficient colorectal cancer screening program based on CT colonography. Gastrointest Endosc. 2011;73(4):AB141.

54. Hur C, Gazelle GS, Zalis ME, et al. An analysis of the potential impact of computed tomographic colonography (virtual colonoscopy) on colonoscopy demand. Gastroenterology. 2004;127:1312–21.

55. Schwartz DC, Dasher KJ, Said A, et al. Impact of a CT colonography screening program on endoscopic colonoscopy in clinical practice. Am J Gastroenterol. 2008;103:346–51.

56. Benson ME, Pier J, Kraft S, et al. Impact of a CT colonography colorectal cancer screening program on optical colonoscopy: 5 year data. Gastrointest Endosc. 2010;71(5):AB129.

57. Ladabaum U, Song K. Projected national impact of colorectal cancer screening on clinical and economic outcomes and health services demand. Gastroenterology. 2005;129:1151–62.

58. Pickhardt PJ, Kim DH. CT colonography (virtual colonoscopy): a practical approach for population screening. Radiol Clin North Am. 2007;45:361–75.

59. Centers for Medicare and Medicaid Services. Cost-effectiveness of CT colonography to screen for colorectal cancer. http://www.cms.gov/determinationprocess/downloads/id58TA.pdf. Accessed 21 Aug 2011.

60. McHugh M, Osei-Anto A, Klabunde CN, Galen BA. Adoption of CT colonography by US hospitals. J Am Coll Radiol. 2011;8(3):169–74.

61. California Technology Assessment Forum. Computed tomographic colonography (virtual colonoscopy) for colorectal cancer screening in average risk individuals. http://www.ctaf.org/files/989_file_VC_final_W.pdf. Accessed 21 Aug 2011.

62. Knudsen AB, Lansdorp-Vogelaar I, Rutter CM, et al. Cost-effectiveness of computed tomographic colonography screening for colorectal cancer in the Medicare population. J Natl Cancer Inst. 2010;102:1238–52.

63. Rockey DC. Computed tomographic colonography: current perspectives and future directions. Gastroenterology. 2009;137:7–17.

64. Mergener K. The role of CT colonography in a colorectal cancer screening program. Gastrointest Endosc Clin North Am. 2010;20(2):367–77.

65. Johnson CD, Chen MH, Toledano AY, et al. Accuracy of CT colonography for detection of large adenomas and cancers. N Engl J Med. 2008;359:1207–17.

66. Pickhardt PJ. CTC interpretation by gastroenterologists: feasible but largely impractical, undesirable, and misguided. Am J Gastroenterol. 2009;104:2932–4.

67. Chin M, Mendelson R, Edwards J, et al. Computed tomographic colonography: prevalence, nature, and clinical significance of extracolonic findings in a community screening program. Am J Gastroenterol. 2005;100:2771–6.

68. Update on CT colonography. Technology Status Evaluation Report. Gastrointest Endosc. 2009;69(3)393–98.

69. Barclay RL, Vicari JJ, Greenlaw RL. Effect of a time-dependent colonoscopic withdrawal protocol on adenoma detection during screening colonoscopy. Clin Gastroenterol Hepatol. 2008;6:1091–8.

CTC Controversies (Radiation Exposure, Extracolonic Findings, Cost-Effectiveness)

7

Andrea Laghi, Franco Iafrate, Maria Ciolina, and Paolo Baldassari

Introduction

CT colonography (CTC) is now in its mature stage. The technique has been consistently standardized [1], different multicenter trials [2–5] and meta-analysis [6] have confirmed the high accuracy in detecting cancer and significant polyps. CTC has completely replaced barium enema in many institutions worldwide, because of its superior diagnostic capability [7], and different indications for its use in current clinical practice have been defined with the agreement of gastroenterologists. CTC is now considered the method of choice to investigate the colon in cases of incomplete colonoscopy (OC) [8] and also in elderly and frail patients [9, 10], where the use of OC might be too risky. Moreover, according to the colorectal cancer (CRC) screening guidelines released in March 2008 by a multidisciplinary joint commission of the American Cancer Society, the US Multi-society Task Force on Colorectal Cancer (comprising three gastroenterology societies), and the American College of Radiology, CTC is also considered one of the preferred CRC screening tests for asymptomatic, average-risk individuals [11]. Unfortunately, especially when the discussion comes to the topic of CRC screening, the debate about the possible use of CTC remains. Other scientific entities, such as the US Preventive Services Task Force (USPSTF) [12], the Asia Pacific Working Group on Colorectal Cancer [13], and the American College of Gastroenterology [14], consider the evidence still insufficient to recommend CTC as a preferred CRC screening test and raise some concerns related to its potential harms. Those concerns were also at the basis of the 2009 decision of the Centers for Medicare and Medicaid (CMS) to not provide reimbursement for screening CTC [15].

Among the potential harms mentioned by the opponents of CTC, the potential biological risks related to radiation exposure, economic and noneconomic impact of detection and management of extracolonic findings, and cost-effectiveness represent the major controversies.

Radiation Exposure

The main potential drawback of screening with CTC is the exposure to ionizing radiation and the consequential theoretical risk of inducing a cancer that is inherent with the technique [16]. The risk is theoretical because there are still many uncertainties with regard to the true effects of ionizing radiation, since there are no markers that unequivocally identify a cancer as being radiation induced as opposed to arising de novo [17].

A. Laghi, M.D. (✉)
Department of Radiological, Oncological and Pathological Sciences, "Sapienza" University of Rome, Via Le Regina Elena 324, 00161 Rome, Italy
e-mail: andrea.laghi@uniroma1.it

F. Iafrate, M.D. • M. Ciolina, M.D. • P. Baldassari, M.D.
Department of Radiological, Oncological and Pathological Sciences, "Sapienza" University of Rome, Rome, Italy

B.D. Cash (ed.), *Colorectal Cancer Screening and Computerized Tomographic Colonography: A Comprehensive Overview*, DOI 10.1007/978-1-4614-5943-9_7, © Springer Science+Business Media New York 2013

Moreover, the largest amount of information about the stochastic effect of ionizing radiation as the reason for increased cancer risk is based on long-term observational studies of survivors of the atomic bombing of Japan in the 1940s. This means that the carcinogenic risk induced by low doses of ionizing radiation has been extrapolated by data collected in populations exposed to very high doses of ionizing radiation using the linear no-threshold (LNT) model [18]. The LNT relationship implies proportionality between dose and cancer risk. This model was introduced in order to facilitate radiation protection, and it works well for high-dose radiation exposures. This is not the case for low doses, where biologic data demonstrate that the body's defense mechanisms against radiation-induced carcinogenesis are multiple and powerful and epidemiological data show that there is no convincing evidence of a carcinogenic effect in humans or experimental animals for doses lower than 100 mGy [19]. Those are the reasons why, according to the Health Physics Society (HPS), "below 5–10 rem [50–100 mSv] (which includes occupational and environmental exposures), risk of health effects are either too small to be observed or are nonexistent" [20]. Nevertheless, the controversy continues to exist. Recently, the French Academy of Sciences and National Academy of Medicine, in a joint report [21], concluded that the LNT hypothesis for assessing the risk associated with low doses "is not based on scientific evidence" [19]. In contrast, the Biological Effects of Ionizing Radiation (BEIR) VII report [22] and that of the International Commission on Radiological Protection (ICRP) [23], largely based on data from Japanese atomic bomb survivors, but also taking into account some of the potential inaccuracies, recommended the use of the LNT model.

Even if the conservative LNT hypothesis is considered to be a valid tool for gauging risk associated with low-dose radiation exposure, the problem of radiation delivery to patients undergoing screening CTC appears to be negligible for several reasons: (1) the mean radiation exposure in screening CTC examinations is low, (2) the benefits associated with screening for CRC outweigh the risks of radiation-induced disease, and (3) epidemiological data from populations of occupational exposures provide an indirect evidence of absence of radiation-induced damage.

Mean Radiation Exposure in Screening CTC Examinations Is Low

Numerous studies have been conducted in order to assess the minimum acceptable dose to be delivered in CTC examinations while maintaining a reasonable image quality [24, 25]. As a result of these studies, it is clear that performance of high-quality CTC with low-dose radiation exposure is possible [26]. In a first European survey, published in 2002 [27], the median effective dose in CTC screening examinations was calculated to be around 8.8 mSv, which subsequently decreased to around 5.6 mSv 6 years later [28]. The theoretical risk of radiation-induced cancer decreased from 0.02% at 8 mSv to around 0.01% at 5 mSv. Recently, updated ESGAR guidelines [29] suggested screening individuals with CTC using ≤50 mAs for both prone and supine positions, excepting overweight patients. With this approach, the radiation dose would be further reduced to a level (around 3.6 mSv) that is slightly higher than annual background radiation, which in Europe is around 2.5–3.0 mSv/year [30].

Further reduction of radiation exposure can now be obtained, thanks to the new iterative reconstruction algorithm available on recent MDCT scanners [31]. This algorithm differs from the current reconstruction method, the filtered back projections, and has the potential to reduce image noise on low-dose images, thereby preserving and enhancing image quality. This method can be modulated according to the percentage of desired dose reduction. As a drawback, the higher the percentage used, the longer (up to more than 30%) is the time required for image reconstruction [32]. In the case of CTC, the use of iterative reconstruction method allows us to achieve a reduction of dose exposure up to 50% [33] (Fig. 7.1).

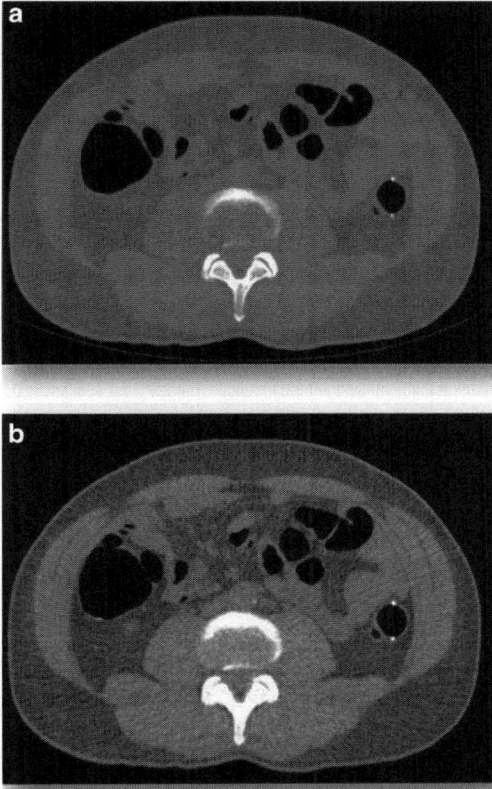

Fig. 7.1 Low-dose CT colonography examination obtained with 120 kVp, 50 mAs, and iterative reconstruction algorithm, 50%: overall dose exposure was 2.76 mSv for both prone and supine scans. Colon (**a**) and abdominal (**b**) windows demonstrate high image quality despite low-dose protocol

Benefits Outweigh Risks

Benefit-risk considerations, when dealing with radiation exposure and subsequent potential biological damage, are mandatory, and even using the upper uncertainty bounds of the risk estimates, the benefit-risk ratio is in favor of CTC screening. An interesting publication [34] recently addressed this issue. The aim of this study was to assess the benefit-risk ratio between cancers prevented and theoretically induced by a CRC screening program using CTC. Results of the study (based on an estimated mean effective dose per CTC examination of 8 mSv in women

and 7 mSv in men and on a screening interval of five years) demonstrated that the estimated number of radiation-related cancers was 150 cases/100,000 individuals screened, compared with the estimated number of CRC prevented by CTC, ranging between 3,580 and 5,190 cases/100,000 individuals screened. The consequent benefit-risk ratio, ranging between 24:1 and 35:1, if considering cancer cases, and becoming even higher if taking into account cancer deaths, was clearly in favor of CTC. Moreover, the authors also calculated the potential impact of radiation-related risk from CT exams performed to follow-up extracolonic findings, demonstrating that this additional radiation exposure does not have any significant impact.

A further improvement of benefit-risk ratio might come from the increased length of time interval between negative CTC exams. If CTC accuracy is confirmed to be quite close to OC, a 10-year interval for CTC can be hypothesized, thus reducing the radiation risks by another 50%. For future discussion, we should also consider the possibility of performing a screening examination once in an individual life, similar to what has been proposed with sigmoidoscopy [35]. In that case, radiation exposure would have a minimal impact, particularly considering that the age of the examination might be at around 58 years, when biological risk is further reduced.

Epidemiological Data from Populations of Occupational Exposures Provide an Indirect Evidence of Absence of Radiation-Induced Damage

Indirect evidence of the very low risk of radiation-induced cancer in patients undergoing CTC originates from studies conducted in selected populations with occupational exposure to radiation risk: airline crews and workers of nuclear plants. For example, airline crews are exposed to an average radiation dose of 5 mSv/year, and an airline pilot has a lifelong exposure close to 80 mSv [36]. A survey of airline pilots in eight European countries found no increase in mortality for radiation-induced cancer over a 30-year

Table 7.1 Classification of extracolonic findings according to C-RADS (CTC Reporting and Data System) [49]

CT Colonography Reporting and Data System (C-RADS)	
E0	Limited exam. Compromised by artifact; evaluation of extracolonic soft tissues is severely limited
E1	Normal exam or anatomic variant. No extracolonic abnormalities visible (a) Anatomic variant: e.g., retroaortic left renal vein
E2	Clinically unimportant finding. No work-up indicated. Examples: (a) Liver and kidney: simple cysts (b) Gallbladder: cholelithiasis without cholecystitis (c) Vertebra: hemangioma
E3	Likely unimportant finding, incompletely characterized. Subject to local practice and patient preference, work-up may be indicated. Examples: (a) Kidney: minimally complex or homogeneously hyperattenuating cysts
E4	Potentially important finding. Communicate to referring physician as per accepted practice guidelines (a) Kidney: solid renal mass (b) Lymphadenopathy (c) Vasculature: aortic aneurysm (d) Lung: nonuniformly calcified parenchymal nodule ≥1 cm

period [37]. Similar findings were observed in nuclear workers in two recently published studies [38, 39]. Thus, at the moment, "whilst there is no level of radiation exposure below which effects do not occur, current evidence indicates that the probability of airline crew or passengers suffering adverse health effects as a result of exposure to cosmic radiation is very low" [40].

Extracolonic Findings

A possible advantage of CTC, but also a challenge, is the detection of extracolonic findings (ECFs) [41]. ECFs represent a mixed blessing. On one hand, they offer the screened individual the reassurance if absent. If detected, however, they can be a source of anxiety, inconvenience, potential complications, and added costs related to additional work-up, particularly for benign and unimportant findings. Care of ECFs should be taken, since with holding or not reviewing scanned regions of the body raises clinical and ethical implications. And the medicolegal consequences of ignoring ECFs would be probably more important than those of responsibly managing them. Responsibility in the management of ECFs is extremely important in order to avoid the risk of practicing defensive medicine, a potential source of further increases in costs and burdens for the healthcare system [42].

Definition and Categorization of ECFs

ECFs could be defined as asymptomatic and unsuspected findings that are unrelated to the colon and incidentally detected during CTC examinations with a potential serious effect on an individual patient's health [43]. This definition excludes findings such as anatomic anomalies and changes related to post-traumatic events or previous surgery. Most ECFs detected during CTC with serious clinical relevance include solid renal mass, hepatic nodules, noncalcified pulmonary nodules (>1 cm), lymphadenopathy, and abdominal aorta aneurysms [43, 44]. To facilitate standardized communication of ECFs identified with CTC, different systems of categorization have been proposed, mainly based on the level of clinical importance [44–48]. In particular, the international Working Group on Virtual Colonoscopy proposed a classification system known as C-RADS (CTC Reporting and Data System) [49], analogous to the well-known Breast Imaging Reporting and Data System (BI-RADS) for mammography [50]. C-RADS classifies ECFs on the basis of their importance and potential need for further work-up (Table 7.1) (Fig. 7.2).

Although most of ECFs do not have any clinical relevance, the ability to definitively characterize incidental findings and to differentiate a benign lesion from a malignancy is often limited, if not impossible, from CTC images. This is due

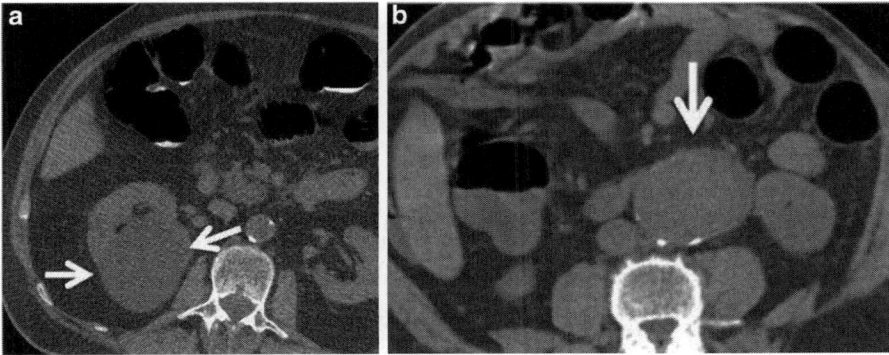

Fig. 7.2 Two examples of extracolonic findings (**a**) E2, simple renal cyst (*arrows*) and (**b**) E4, abdominal aortic aneurysm (*arrow*)

to the lack of routine injection of intravenous contrast medium and the use of low-dose technique with CTC, resulting in wide variability of detection and characterization of ECFs among radiologists [51].

Prevalence of ECFs

The prevalence of ECFs is variable. It has been reported to range between 5% [52] and 25% [53] if only major findings are considered, but if also including minor or moderate ECFs, it is much higher, increasing to 60–70% [54]. This discrepancy may be related to differences in patient selection, definitions, and reporting thresholds of extracolonic abnormalities. In general, older patients have a higher frequency of ECFs [55]. This is also true in symptomatic patients compared with asymptomatic patients [56, 57]. It should be clear, however, that most ECFs will ultimately prove to be of little or no clinical relevance; thus, recommendations for further diagnostic work-up must be carefully considered.

ECF-Related Costs and Benefits

The major issue concerning ECFs is the extra time necessary for reporting and the costs induced by unnecessary investigations of common benign abnormalities. The reporting of suspicious ECFs may lead to additional examinations, necessary for better characterization, potentially inducing a "cascade effect" of additional exams [51]. Additional procedures result in increased costs and risks of morbidity (and rarely mortality) due to invasive diagnostic examinations and surgical interventions.

Some studies have recently estimated costs and benefits of CTC including detection of ECFs. In the prospective study of Xiong et al. [58], an average cost of $297 per patient, considering not only initial diagnostic costs but also all downstream expenses (e.g., interventional procedures, surgery, and hospitalizations), was calculated. The estimated overall cost was 46% greater than the value of CTC examination. This figure is quite distant from the results obtained in two previous studies that estimated the cost of ECFs to be $28 [44] and $67 [45], respectively, per patient. Differences among these studies are mainly related to the calculation of downstream costs, in particular surgical procedures, accounting for 87% of the total amount.

However, ECFs can also be considered a potential benefit (i.e., detection of unsuspected abdominal aortic aneurysm or renal cancer at a curable stage) that improves the overall cost-effectiveness of CTC. It should not be forgotten that extracolonic cancers are more frequent than CRC. In a screening of average-risk population, extracolonic malignancies are encountered in 1/250 patients, whereas the expected prevalence of CRC is around 1/400–500 individuals [42].

In a study published by Hassan et al. [59], a cost-effectiveness analysis on a simulated average-risk population of 100,000 subjects was performed, comparing CTC, including the detection of ECF, and OC both with and without abdominal ultrasonography for abdominal aortic aneurysm detection. Results of the model demonstrated that when detection of ECFs were considered in addition to CRC, CTC is a dominant screening strategy (i.e., more effective and less expensive) compared with both OC and OC with 1-time ultrasonography.

Management of ECFs

The most important task for radiologists approaching CTC is to report clinically relevant ECFs, avoiding misdiagnosis of severe disease and taking into account the need for limiting a possible increase of costs related to excessive recommendations for additional imaging. This can be achieved if experienced abdominal radiologists, trained in CT interpretation, are used for interpreting and reporting. In a recent study [60], trained radiologists had similar rate of recommendations for additional imaging (6.0% and 4.4%, respectively) in two populations of patients (seniors and nonseniors) with a clear difference in the number of ECFs (74% versus 55%). In other words, it is not the prevalence of ECFs that is implicated with the rate of recommendations, but rather the experience of the readers. The consequences of a low rate of recommendations for additional imaging are obvious.

Cost-Effectiveness

Reasons for discussing cost-effectiveness have their basis in the fact that before a test is adopted for screening, in this particular case CRC screening, cost-effectiveness must be demonstrated. Given the large budget deficits most countries currently face, it is of great importance that resources be used efficiently and that any new options for CRC screening be cost-effective. In fact, while many available tests are variously effective for the detection of CRC and its precursors, there are still many uncertainties about relative cost-effectiveness [61]. This has resulted in a wide variety of screening strategies being offered worldwide and also in conflicting data among guidelines published by different authorities. The case of CTC is emblematic: on the one hand, according to multidisciplinary joint commission of the American Cancer Society, the US Multi-society Task Force on Colorectal Cancer, and the American College of Radiology, CTC is recommended as a potential CRC screening test in average-risk individuals [11]. Conversely, the adoption of CTC is considered not supported by sufficient evidence according to the guidelines from USPSTF [12]. These different opinions underscore the fact that cost analysis is a very difficult task, especially in the absence of real data, and necessarily based only on mathematical models.

Among the seven studies published in the literature [62–68], only two are in favor of CTC, demonstrating that CTC was dominant (i.e., less expensive and more effective) over flexible sigmoidoscopy and cost effective compared with OC (i.e., showing a favorable incremental cost-effectiveness ratio, ICER). However, a subsequent review of the literature [69] pointed out the profound differences among the different models used in these studies, as well as the weakness of this mathematical approach, where a minimal variation of a single input may completely alter the final results. As an example, if the cost ratio between CTC and OC is ≤70%, the model is usually in favor of CTC. If, however, the cost of CTC is higher than 80% of the cost of OC, then OC is the most cost-effective method.

Other variables, with the potential to deeply affect models and consequent evaluation of effectiveness, should be taken into consideration: natural history assumptions related to colorectal polyps and population screening adherence rate. The key feature of natural history is the dwell time of preclinical disease: dwell time of CRC vary from 8 to 25 years across models and help explain differences in projected screening effectiveness [70]. Another very important issue, screening adherence rate, is rarely taken into account in cost-effectiveness models [69]. If it is considered, it is typically considered with a baseline of 100% with subsequent reduced screening adherence scenarios hypothesized and applied equally to all screening tests [71]. As we all know, this is absolutely not true, as shown by recent published data of the COCOS trial, demonstrating a clear advantage of CTC over OC in terms of the screening adherence rate of the invited population of screening individuals [72]. Adherence rate is one of the major variables affecting the positive outcome of a screening program, since low adherence may dilute the benefits of a very accurate test, making it less efficient in terms of cancer prevention compared with a test with lower accuracy but higher penetration in the population. As an example, if we consider the efficiency of a screening program in preventing cancer as the product between efficacy of the test and adherence, OC, with an efficacy of around 85%, would prevent exactly 85% of the cancer in the screened population only if each single individual would be part of the program (adherence = 100%). But if adherence drops to 9%, the efficiency of a program using OC would be 7.6% (efficiency of OC = efficacy, 85% × adherence, 9%). This means that if we use a less effective test (e.g., FOBT with a reported efficacy in CRC cancer of around 16–33%) but with higher adherence (e.g., 50%), the overall efficiency of a FOBT program would be 16%, more than two times higher than the OC program and at a definitely lower cost.

Finally, unequivocal data, at least in Europe, are almost impossible to collect, because of the differences in the multitude of healthcare systems, reimbursement, cost of equipment, and personnel, all of which are additional important variables affecting the final outcome of cost-effectiveness. Thus, cost-effective analyses remain an important tool in the hands of policy makers, but their results do not speak for themselves. There are important uncertainties due to the inherent theoretical assumptions of these analyses and to the difficulties in quantifying benefits and harms of each individual test [73].

Conclusions

Biological risks related to radiation exposure, economical and noneconomical impact of detection and management of ECFs, and cost-effectiveness represent the major controversies of CTC and its positioning as an acceptable CRC screening modality. While additional data has become available that has clarified some of these issues, the discussion and uncertainty around all three issues still exists. Additional evidence geared toward providing more definitive estimates of the direction and magnitude of these issues is needed. Given the data that has accumulated over the last decade, it is likely that additional analyses will continue to support CTC as a viable and acceptable CRC screening modality.

Key Points

- Major controversies of CTC are represented by biological risks of radiation exposure, impact of detection and management of extracolonic findings, and cost-effectiveness.
- Carcinogenic risk of low-dose radiation exposure is still under debate, but the amount of radiation delivered during screening CTC examination is low, and it will become even lower with advances in CT technology.
- The benefit-risk ratio of using CTC as a CRC screening test has been estimated to range between 25:1 and 35:1, thus in clear favor of CTC.
- Indirect evidence derived from selected populations with occupational exposure to radiation risk indicates that the probability of adverse health effects as a result of exposure to ionizing radiation is extremely low.
- Extracolonic findings have high prevalence, but only a minority have clinical relevance; they are more common in symptomatic and elderly patients.
- Extracolonic findings represent not only an extra cost (due to recommendations for additional imaging and/or follow-up), but they can

be considered a unique opportunity to improve cost-effectiveness of screening CTC.

- The most important task for CT colonographers is to report clinically relevant extracolonic findings, avoiding misdiagnoses of severe diseases and limiting excessive recommendations for additional imaging.
- Cost-effective analyses are an important instrument in the hands of policy makers, but their results do not speak for themselves. There are important uncertainties due to theoretical assumptions and to the difficulties in quantifying benefits and harms of each single test.

References

1. Taylor SA, Laghi A, Lefere P, et al. European Society of Gastrointestinal and Abdominal Radiology (ESGAR): consensus statement on CT colonography. Eur Radiol. 2007;17:575–9.
2. Johnson CD, Chen MH, Toledano AY, et al. Accuracy of CT colonography for detection of large adenomas and cancers. N Engl J Med. 2008;359:1207–17.
3. Regge D, Laudi C, Galatola G, et al. Diagnostic accuracy of computed tomographic colonography for the detection of advanced neoplasia in individuals at increased risk of colorectal cancer. JAMA. 2009;301: 2453–61.
4. Graser A, Stieber P, Nagel D, et al. Comparison of CT colonography, colonoscopy, sigmoidoscopy and faecal occult blood tests for the detection of advanced adenoma in an average risk population. Gut. 2009;58:241–8.
5. Halligan S, Lilford RJ, Wardle J, et al. Design of a multicentre randomized trial to evaluate CT colonography versus colonoscopy or barium enema for diagnosis of colonic cancer in older symptomatic patients: the SIGGAR study. Trials. 2007;8:32–41.
6. Chaparro M, Gisbert JP, del Campo L, et al. Accuracy of computed tomographic colonography for the detection of polyps and colorectal tumors: a systematic review and meta-analysis. Digestion. 2009;80:1–17.
7. Sosna J, Sella T, Sy O, et al. Critical analysis of the performance of double-contrast barium enema for detecting colorectal polyps ≥6 mm in the era of CT colonography. Am J Roentgenol. 2008;190:374–85.
8. AGA Clinical Practice and Economics Committee. Position of the American Gastroenterological Association (AGA) Institute on computed tomographic colonography. Gastroenterology. 2006;131:1627–8.
9. Iafrate F, Hassan C, Zullo A, et al. CT colonography with reduced bowel preparation after incomplete colonoscopy in the elderly. Eur Radiol. 2008;18:1385–95.
10. Keeling AN, Slattery MM, Leong S, et al. Limited-preparation CT colonography in frail elderly patients: a feasibility study. Am J Roentgenol. 2010;194:1279–87.
11. Levin B, Lieberman DA, McFarland B, et al. Screening and surveillance for the early detection of colorectal cancer and adenomatous polyps, 2008: a joint guideline from the American Cancer Society, the US Multi-Society Task Force on Colorectal Cancer, and the American College of Radiology. CA Cancer J Clin. 2008;58:130–60.
12. U.S. Preventive Services Task Force. Screening for colorectal cancer: U.S. Preventive Services Task Force recommendation statement. Ann Intern Med. 2008;149:627–37.
13. Sung JJ, Lau JY, Young GP, et al. Asia Pacific consensus recommendations for colorectal cancer screening. Gut. 2008;57:1166–76.
14. Rex DK, Johnson DA, Anderson JC, et al. American College of Gastroenterology guidelines for colorectal cancer screening 2009. Am J Gastroenterol. 2009;104:739–50.
15. Mitka M. Virtual colonoscopy dealt set back with rejection for coverage by medicare. JAMA. 2009;301: 1327–8.
16. Brenner DJ, Georgsson MA. Mass screening with CT colonography: should the radiation exposure be of concern? Gastroenterology. 2005;129:328–37.
17. Amis ES. CT radiation dose: trending in the right direction. Radiology. 2011;261:5–8.
18. Little MP, Wakeford R, Tawn EJ, et al. Risks associated with low doses and low dose rates of ionizing radiation: why linearity may be (almost) the best we can do. Radiology. 2009;251:6–12.
19. Tubiana M, Feinendegen LE, Yang C, et al. The linear no-threshold relationship is inconsistent with radiation biologic and experimental data. Radiology. 2009;251:13–22.
20. Health Physics Society (HPS), editor. Ionizing radiation-safety standards for the general public: Position Statement of the Health Physics Society. McLean: Health Physics Society; 2003. p. 1–3.
21. Tubiana M, Aurengo A, Averbeck D, et al. Dose–effect relationships and the estimation of the carcinogenic effects of low doses of ionizing radiation. Academy of Medicine (Paris) and Academy of Science (Paris) Joint Report No. 2, 30 Mar 2005
22. National Research Council, Committee to assess health risks from exposure to low levels of ionizing radiation. Health risks from low levels of ionizing radiation: BEIR VII, Phase 2. Washington, DC: The National Academies Press; 2006
23. International Commission on Radiological Protection. Low-dose extrapolation of radiation-related cancer risk. Publication 99. Amsterdam, the Netherlands: Elsevier; 2006.
24. van Gelder RE, Venema HW, Florie J, et al. CT colonography: feasibility of substantial dose reduction–comparison of medium to very low doses in identical patients. Radiology. 2004;232:611–20.

25. van Gelder RE, Venema HW, Serlie IW, et al. CT colonography at different radiation dose levels: feasibility of dose reduction. Radiology. 2002;224:25–33.
26. Iannaccone R, Laghi A, Catalano C, et al. Detection of colorectal lesions: lower-dose multi-detector row helical CT colonography compared with conventional colonoscopy. Radiology. 2003;229:775–81.
27. Jensch S, van Gelder RE, Venema HW, et al. Effective radiation doses in CT colonography: results of an inventory among research institutions. Eur Radiol. 2006;16:981–7.
28. Liedenbaum MH, Venema HW, Stoker J. Radiation dose in CT colonography—trends in time and differences between daily practice and screening protocols. Eur Radiol. 2008;18:2222–30.
29. Neri E, Halligan S, Hellstrom M, et al. (2012) The second ESGAR consensus statement on CT colonography. Eur Radiol. 2012 Sep. 15 [Epub ahead of print].
30. Thorne MC. Background radiation: natural and manmade. J Radiol Prot. 2003;23:29–42.
31. May MS, Wüst W, Brand M, et al. Dose reduction in abdominal computed tomography: intraindividual comparison of image quality of full-dose standard and half-dose iterative reconstructions with dual-source computed tomography. Invest Radiol. 2011;46:465–70.
32. Sagara Y, Hara AK, Pavlicek W, et al. Abdominal CT: comparison of low-dose CT with adaptive statistical iterative reconstruction and routine-dose CT with filtered back projection in 53 patients. Am J Roentgenol. 2010;195:713–9.
33. Flicek KT, Hara AK, Silva AC, et al. Reducing the radiation dose for CT colonography using adaptive statistical iterative reconstruction: A pilot study. Am J Roentgenol. 2010;195:126–31.
34. Berrington de González A, Kim KP, Knudsen AB, et al. Radiation-related cancer risks from CT colonography screening: a risk-benefit analysis. Am J Roentgenol. 2011;196:816–23.
35. Atkin WS, Edwards R, Kralj-Hans I, et al. Once-only flexible sigmoidoscopy screening in prevention of colorectal cancer: a multicentre randomised controlled trial. Lancet. 2010;375:1624–33.
36. Hammer GP, Blettner M, Zeeb H. Epidemiological studies of cancer in aircrew. Radiat Prot Dosimetry. 2009;136:232–9.
37. Zeeb H, Blettner M, Langner I, et al. Mortality from cancer and other causes among airline cabin attendants in Europe: a collaborative cohort study in eight countries. Am J Epidemiol. 2003;158:35–46.
38. Guerins S, Richard G, Biau A, et al. Cancer mortality among French nuclear contract workers. Am J Ind Med. 2009;52:916–25.
39. Jeong M, Jin YW, Yang KH, Ann YO, Cha CY. Radiation exposure and cancer incidence in a cohort of nuclear power industry workers in the Republic of Korea, 1992–2005. Radiat Environ Biophys. 2010; 49:47–55.
40. Bagshaw M. Cosmic radiation in commercial aviation. Travel Med Infect Dis. 2008;6:125–7.
41. Ginnerup Pedersen B, Rosenkilde M, Christiansen TE, et al. Extracolonic findings at computed tomography colonography are a challenge. Gut. 2003;52:1744–7.
42. Pickhardt PJ, Hanson ME, Vanness DJ, et al. Unsuspected extracolonic findings at screening CT colonography: clinical and economic impact. Radiology. 2008;249:151–9.
43. Berland LL. Incidental extracolonic findings on CT colonography: the impending deluge & its implications. J Am Coll Radiol. 2009;6:14–20.
44. Hara AK, Johnson CD, MacCarty RL, et al. Incidental extracolonic findings at CT colonography. Radiology. 2000;215:353–7.
45. Gluecker TM, Johnson CD, Wilson LA, et al. Extracolonic findings at CT colonography: evaluation of prevalence and cost in a screening population. Gastroenterology. 2003;124:911–6.
46. Rajapaksa R, Macari M, Bini EJ. Prevalence and impact of extracolonic findings in patients undergoing CT colonography. Am J Gastroenterol. 2002;97:S111–2.
47. Edwards JT, Wood CJ, Mendelson RM, et al. Extracolonic findings at virtual colonoscopy: implications for screening programs. Am J Gastroenterol. 2001;96:3009–12.
48. Yee J, Kumar NN, Godara S, et al. Extracolonic abnormalities discovered incidentally at CT colonography in a male population. Radiology. 2005;236:519–26.
49. Zalis ME, Barish MA, Choi JR, et al. CT colonography reporting and data system: a consensus proposal. Radiology. 2005;236:3–9.
50. American College of Radiology. Breast imaging reporting and data system (BI-RADS). 3rd ed. Reston: Auflage; 1998.
51. Yee J, Sadda S, Aslam R, Yeh B. Extracolonic findings at CT colonography. Gastrointest Endosc Clin N Am. 2010;20:305–22.
52. Pickhardt PJ, Taylor AJ. Extracolonic findings identified in asymptomatic adults at screening CT Colonography. Am J Roentgenol. 2006;186:718–28.
53. Spreng A, Netzer P, Mattich J, et al. Importance of extracolonic findings at IV contrast medium-enhanced CT colonography versus those at non-enhanced CT colonography. Eur Radiol. 2005;15:2088–95.
54. Siddiki H, Fletcher JG, McFarland B, et al. Incidental findings in CT Colonography: literature review and survey of current research practice. J Law Med Ethics. 2008;36:320–31.
55. Ng CS, Doyle TC, Courtney HM, et al. Extracolonic findings in patients undergoing abdomino-pelvic CT for suspected colorectal carcinoma in the frail and disabled patient. Clin Radiol. 2004;59:421–30.
56. Hellstrom M, Svensson MH, Lasson A. Extracolonic and incidental findings on CT colonography (virtual colonoscopy). Am J Roentgenol. 2004;182:631–8.
57. Kim YS, Kim N, Kim SY, et al. Extracolonic findings in an asymptomatic screening population undergoing intravenous contrast-enhanced computed tomography colonography. J Gastroenterol Hepatol. 2008; 23:e49–57.

58. Xiong T, McEvoy K, Morton DG, et al. Resources and costs associated with incidental extracolonic findings from CT colonography: a study in a symptomatic population. Br J Radiol. 2006;79:948–61.

59. Hassan C, Pickhardt P, Laghi A, et al. Computed tomographic colonography to screen for colorectal cancer, extracolonic cancer, and aortic aneurysm: model simulation with cost effectiveness analysis. Arch Intern Med. 2008;168:696–705.

60. Macari M, Nevsky G, Bonavita J, et al. CT colonography in senior versus nonsenior patients: extracolonic findings, recommendations for additional imaging, and polyp prevalence. Radiology. 2011;259:767–74.

61. Lansdorp-Vogelaar I, Knudsen AB. Brenner H. Cost-effectiveness of colorectal cancer screening. Epidemiol Rev. 2011;33:88–100.

62. Sonnenberg A, Delcò F, Bauerfeind P. Is virtual colonoscopy a cost-effective option to screen for colorectal cancer? Am J Gastroenterol. 1999;94:2268–74.

63. Ladabaum U, Song K, Fendrick AM. Colorectal neoplasia screening with virtual colonoscopy: when, at what cost, and with what national impact? Clin Gastroenterol Hepatol. 2004;2:554–63.

64. Vijan S, Hwang I, Inadomi J, et al. The cost-effectiveness of CT colonography in screening for colorectal neoplasia. Am J Gastroenterol. 2007;102:380–90.

65. Pickhardt PJ, Hassan C, Laghi A, et al. Cost-effectiveness of colorectal cancer screening with computed tomography colonography: the impact of not reporting diminutive lesions. Cancer. 2007;109:2213–21.

66. Lin OS, Kozarek RA, Schembre DB, et al. Risk stratification for colon neoplasia: screening strategies using colonoscopy. Gastroenterology. 2006;131:1011–9.

67. Heitman SJ, Manns BJ, Hilsden RJ, et al. Cost-effectiveness of computerized tomographic colonography versus colonoscopy for colorectal cancer screening. CMAJ. 2005;173:877–81.

68. Hassan C, Zullo A, Laghi A, et al. Colon cancer prevention in Italy: cost-effectiveness analysis with CT colonography and endoscopy. Dig Liver Dis. 2007;39:242–50.

69. Mavranezouli I, East JE, Taylor SA. CT colonography and cost-effectiveness. Eur Radiol. 2008;18:2485–97.

70. van Ballegooijen M, Rutter CM, Knudsen AB, et al. Clarifying differences in natural history between models of screening: the case of colorectal cancer. Med Decis Making. 2011;31:540–9.

71. Vanness DJ, Knudsen AB, Lansdorp-Vogelaar I, et al. Comparative economic evaluation of data from the ACRIN National CT colonography trial with three cancer intervention and surveillance modelling network microsimulations. Radiology. 2011;261:487–98.

72. Stoop EM, de Haan MC, de Wijkerslooth TR, et al. Participation and yield of colonoscopy versus non-cathartic CT colonography in population-based screening for colorectal cancer: a randomised controlled trial. Lancet Oncol. 2012;13:55–64.

73. Harris R. Speaking for the evidence: colonoscopy vs. computed tomographic colonography. J Natl Cancer Inst. 2010;102:1212–14.

CTC Pitfalls/Limitations

8

Donald W. Jensen and Duncan Barlow

Introduction

There are numerous pitfalls and artifacts in computed tomography colonography (CTC) interpretation. One must be cognizant of these in order not to overcall pathology and refer patients for unnecessary optical colonoscopies (OC). This chapter will demonstrate the most common pitfalls and artifacts associated with CTC interpretation and provide ways to best analyze and accurately assess these findings. At a minimum, a combined 3-D and 2-D analysis is required to adequately analyze and accurately interpret a CTC. In order to minimize artifacts, one must start with the best 3-D model possible. Many interpretation pitfalls and image artifacts can be avoided when attention is paid to proper patient preparation and image acquisition. A diagnostic quality CTC requires an adequate bowel cleansing prep, stool and fluid tagging with barium and water-soluble contrast agents, adequate patient hydration, mechanical CO_2 insufflation of the colon, and optimal distension of all colon segments (Fig. 8.1a–d).

The artifacts associated with CTC interpretation can be considered in three major categories: (a) bowel preparation-related artifacts, (b) imaging-related pitfalls and artifacts, and (c) anatomical variants. Preparation-related pitfalls and artifacts include retained stool and fluid, retained dense and dilute contrast, and problems related to detection and measuring of submerged polyps. Imaging-related artifacts include segmental spasm, air–fluid interface artifact, electronic cleansing artifact, respiratory motion artifact, image noise or quantum mottle artifact, spray artifact, and data dropout. Anatomical variants include extrinsic compression effects from adjacent structures, stool-filled diverticula, flat and pedunculated polyps, lipomas, rectal veins, hemorrhoids, and variations of the ileocecal valve and appendix. Each of these will be addressed below.

Preparation-Related Pitfalls and Artifacts

All bowel preparations leave behind residual stool and fluid in the colon. Depending on the length and redundancy of the colon, this stool and fluid contamination may be significant. It is imperative that patients understand the significance of following the bowel preparation and stool tagging instructions so that optimal cleansing and tagging can be accomplished. The majority of retained stool and fluid can be adequately tagged and electronically subtracted in most patients. When there is significant stool and fluid contamination present, there may not be complete tagging and electronic cleansing.

D.W. Jensen, M.D. • D. Barlow, M.D. (✉)
Department of Gastroenterology, Walter Reed National Military Medical Center, Bethesda, MD, USA
e-mail: duncans@mcw.edu

B.D. Cash (ed.), *Colorectal Cancer Screening and Computerized Tomographic Colonography: A Comprehensive Overview*, DOI 10.1007/978-1-4614-5943-9_8, © Springer Science+Business Media New York 2013

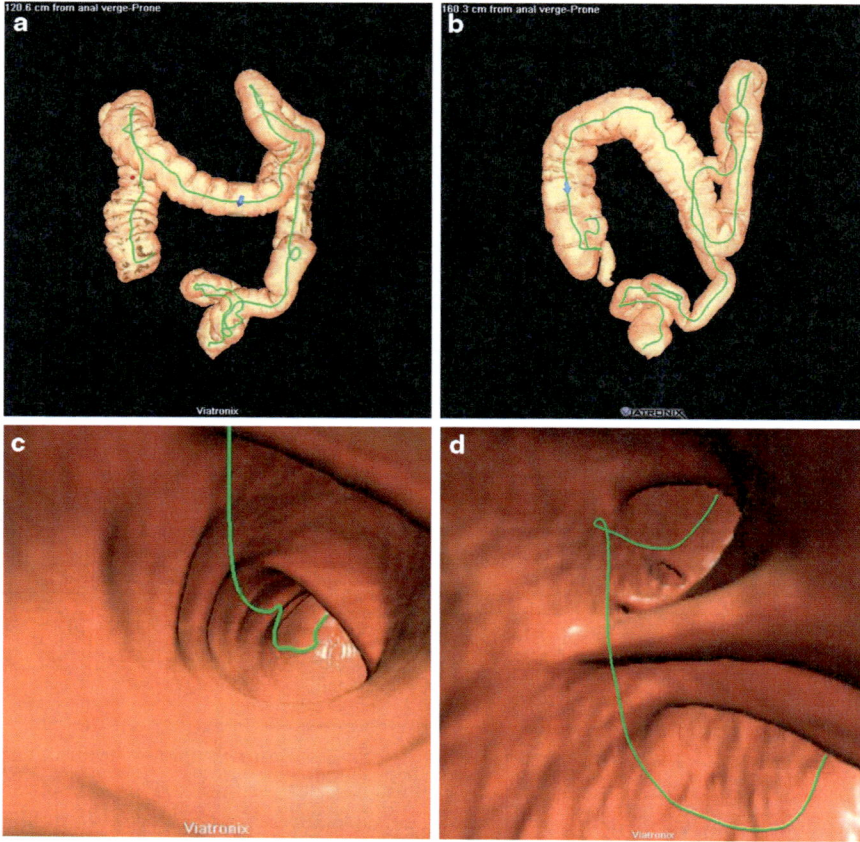

Fig. 8.1 Images (**a**) and (**b**) are normal supine and prone overviews of the colon, demonstrating complete distention from the rectum to cecum. Images (**c**) and (**d**) are normal 3-D endoluminal images demonstrating a smooth mucosal surface with essentially no contamination or adherent stool/barium

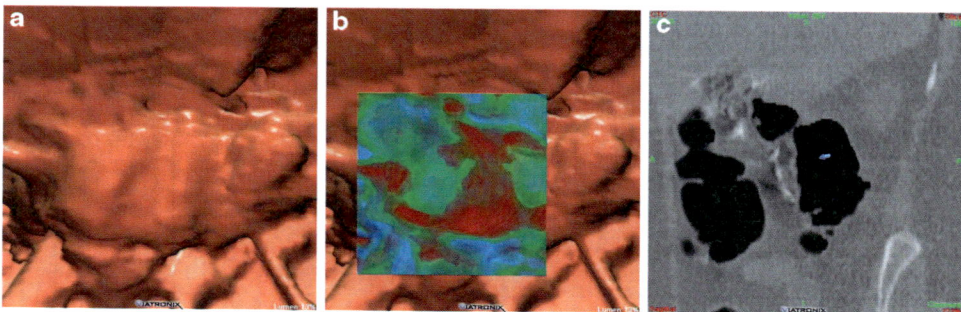

Fig. 8.2 Images (**a**)–(**c**) demonstrate a large collection of stool which contains multiple pockets of air and fecal fat giving it a heterogeneous appearance on the 2-D source and attenuation color window mapping images

Large collections of stool contain small pockets of air and fecal fat that can be easily visualized on 2-D source images and attenuation color mapping (Fig. 8.2a–c). Even moderate-sized stool balls demonstrate this heterogeneous attenuation on 2-D source images and color mapping (Fig. 8.3a–c). Smaller stool balls, however, may not contain significant collections of air or fecal

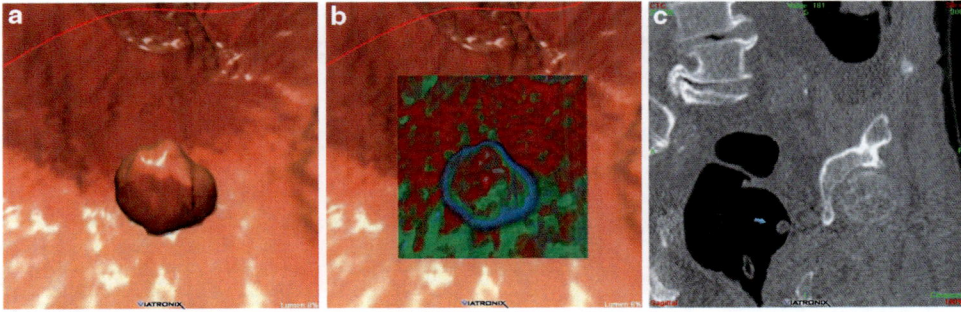

Fig. 8.3 Images (**a**)–(**c**) demonstrate a moderate-sized stool ball containing air and fecal fat also giving it a heterogeneous appearance on the 2-D source and attenuation color window mapping images

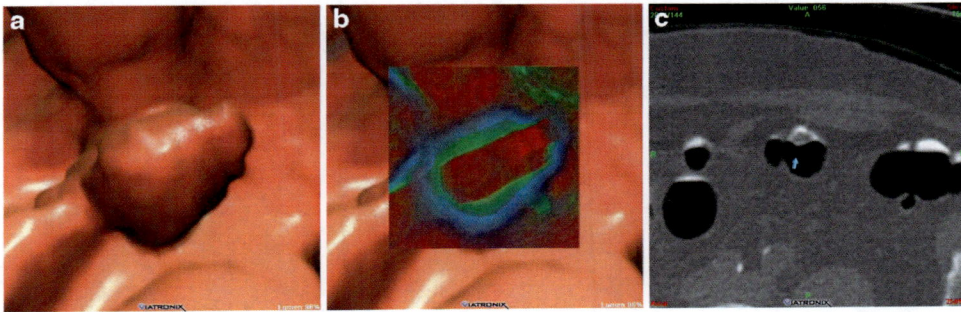

Fig. 8.4 Images (**a**)–(**c**) demonstrate a dense stool ball without internal collections of air and fecal fat which shows the characteristic angulated, squared, or facetted contour of stool

fat and therefore can mimic polyps. To distinguish these small stool balls from true polyps, one must look to the contour and mobility of the lesions in question. Stool balls have an angulated, squared, or facetted contour (Fig. 8.4a–c), and, unless adherent to the colon wall, fall to the dependent portion of the colon on prone and supine views (Fig. 8.5a–d). Figure 8.6a–h demonstrates varying degrees of stool contamination found on CTC.

Retained fluid within the colon can also significantly impair visualization of the colon wall and degrade polyp detection. When there is significant retained fluid present, oral contrast agents will be diluted down to a point below the cutoff for electronic cleansing. As a result, this dilute and tagged fluid will not be subtracted out. This can mask the dependent colon wall on the 3-D endoluminal views. Imaging of the colon in the prone and supine positions is performed in order to shift the dilute fluid to opposing dependent walls or to different segments of colon. This allows for visualization of the colon surface on at least one view (Fig. 8.7a–d). When diluted fluid fills the entire lumen of the colon, 3-D endoluminal visualization of the involved segment cannot be performed. With prone and supine imaging, however, the dilute fluid will typically shift and allow adequate visualization of the colon lumen on at least one view (Fig. 8.8a–f). If there is adequate luminal distension by the residual tagged fluid, the 2-D source CT images can be used to evaluate for polyps or masses. The 2-D source images should be viewed with the electronic cleansing algorithm turned off. Then, just like with solid column barium enema, polyps or masses will be visible as filling defects in the fluid pool on the 2-D CT images (Fig. 8.9a, b).

Dense contrast collections may also decrease sensitivity for polyp detection. Droplets of desiccated barium can adhere to the colon wall and mimic sessile polyps on the endoluminal views. These droplets are usually seen in patients who

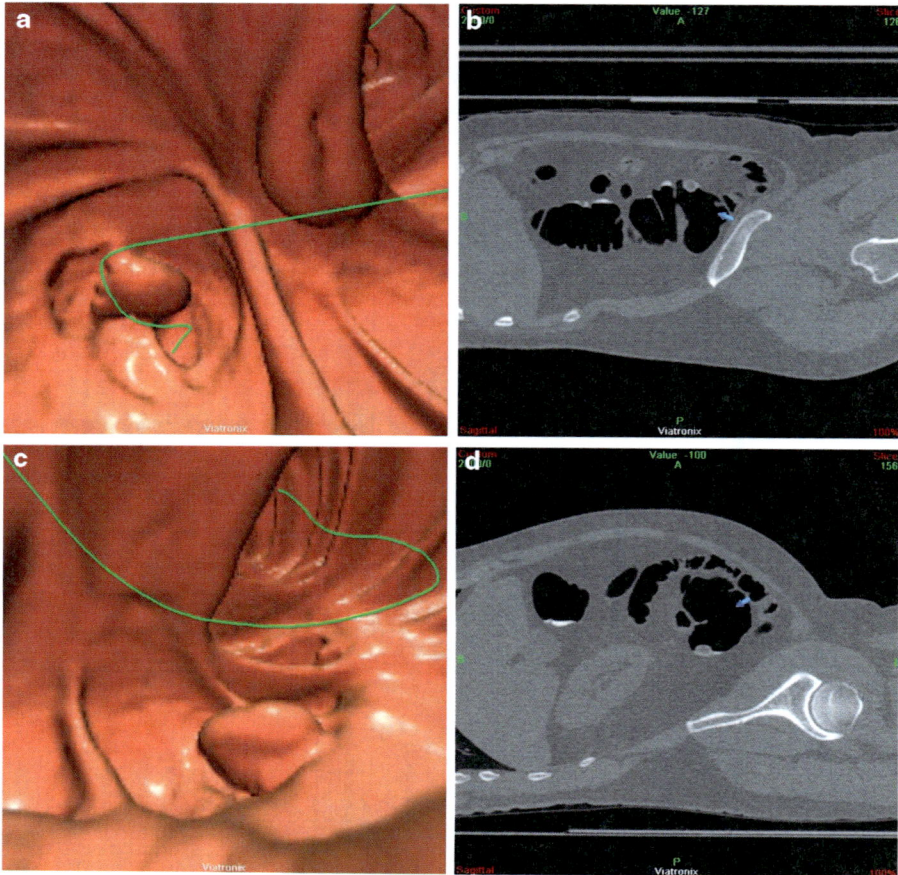

Fig. 8.5 Images (**a**)–(**d**) demonstrate a mobile stool ball in the cecum

did not maintain adequate hydration during the bowel preparation or who did not take the water-soluble contrast agent with the barium tagging agent. The water-soluble contrast agent is hyperosmolar and serves as a wetting agent in the colon, thereby preventing desiccation of the barium droplets on the colon surface. Desiccated barium droplets can be differentiated from true polyps by their high density on both the 2-D source images and colon window images. They make interpretation difficult only due to their increased number (Fig. 8.10a–c). Contrast tagged fluid surrounding submerged polyps can complicate detection and analysis of polyps. The electronic cleansing algorithms are not complete. They can distort the surface of the colon wall or polyp that abuts the tagged fluid. Due to this subtraction artifact, the surface of a submerged polyp may be irregular on the 3-D endoluminal views, mimicking the surface of stool. Polyps will maintain their normal smooth contour on the non-submerged endoluminal view. Evaluation of submerged polyps can be facilitated by again turning the subtraction algorithm off on the 2-D source images. The polyp will be seen as a filling defect in the tagged fluid on the 2-D source images (Fig. 8.11a–d).

Polyp measurement is best obtained on the 3-D endoluminal images with the polyp free from surrounding tagged fluid (i.e., on the nondependent wall of the colon). Polyp measurements should be taken perpendicular to the base of the polyp and colon wall. Measurements taken of submerged polyps on the 3-D endoluminal views will underestimate the true size of the polyp (Fig. 8.12a, b).

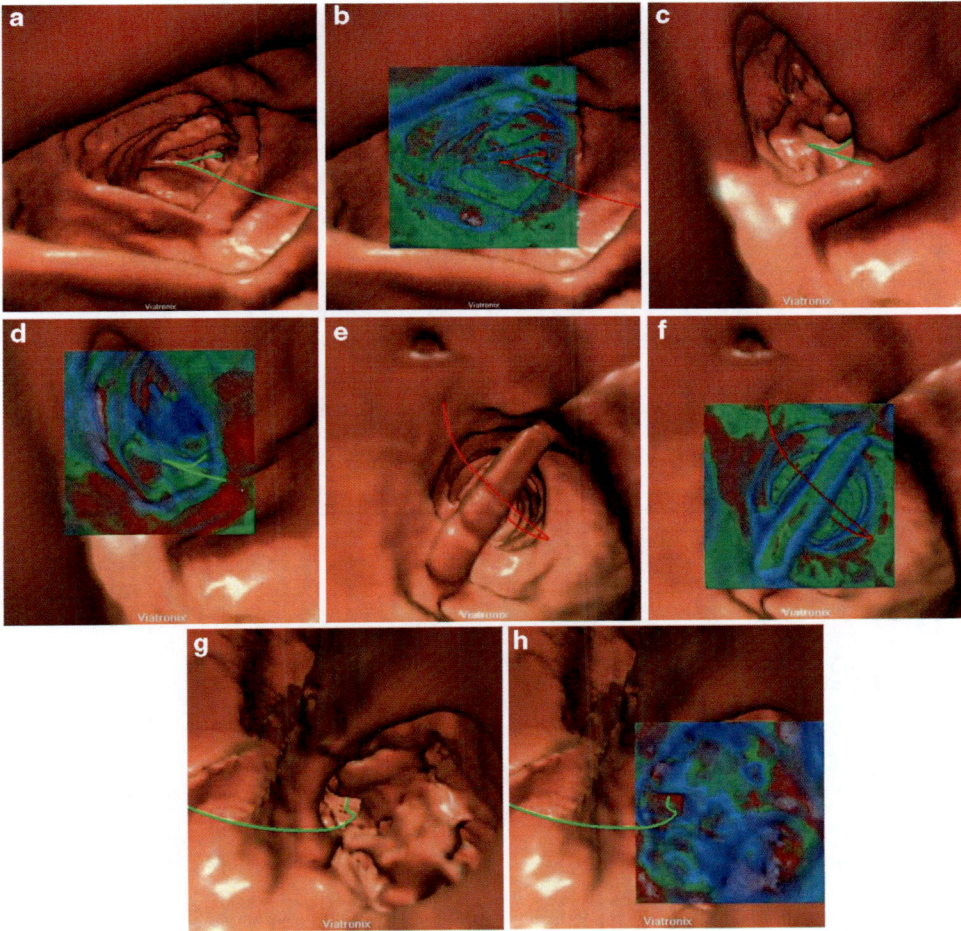

Fig. 8.6 Images (**a**)–(**h**) demonstrate varying degrees of stool contamination found on CTC

Preparation-related pitfalls and imaging artifacts can best be minimized with the utilization of a proper cathartic bowel preparation, stool and fluid tagging with electronic cleansing, and imaging the patient in the prone and supine positions. However, when faced with significant residual stool or fluid and contrast contamination, one can utilize the characteristic morphology and density of stool and dense contrast coupled with the physics of prone and supine positioning to help differentiate true polyps from contamination. Using the 2-D source images with the cleansing algorithm turned off can help in detecting polyps when there is complete filling of the colon lumen by tagged fluid. Finally, by understanding the effects of residual fluid on submerged polyps, one can accurately identify and measure these lesions.

Imaging-Related Pitfalls and Artifacts

There are multiple pitfalls and artifacts related to the actual imaging of the CTC patient. Some of these artifacts and pitfalls can be minimized with proper imaging techniques. Others are the inevitable by-product of the standard low-dose technique used for this screening study and the imaging properties of CT. Luminal narrowing, segmental collapse, air–fluid interface artifact,

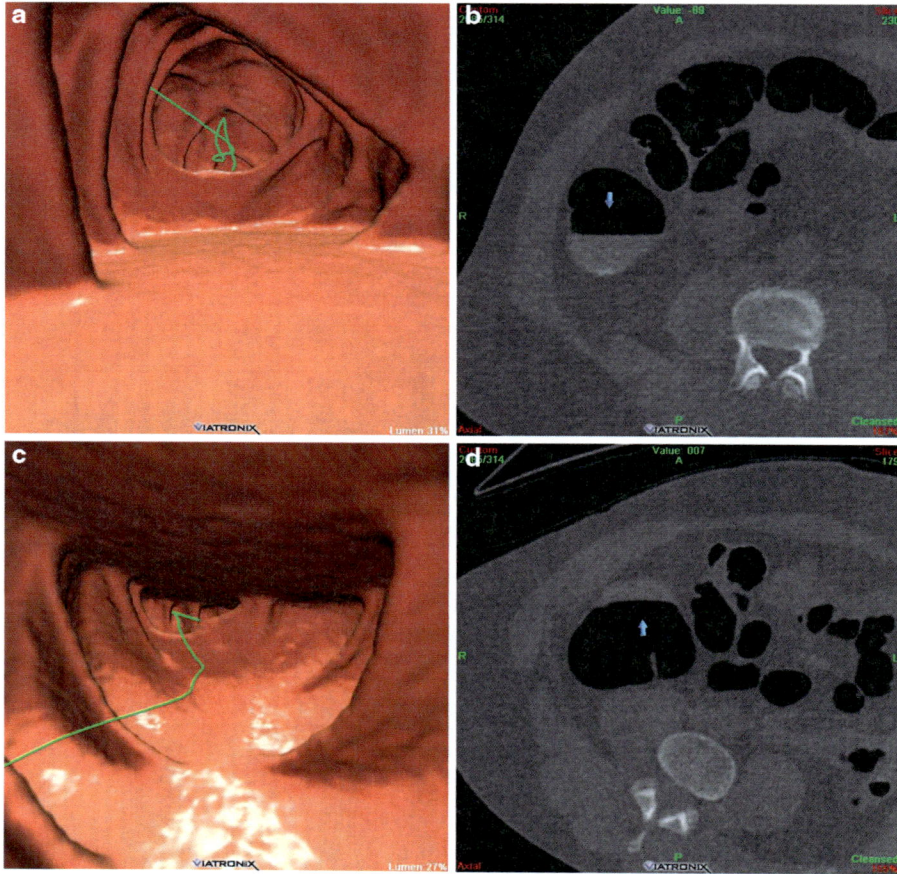

Fig. 8.7 Images (**a**)–(**d**) demonstrate the utility of prone and supine imaging. Dilute non-subtracted fluid is shifted to the opposing walls of the colon, allowing for visualization of the colon surface on at least one view

electronic cleansing or subtraction artifact, image noise artifact, spray artifact, and data dropout are the major imaging-related pitfalls and artifacts. Each of these will be addressed below.

Adequate colon distension is critical for proper 3-D model building. Inadequate distension leads to luminal narrowing or frank segmental collapse. Luminal narrowing produces thickening of the colonic folds, which, if focal enough, can mimic a polyp. This is especially true when evaluating for polyps on the 2-D source images. True fold thickening, in contrast to adherent stool/barium or a sessile polyp, should be uniform in caliber and smooth. It is usually found on the inside curve of a flexure or a turn of the sigmoid or transverse colon

(Fig. 8.13a–f). Segmental narrowing can result from spasm, colon cancer, diverticulosis, scarring from prior surgery, radiation, or inflammation (Fig. 8.14a–f). Figure 8.15a, b demonstrates a stent placed across a known colon cancer in the descending colon. Suboptimal distension of the colon requires an intense 3-D and 2-D analysis of the involved segments to exclude underlying polyps or masses.

Frank collapse secondary to focal spasm results in total loss of visualization of the colon lumen on both the 3-D and 2-D images. Significant polyps or masses cannot be excluded from these segments. If the segmental collapse involves the same segment on both the supine and prone series, then this constitutes an incomplete CTC

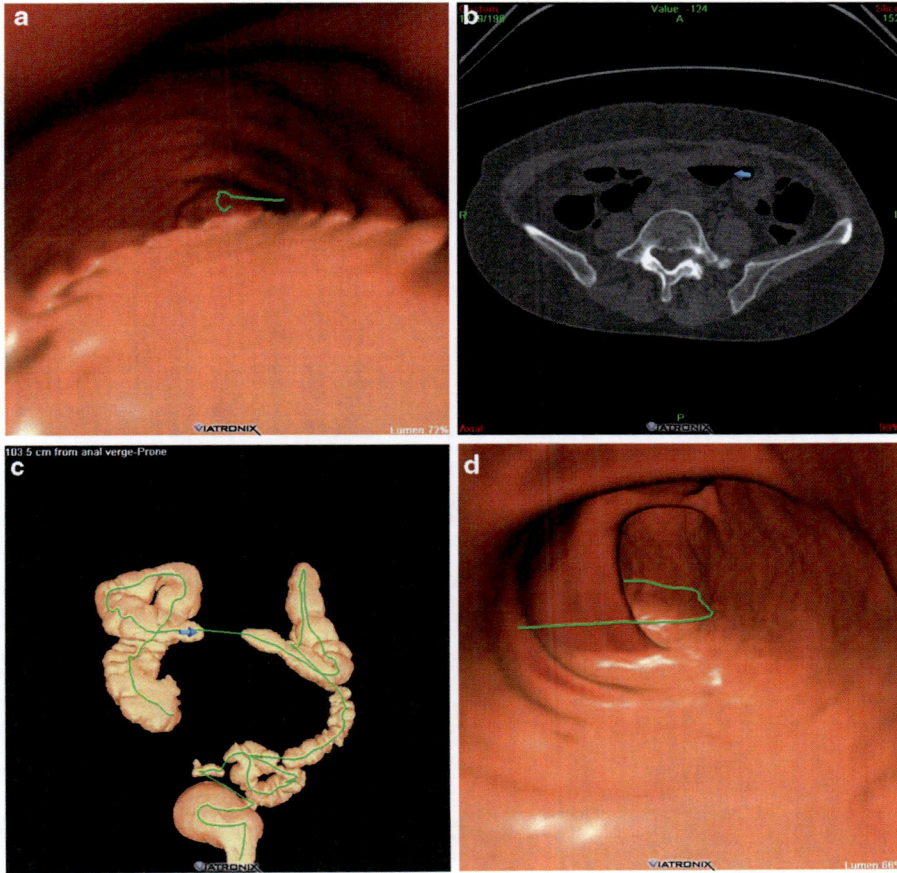

Fig. 8.8 Images (**a**)–(**d**) demonstrate the problem with significant dilute fluid filling the entire lumen of the colon. In the prone position, fluid fills the mid-transverse colon preventing 3-D endoluminal visualization of that segment. In the supine position, the fluid moves to the ascending or descending colon, allowing for 3-D endoluminal visualization of the mid-transverse colon

(Fig. 8.16a, b). Tailoring the exam to the patient's anatomy can minimize luminal narrowing and segmental collapse. Obtaining a scout image or representative preliminary slices through the abdomen and pelvis prior to scanning the patient allows the CT technologist to verify maximal distention of the colon. Review of the scout images may also result in the detection of pathology outside of the colon (Fig. 8.17a–d). If narrowed or collapsed segments are identified on the scout view or preliminary slices, placing the patient in a decubitus or oblique position and re-insufflating the colon may adequately distend the narrowed or collapsed segments identified (Fig. 8.18a–f).

Large air–fluid levels in the colon can lead to an air–fluid interface artifact within the lumen of the colon that can obscure portions of the colon wall. Manual fly-through both above and below this artifact on the 3-D views, as well as careful analysis of the 2-D source images, is required to adequately evaluate the involved segment (Fig. 8.19a–d). Stool and fluid cleansing algorithms, in addition to distorting the contour of submerged polyps, can produce irregularities in the colon wall itself. Electronically cleansed pools of fluid leave a "bathtub ring" type of irregularity on the dependent wall of the colon (Fig. 8.20a–d). Thin folds submerged in tagged

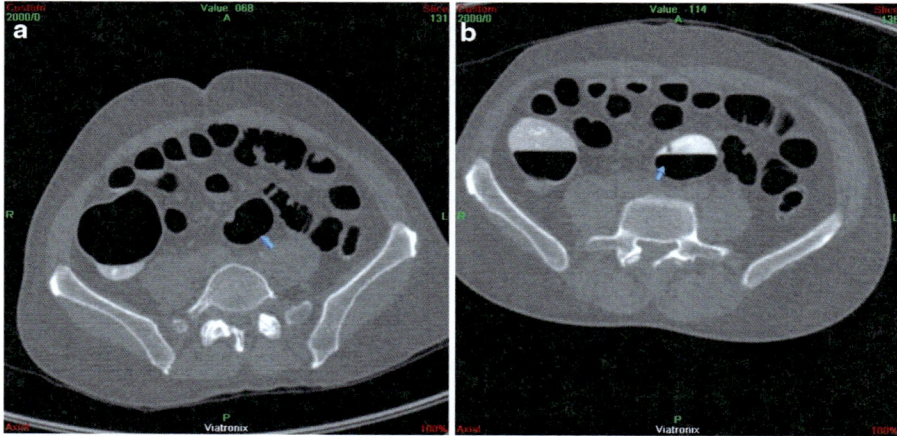

Fig. 8.9 Images (**a**) and (**b**) demonstrate the benefit of evaluating fluid-filled segments of bowel on the 2-D source images with the electronic cleansing algorithm turned off. Polyps or masses can be seen as persistent filling defects in the fluid pool on these 2-D images

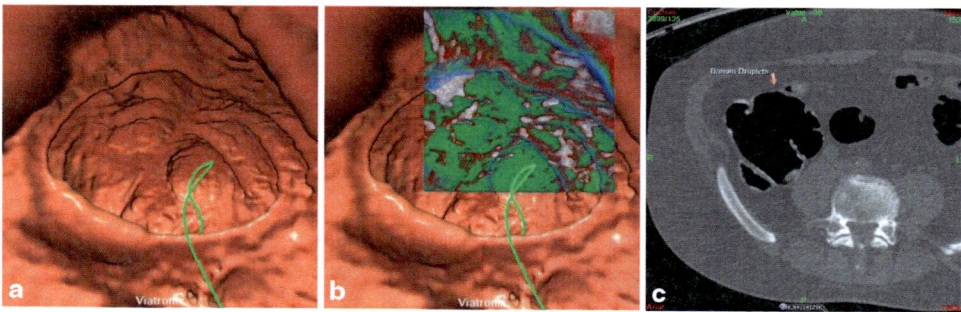

Fig. 8.10 Images (**a**)–(**c**) demonstrate desiccated barium droplets carpeting the mucosal surface of the cecum. Their high density can be easily seen on the color window and 2-D source images

fluid can have significant erosions of the apex of the fold (Fig. 8.21a–d). If tagged fluid is present in adjacent segments of bowel, the contiguous walls may be subtracted out together producing a communicating hole between the two segments of the bowel. When present, a manual fly-through of the excluded segment of the bowel is required (Fig. 8.22a–c). These electronic cleansing artifacts are positional in nature, involving the dependent portions of bowel, and therefore should not be persistent on both the supine and prone views.

With today's multi-slice CT scanners, imaging of the abdomen and pelvis can usually be obtained during a single breath hold. However, in some patients with underlying respiratory or cardiovascular conditions, imaging in the supine or prone positions may be problematic. Significant tachypnea can result in a stair-stepping artifact involving those bowel segments and solid organs adjacent to the diaphragm. This can be pronounced on the 3-D images as well as the 2-D sagittal- and coronal-formatted images. The axial 2-D images source images will show the least motion artifact (Fig. 8.23a–c).

CTC utilizes a low-dose technique to obtain the source CT data that is used to build the 3-D model. This low-dose technique, coupled with the large body habitus of the average patient, results in a decrease in the signal to noise ratio of the source images. This produces a mottled irregularity to the 2-D source images as well as the colon surface on the 3-D endoluminal images. On the 2-D source images, this image noise, or

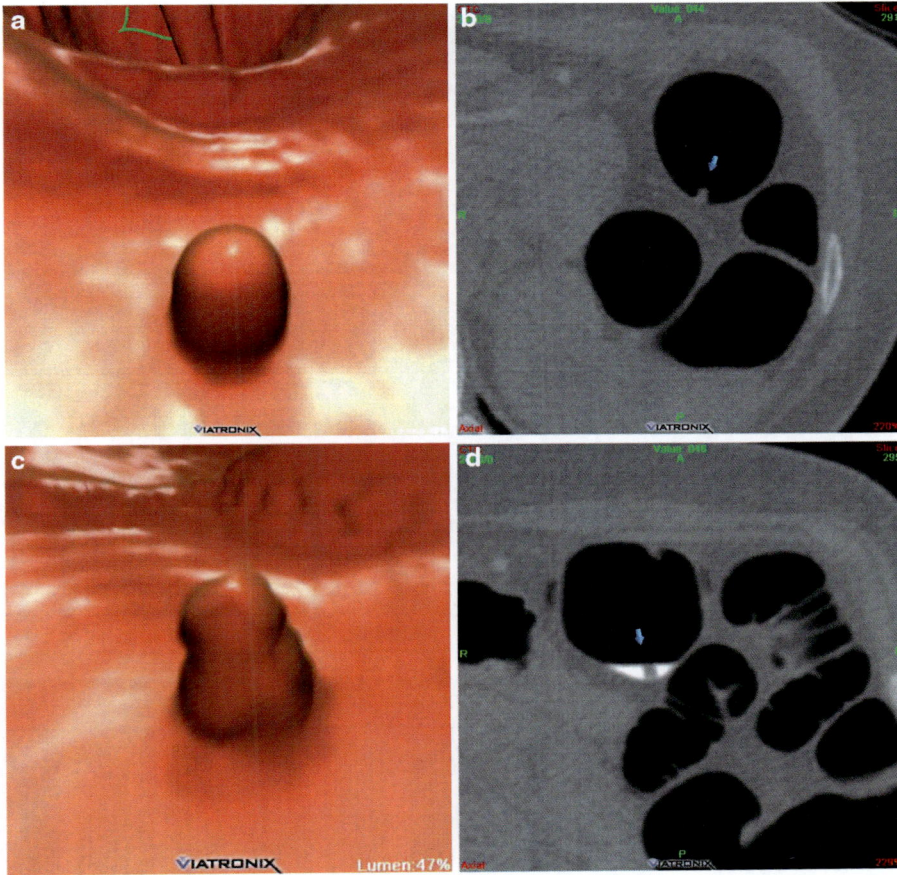

Fig. 8.11 Images (**a**)–(**d**) demonstrate the effect of the electronic cleansing algorithm on the surface contour of submerged polyps. Images (**a**) and (**b**) show the smooth surface contour of a non-submerged sessile polyp. Images (**c**) and (**d**) show the same polyp submerged in contrast. Note the irregular surface contour of the polyp on the 3-D endoluminal images

quantum mottle, is manifested to a greater extent on the narrow soft tissue windows. It is recommended that the 2-D images be evaluated on the wider bone windows (Fig. 8.24a–d).

Spray artifact from retained metal hardware can degrade both the 3-D endoluminal and 2-D source images. Hip prostheses, Harrington rods, and spinal fusion hardware can produce significant spray artifact, limiting visualization of the bowel and adjacent structures in the abdomen and pelvis. As with image noise, spray artifact is less pronounced on the 2-D images when viewed with the wider bone windows (Fig. 8.25a–c).

Data dropout occurs when portions of the colon are not included in the 2-D CT data set. This usually involves the flexures or the rectum. Data dropout appears as a black region devoid of any mucosal detail in the 3-D colon model. This artifact can be avoided with proper imaging of the entire abdomen and pelvis from the dome of the diaphragm to the pubic symphysis. It is also unusual for it to be present on both the prone and supine views (Fig. 8.26a–f).

As with patient preparation, the actual imaging of the CTC patient can be problematic, resulting in imaging pitfalls and artifacts. Adequate colonic distension is critical to the production of a diagnostic quality CTC study. The mechanical CO_2 insufflator has revolutionized CTC imaging. Slow and gentle CO_2 insufflation, coupled with maintaining a steady state luminal pressure of 25 psi during the exam, has significantly reduced

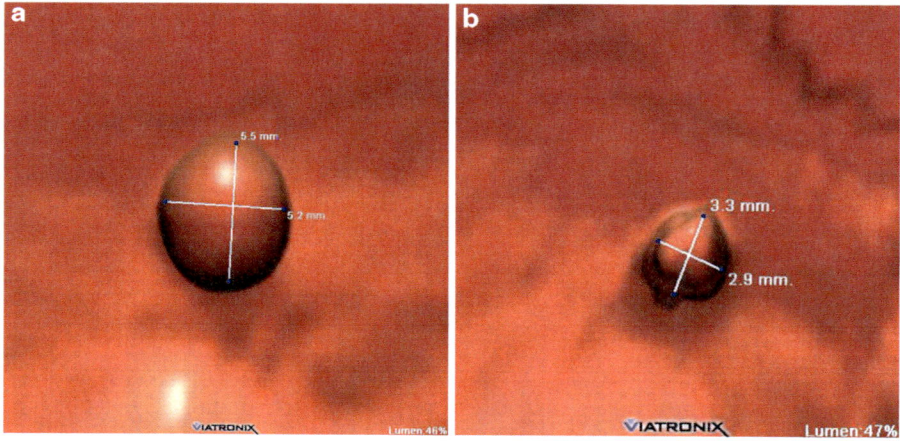

Fig. 8.12 The electronic cleansing algorithm will also distort the size of submerged polyps. Image (**a**) shows the measurements taken of a 5-mm sessile polyp on a nondependent wall of the colon. Image (**b**) shows the measurements taken on the same polyp submerged in retained fluid. The measurements taken on a submerged polyp greatly underestimate the actual size of that polyp

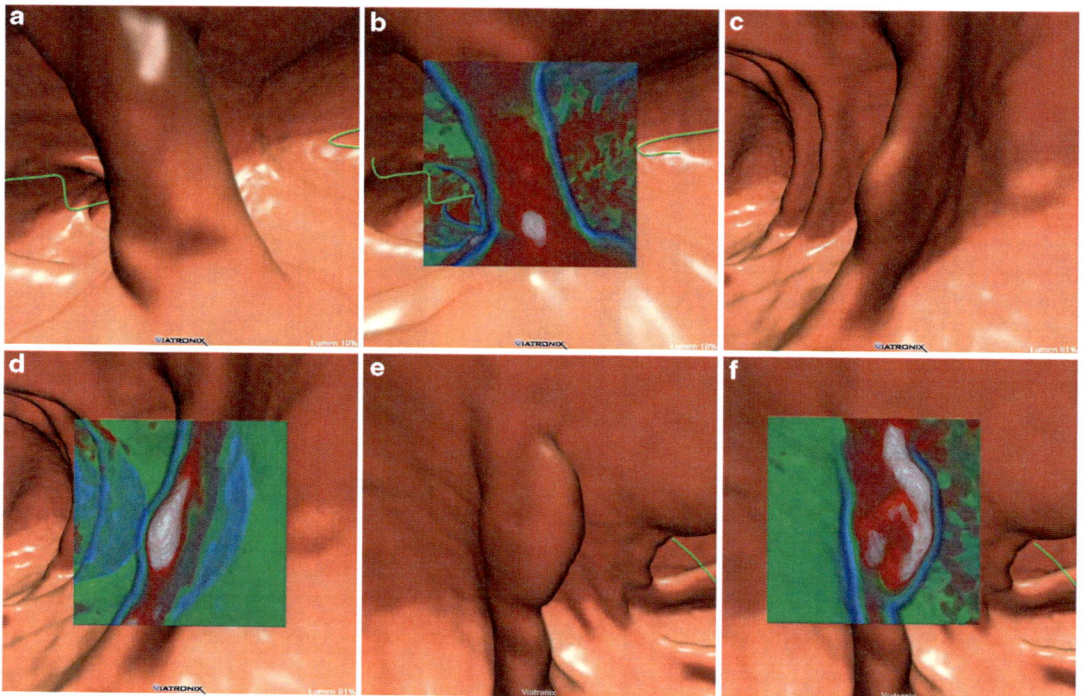

Fig. 8.13 Luminal narrowing can produce wall thickening which is usually uniform in caliber as demonstrated on images (**a**) and (**b**). Focal wall thickening can be the result of adherent barium/stool (images **c** and **d**) or a sessile polyp (images **e** and **f**)

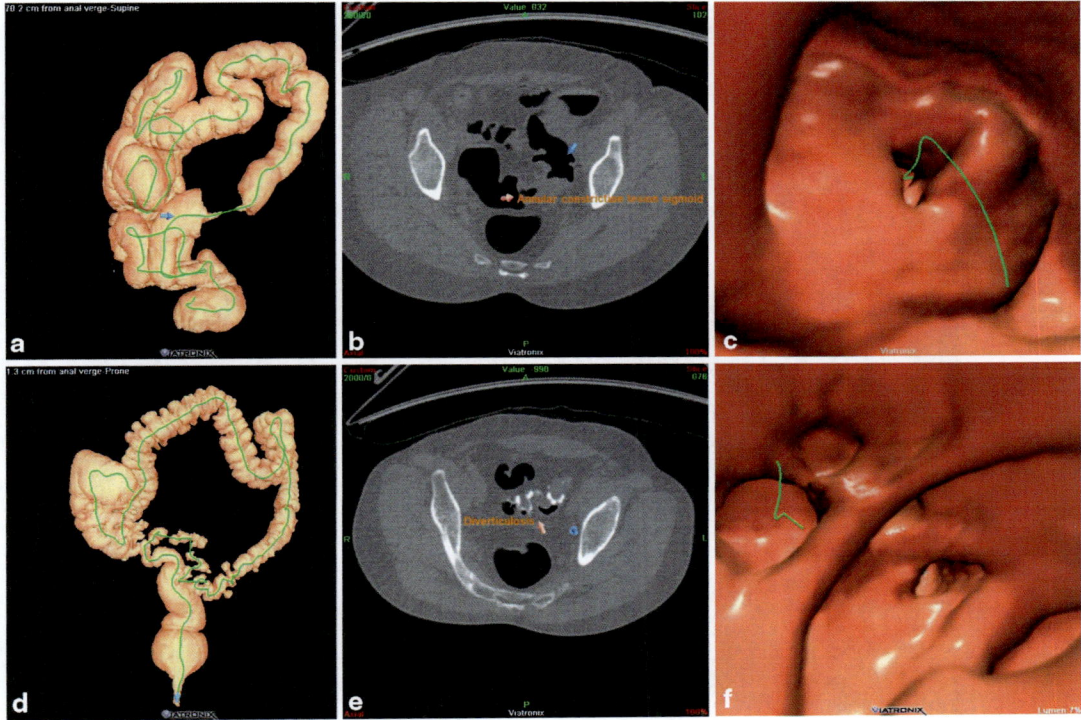

Fig. 8.14 Two examples of segmental narrowing. Images (**a**)–(**c**) demonstrate an annular constricting mass with overhanging edges in the distal sigmoid colon that turned out to be an adenocarcinoma. Images (**d**)–(**f**) demonstrate segmental narrowing in the sigmoid colon secondary to diverticulosis with secondary muscular hypertrophy and spasm

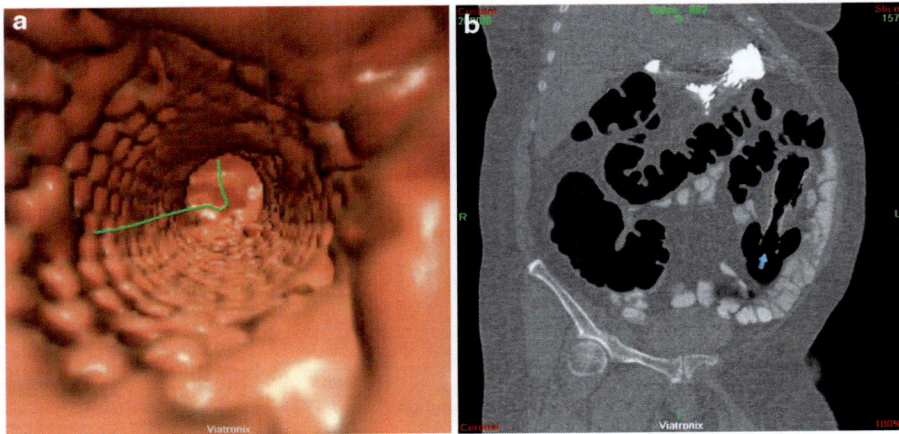

Fig. 8.15 Images (**a**) and (**b**) demonstrate an indwelling colon stent, placed across a annular constricting mass in the descending colon

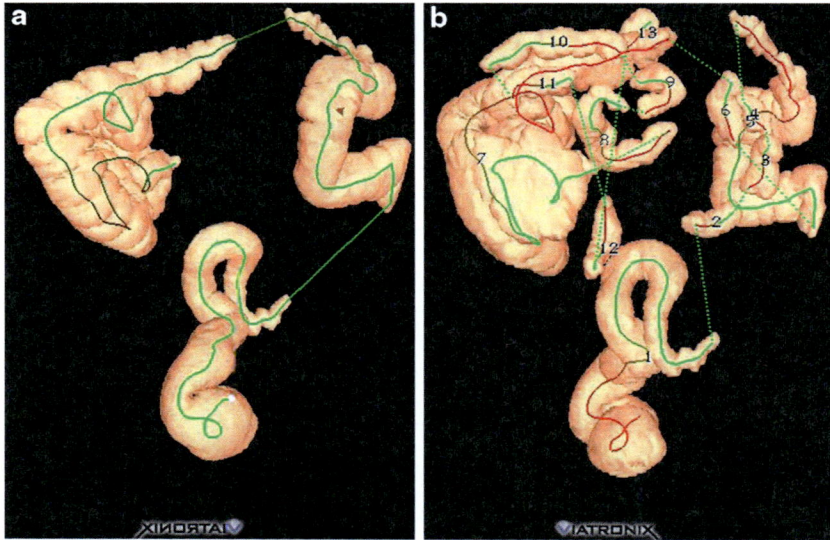

Fig. 8.16 Images (**a**) and (**b**) demonstrate segmental collapse of the colon on both the supine and prone series resulting in non-visualization of the transverse and sigmoid colon. This constitutes an incomplete CTC

the incidence of luminal narrowing or frank segmental collapse. Targeting narrowed or collapsed segments on the scout or preliminary views and aggressively distending those segments through the use of decubitus patient positioning can also decrease the incidence of segmental narrowing or collapse. Air–fluid interface artifact, electronic cleansing artifact, image noise artifact, spray artifact, and data dropout artifact are the by-products of the 3-D model building software algorithms and low-dose CT imaging technique used in CTC. They must be understood and recognized as imaging artifacts in order to adequately interpret a CTC study.

Anatomical Variant Pitfalls and Artifacts

No two patients are the same. There are numerous anatomical variants that can mimic pathology on 3-D endoluminal images. It is important to recognize these anatomical variants when evaluating the colon for pathology. Essentially, any structure in the abdomen or pelvis that abuts the colon can cause mass effect on the bowel wall and can be mistaken for pathology on the

endoluminal views. Diverticular disease can simulate sessile polyps. Flat polyps are a variant of sessile polyps, which are especially difficult to detect on both CTC and OC. Pedunculated polyps can be mistaken for mobile stool if their stalk is long and inconspicuous. Benign lipomas of the colon can look identical to sessile polyps on 3-D endoluminal views. Rectal veins, anal papillae, and internal hemorrhoids can produce mucosal defects in the rectum that can be mistaken for intracolonic neoplasia. Finally, variations in contour and configuration of the appendix and ileocecal valve can represent normal variants or true pathology. Examples of each of these cases will be discussed below.

Extrinsic compression of the colon by any of the adjacent structures in the abdomen and pelvis can produce a mass effect on the bowel wall resulting in a pseudopolyp or mass on the 3-D endoluminal views. Rib ends (Fig. 8.27a, b), the sacrum (Fig. 8.28a, b), the iliac arteries (Fig. 8.29a–c), uterine fibroids (Fig. 8.30a–c), small bowel (Fig. 8.31a–c), and even a calcified gallstone (Fig. 8.32a–c) have been shown to produce such extrinsic compression artifacts on the colon wall. Extrinsic compression by foreign bodies such as surgical clips (Fig. 8.33a, b), a

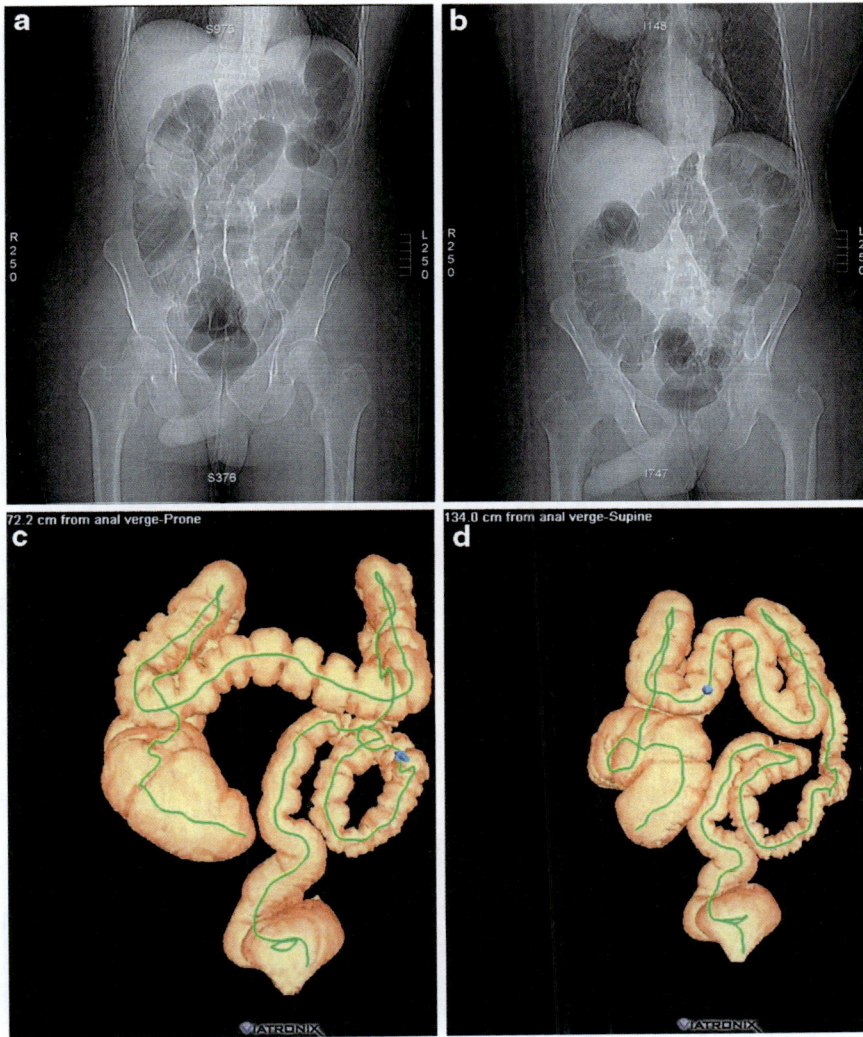

72.2 cm from anal verge-Prone

134.0 cm from anal verge-Supine

Fig. 8.17 Images (**a**) and (**b**) are scout images from a CTC which demonstrate adequate CO_2 distension of the entire colon on both the prone and supine series. Obtaining scout images or representative preliminary slices through the abdomen and pelvis prior to imaging the patient helps to guarantee maximal distension of the colon during imaging. Review of the scout images may also detect pathology outside of the colon. The supine scout on this patient demonstrates a clinically occult right upper lobe pulmonary mass. Images (**c**) and (**d**) demonstrate a diagnostic quality 3-D model of the colon on both the prone and supine series. The colon is adequately inflated on both views, and a continuous virtual flight path (demarcated by the *green line*) has been established from the rectum to the cecum on both the prone and supine series

granulation tissue in a suture line (Fig. 8.34a–c), a vaginal tampon (Fig. 8.35a, b), and a rectal tube (Fig. 8.36a, b) can produce similar pseudopolyp or mass-like artifacts on the 3-D endoluminal views. Endoluminal views of a pedunculated polyp (Fig. 8.37a, b), a sessile polyp (Fig. 8.37c, d), and a flat polyp (Fig. 8.37e, f) are shown for comparison. Correlation with the 2-D CT images is required to exclude extrinsic compression by an adjacent structure as the etiology of these polyps or masses on the 3-D endoluminal images.

There are many conditions associated with a prepared colon that can mimic polyps.

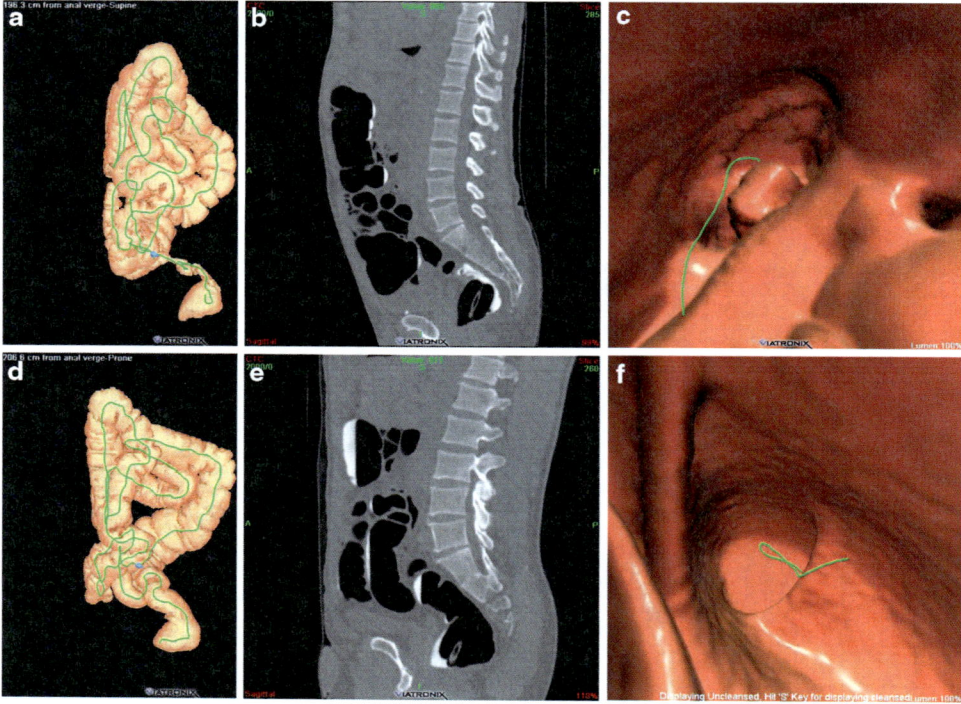

Fig. 8.18 Images (**a**)–(**f**) demonstrate the benefit of oblique or decubitus positioning. The rectosigmoid junction is partially collapsed on the supine series. Imaging the patient in an oblique decubitus position allows for adequate distension and therefore visualization of that segment of colon

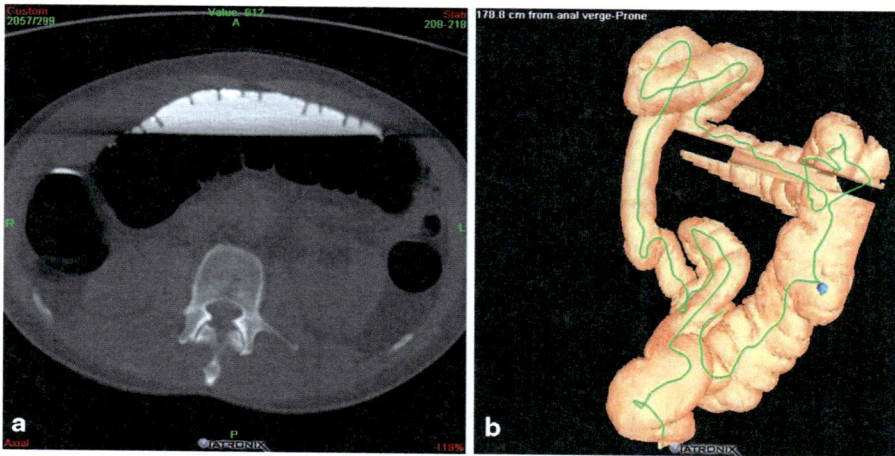

Fig. 8.19 Images (**a**)–(**b**) demonstrate an air/fluid interface artifact in the transverse colon

These include dense adherent stool (Fig. 8.38a–c), air bubbles trapped under contrast (Fig. 8.39a–c), tagged stool in a barium pool (Fig. 8.40a–c), and residual ingested material (Fig. 8.41a–d). Even submucosal air-filled cysts as seen in pneumatosis cystoides intestinalis (Fig. 8.42a–c) can simulate polyps in the prepared colon. These entities can usually be differentiated from true polyps by density analysis and correlation with the 2-D source images.

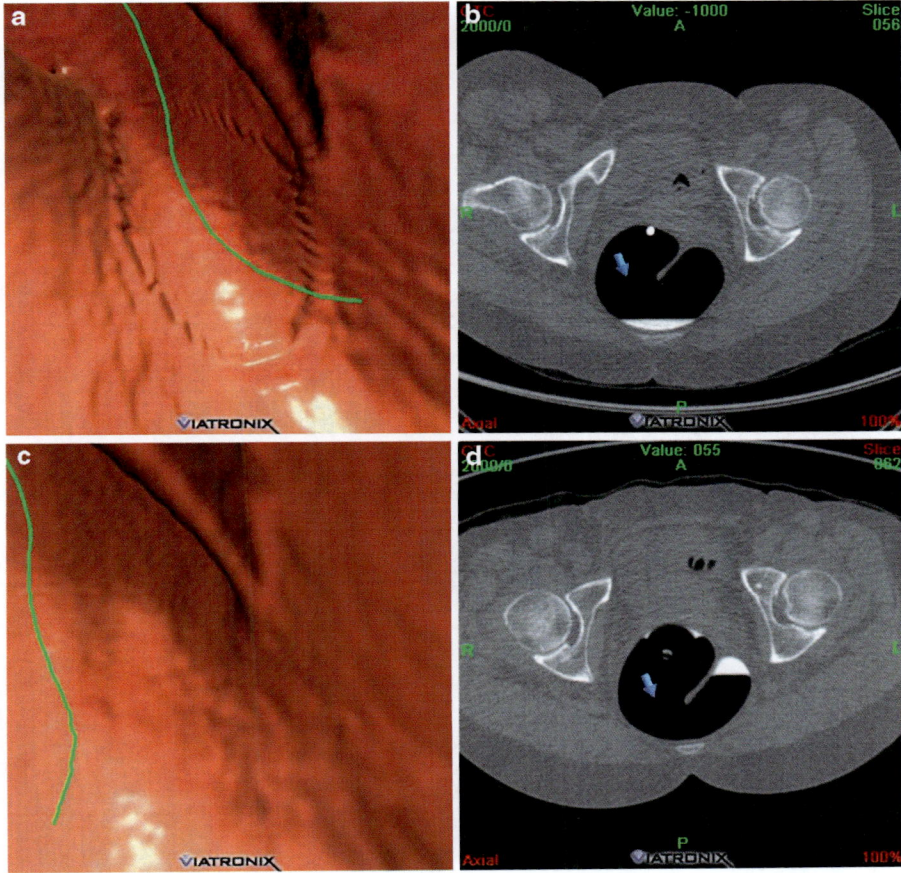

Fig. 8.20 Images (**a**)–(**d**) demonstrate the characteristic "bathtub ring"-type artifact produced by the electronic cleansing algorithm. This artifact is seen on the posterior wall of the rectum with the patient in the supine position. Rolling the patient into the prone position shifts the tagged fluid into the proximal sigmoid colon. The posterior wall of the rectum in the prone position demonstrates the normal smooth colonic mucosa with clearing of the ring artifact

Diverticular disease is endemic in the CRC screening population. It usually involves the descending and sigmoid colon and can be rather extensive in these segments. Stool-filled diverticula can mimic sessile polyps (Fig. 8.43a–c). Correlation with the 2-D CT images as well as density interrogation, however, can usually differentiate these lesions from true polyps. The retained stool in the diverticulum will contain dense contrast as well as low-density fecal fat and air bubbles. Its location in a diverticulum can be confirmed on the appropriate 2-D CT images.

Flat polyps, given their diminutive height above the colon wall, are difficult to identify on both CTC and OC. Flat polyps appear as subtle mucosal irregularities on the 3-D endoluminal views. Varying the artificial light source and correlation with the 2-D CT views can help in detecting the subtle lesions (Fig. 8.44a–d).

Mobility in positioning on the prone and supine views is one of the characteristics of stool. Pedunculated polyps on long stalks can also demonstrate such mobility and therefore be mistaken for stool if the stalk is not recognized (Fig. 8.45a–c). Whenever dealing with mobile lesions in the colon, always consider the pedunculated polyp and look for the diminutive stalk on both the 3-D and 2-D images.

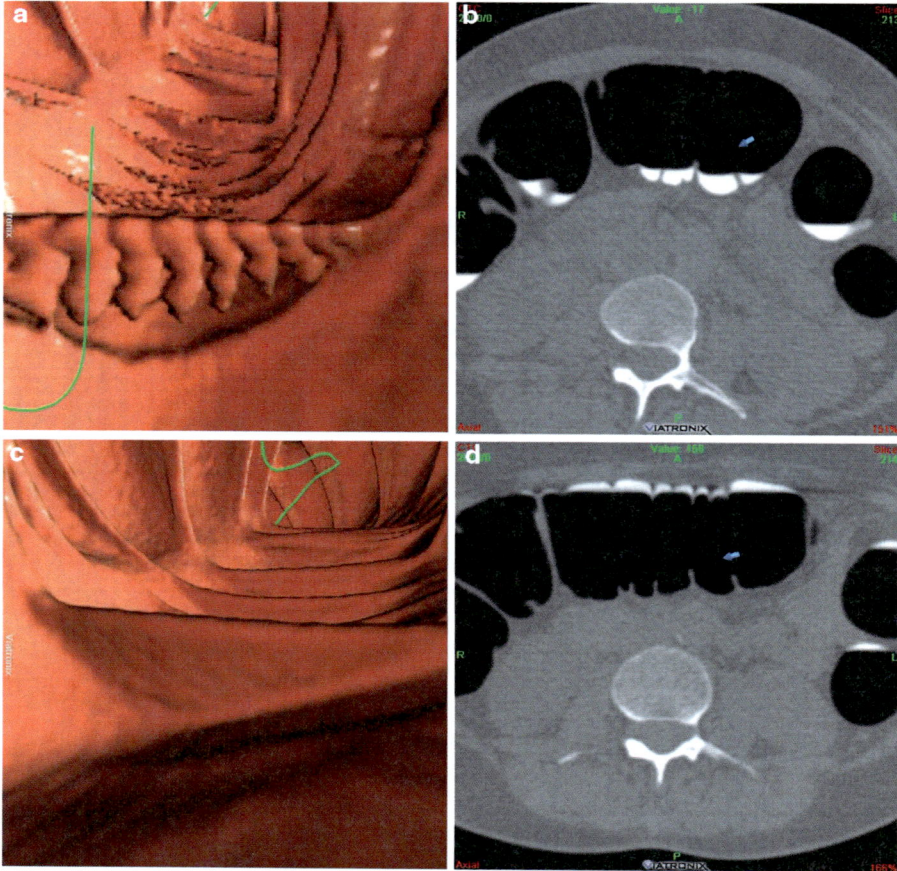

Fig. 8.21 When there is tagged fluid on both sides of a thin fold, the electronic cleansing algorithm can create significant distortion of that fold as seen in images (**a**) and (**b**). Images (**c**) and (**d**) demonstrate those same folds without adjacent fluid or distortion

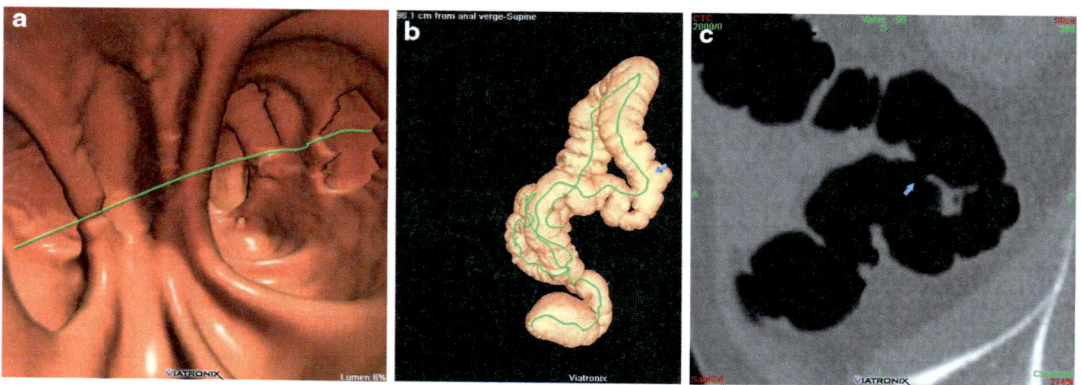

Fig. 8.22 Images (**a**)–(**c**) demonstrate a communicating hole between adjacent segments of bowel secondary to electronic cleansing artifact. The bypassed segment of the colon must be evaluated with a manual fly-through on the 3-D model

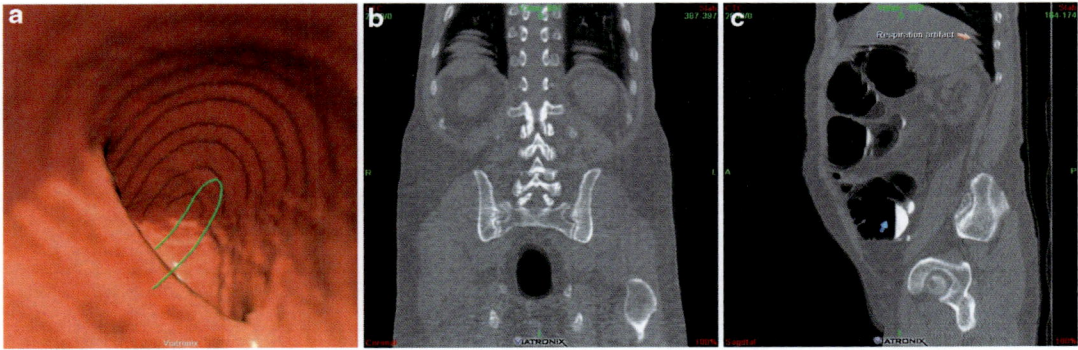

Fig. 8.23 Images (**a**)–(**c**) demonstrate stair step-like artifact secondary to respiratory motion. This artifact is more pronounced on the 3-D endoluminal images and the coronal- and sagittal- reformatted images

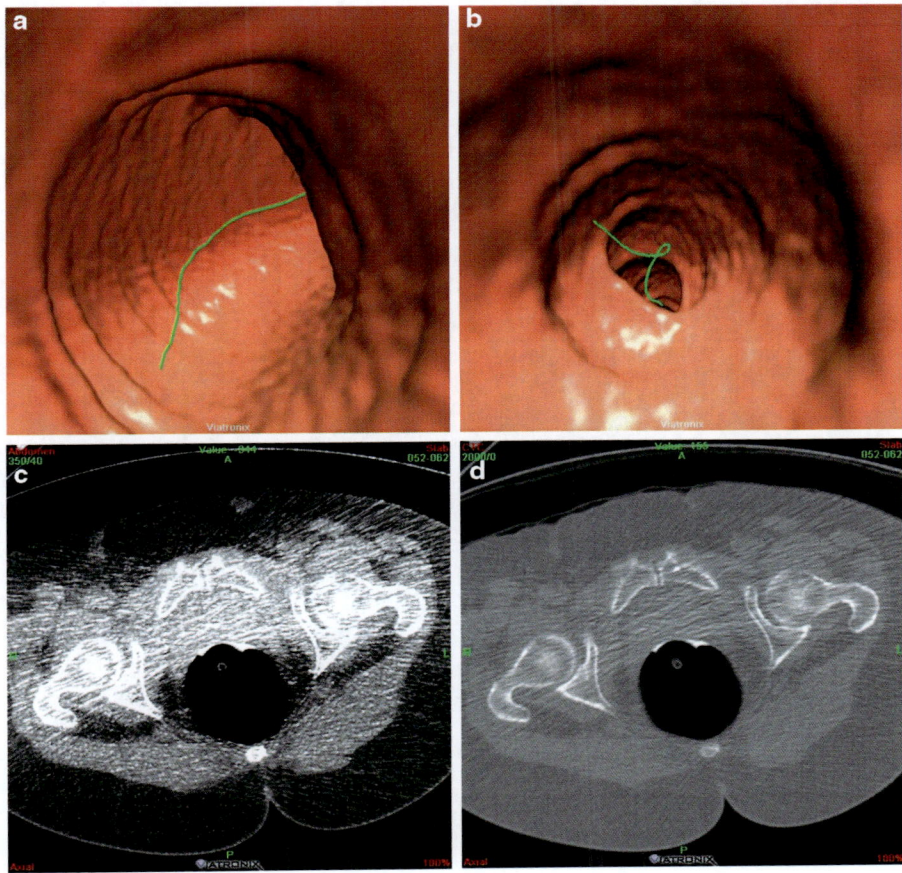

Fig. 8.24 Images (**a**) and (**b**) show a mottled irregularity to the surface of the colon on the 3-D endoluminal views which is the result of increased image noise associated with the low-dose imaging of CTC. Image (**c**) demonstrates the same image noise or quantum mottle on the 2-D source images. Image noise can be decreased on the 2-D images through the use of wider windows as seen in image (**d**)

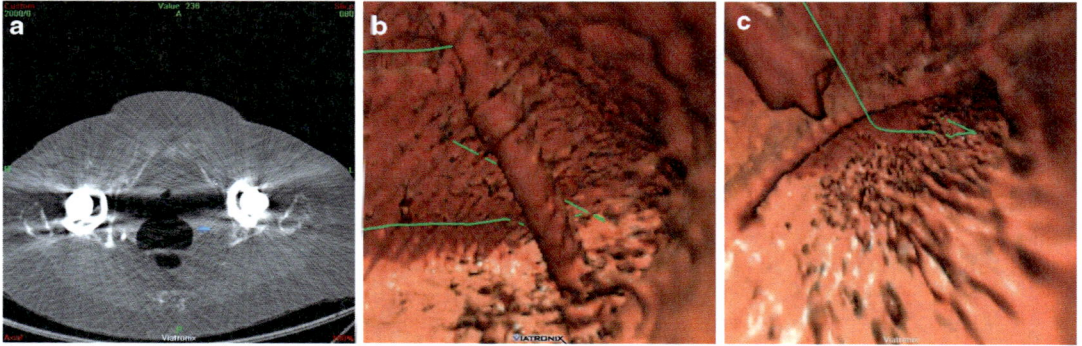

Fig. 8.25 Spray artifact from hip replacements can severely degrade the 3-D endoluminal views of the rectum as well as the adjacent pelvic structures on the 2-D source images, as seen in images (**a**)–(**c**). Spray artifact, like image noise, is less pronounced on the 2-D source images when viewed with wider windows

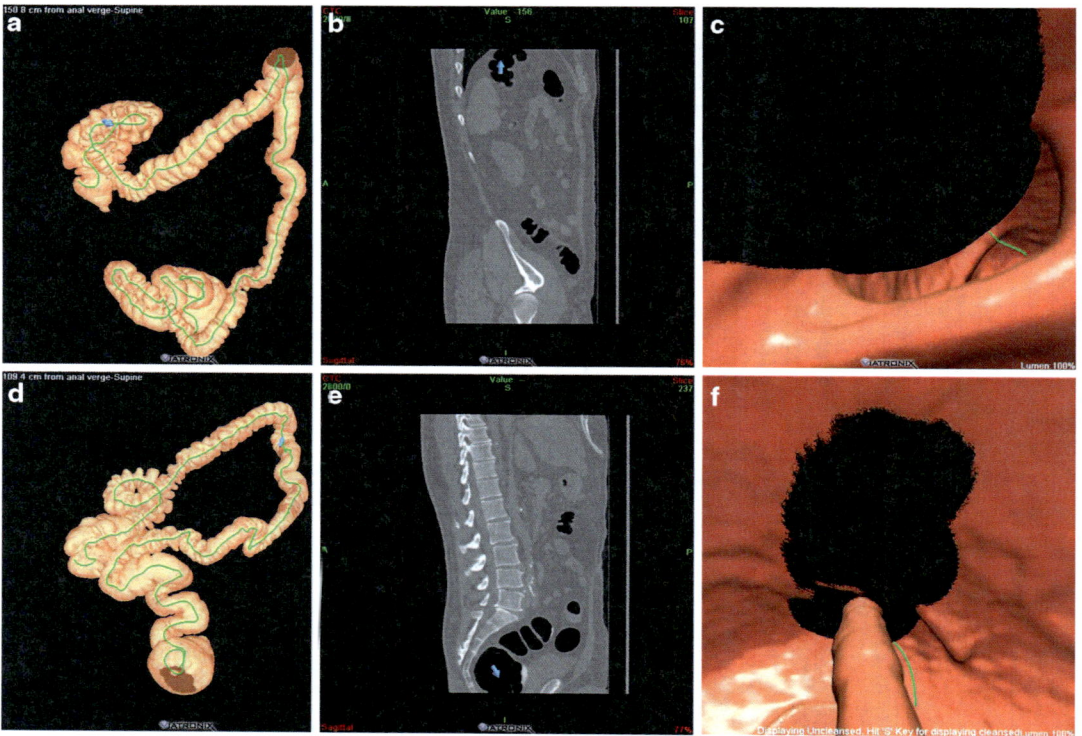

Fig. 8.26 Data dropout which is manifested as a black area devoid of mucosal detail is demonstrated on images (**a**)–(**f**). It usually involves the colon flexures or the rec-tum. It is the result of portions of the colon not being included in the 2-D data set

Lipomas of the colon are benign entities that do not require removal. They can mimic polyps on the 3-D endoluminal images. Lipomas are usually sessile in nature. Given their soft consistency, they may show different degrees of prominence on the supine and prone images. They will demonstrate uniform fat attenuation with Hounsfield units of -75 to -125 on the 3-D and 2-D images (Fig. 8.46a–c). Density interrogation can usually differentiate a lipoma from a sessile polyp.

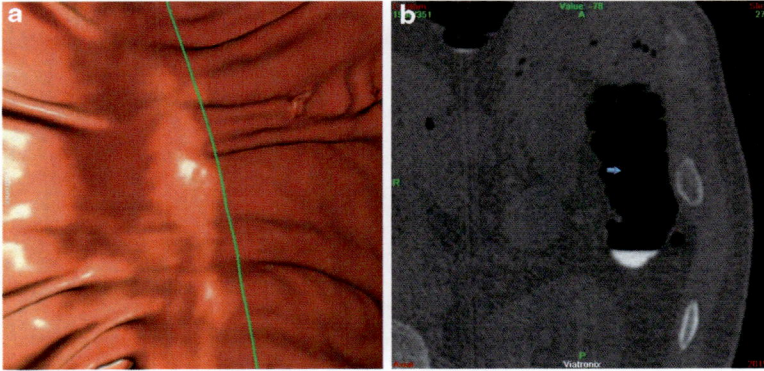

Fig. 8.27 Extrinsic compression of the splenic flexure by an adjacent rib end produces a pseudo flat polyp on the 3-D endoluminal view, as seen in images (**a**) and (**b**)

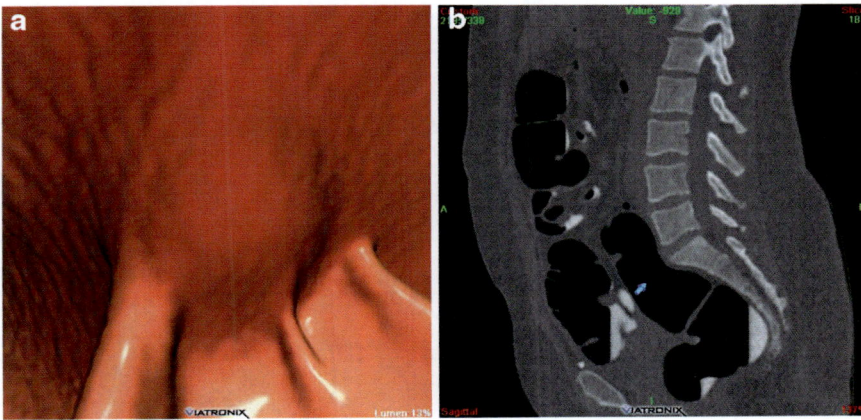

Fig. 8.28 Images (**a**) and (**b**) demonstrate extrinsic compression on the posterior wall of the rectum by the sacral promontory, which produces a pseudo flat polyp on the 3-D endoluminal view

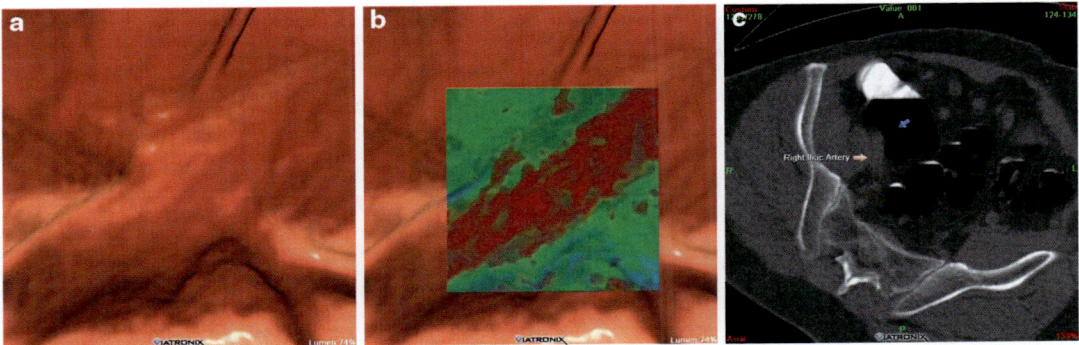

Fig. 8.29 The aorta and iliac arteries can produce extrinsic compression on adjacent segments of colon in the abdomen and pelvis, which in turn can mimic pathology on the 3-D endoluminal views. Images (**a**)–(**c**) show extrinsic compression on the lateral wall of the cecum by the right external iliac artery, which produces a pseudo flat polyp on the 3-D endoluminal view

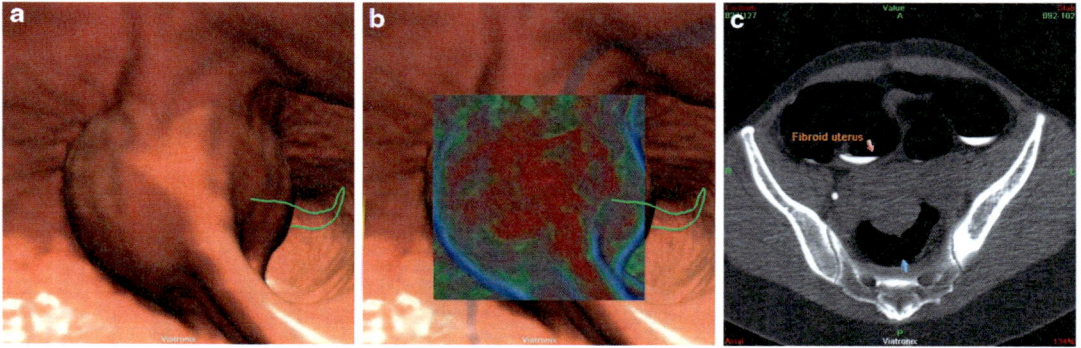

Fig. 8.30 Exophytic uterine fibroids can compress the adjacent colon and produce pseudo lesions on the 3-D endoluminal views. Images (**a**)–(**c**) demonstrate a serosal uterine fibroid producing a pseudo sessile polyp at the base of a fold in the sigmoid colon

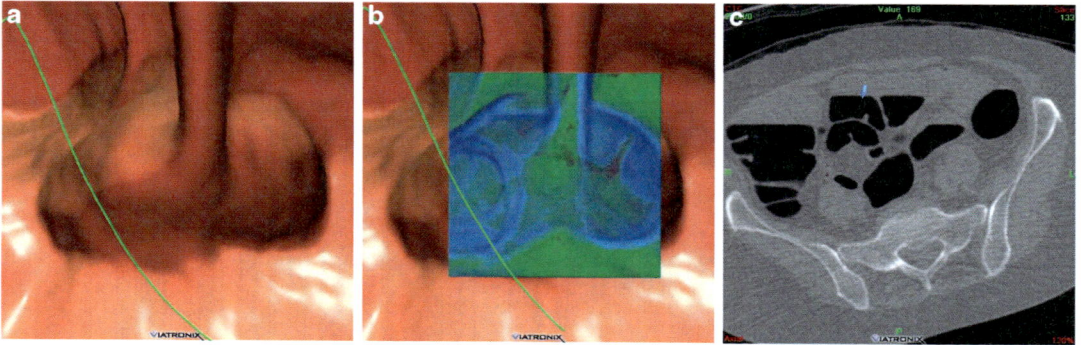

Fig. 8.31 Fluid- or gas-filled segments of small bowel can produce extrinsic compression on adjacent segments of colon. Images (**a**)–(**c**) demonstrate a pseudo sessile polyp in the sigmoid colon secondary to extrinsic compression by an adjacent gas-filled segment of the small bowel

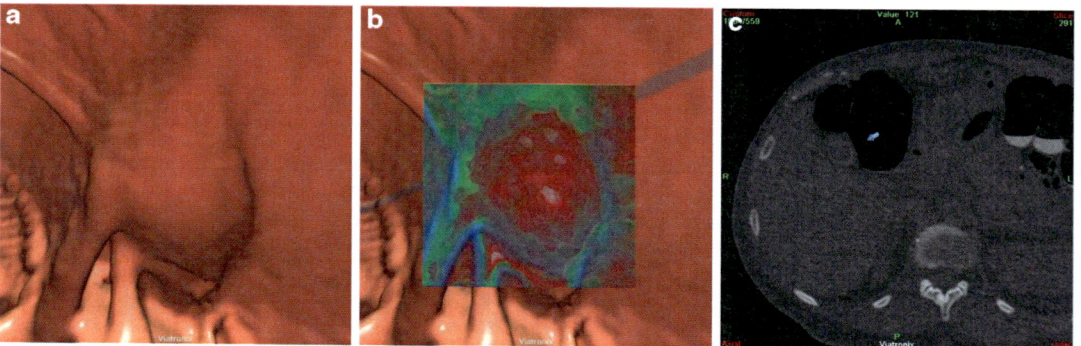

Fig. 8.32 Images (**a**)–(**c**) demonstrate a pseudo sessile polyp in the hepatic flexure secondary to extrinsic compression by a calcified gallstone in the gallbladder lumen

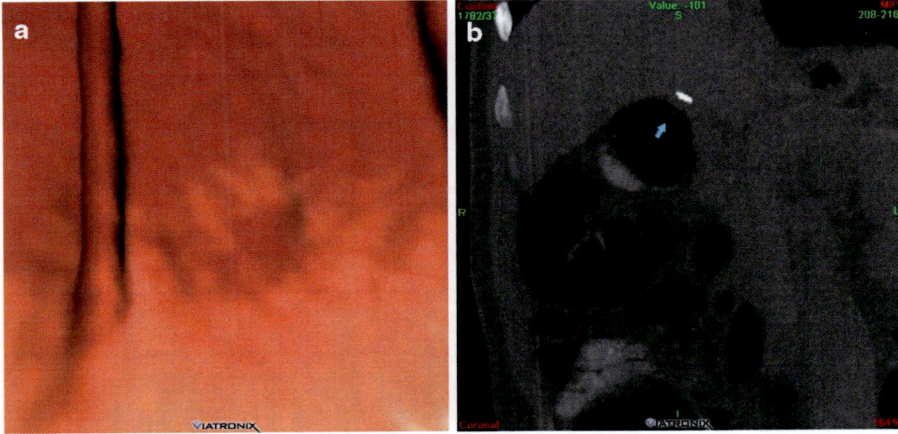

Fig. 8.33 Foreign bodies within the abdomen or pelvis can produce extrinsic compression on the bowel. Images (**a**) and (**b**) demonstrate a pseudo flat polyp in the hepatic flexure secondary to surgical clips from a prior cholecystectomy

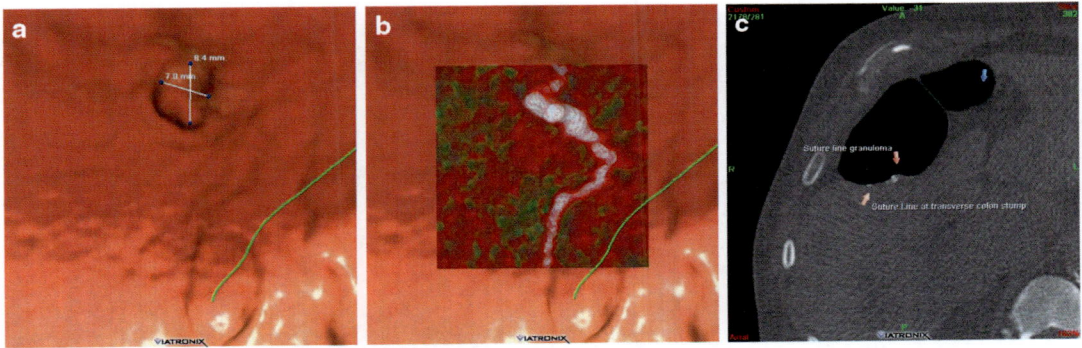

Fig. 8.34 Granulation tissue in the postoperative colon can produce pseudo polyps or masses on the 3-D endoluminal views. Images (**a**)–(**c**) demonstrate a pseudo sessile polyp in the transverse colon secondary to granulation tissues associated with a suture line. The patient was status post right hemicolectomy

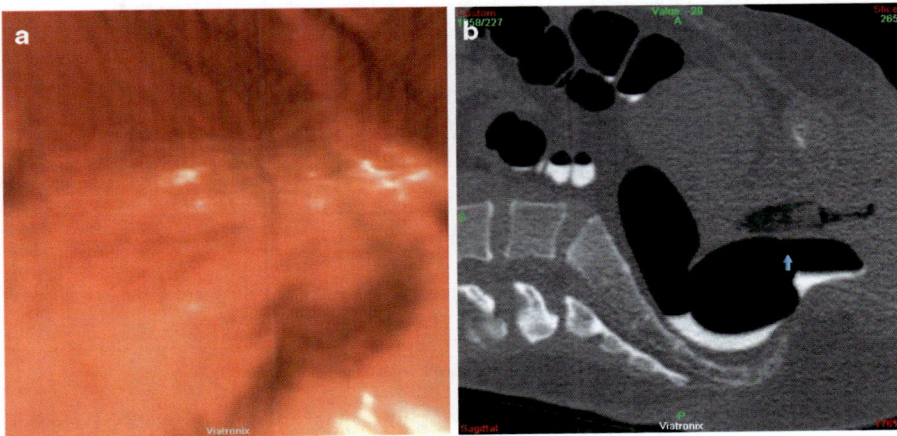

Fig. 8.35 Images (**a**)–(**b**) demonstrate a pseudo flat polyp secondary to extrinsic compression on the anterior wall of the rectum by a vaginal tampon

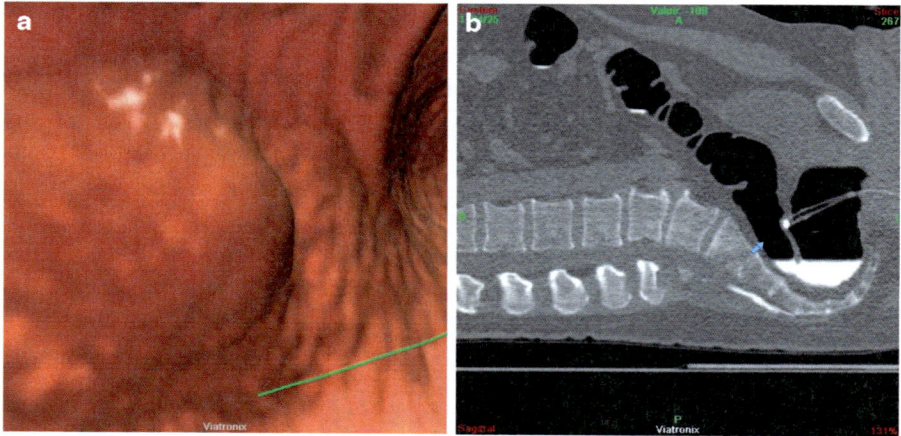

Fig. 8.36 The rectal tube, required for CO_2 insufflation of the colon, can sometimes simulate pathology at the level of the rectosigmoid junction. Images (**a**) and (**b**) demonstrate a pseudo flat polyp on the 3-D endoluminal views of the rectosigmoid junction due to compression from the rectal tube

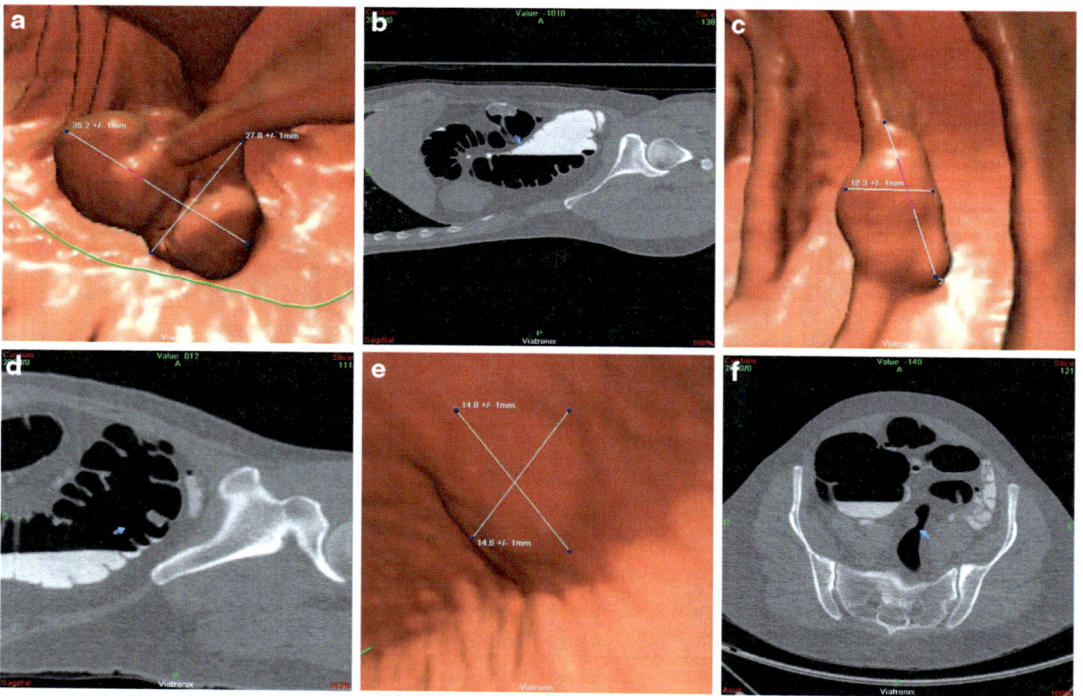

Fig. 8.37 3-D and 2-D images of a pedunculated polyp (images **a** and **b**), a sessile polyp (images **c** and **d**) and a flat polyp (images **e** and **f**) are submitted for comparison to the pseudo lesions shown above and below

Prominent veins, anal papillae, and internal hemorrhoids are anatomical variants found in the rectum. The isolated rectal vein can usually be differentiated from a polyp or rectal fold by its torturous and bifurcating nature (Fig. 8.47). Anal papillae are small skin tags that are typically found abutting the rectal catheter as it traverses the anus (Fig. 8.48). Internal hemorrhoids are dilated veins

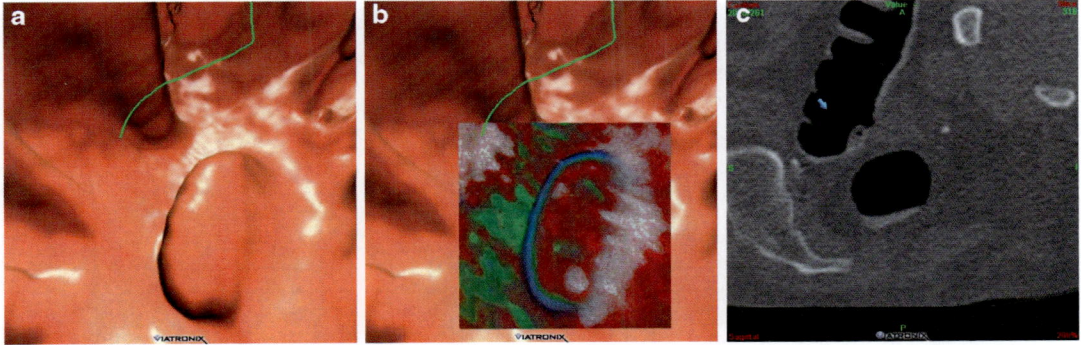

Fig. 8.38 Dense adherent stool can mimic polyps on the 3-D endoluminal images. Adherent stool will not change positions on the prone and supine images. It can be differentiated from a true polyp by the presence of internal fat and air. Images (**a**)–(**c**) demonstrate small pockets of fecal fat and air within the adherent stool on density analysis and on the corresponding 2-D source images

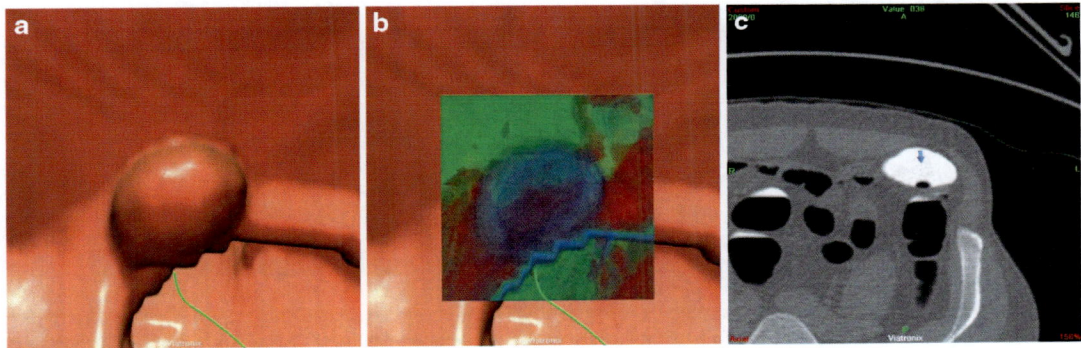

Fig. 8.39 Small air bubbles that become trapped under collections of contrast can mimic smooth sessile polyps. Images (**a**)–(**c**) demonstrate a small bubble in the descending colon. These air bubbles can be differentiated from true polyps with the help of density analysis and correlation with the 2-D source images

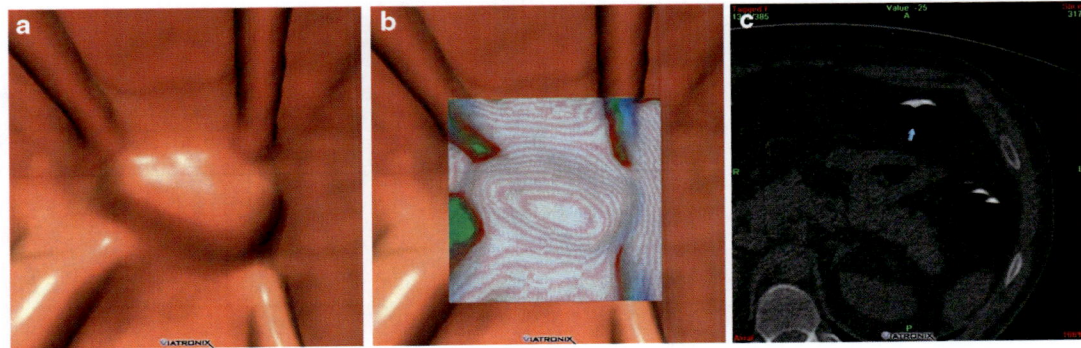

Fig. 8.40 Images (**a**)–(**c**) demonstrate tagged stool floating on a pool of contrast which mimics a sessile polyp between two folds in the transverse colon. Density analysis and correlation with the corresponding 2-D source image reveal the true composition of this pseudo polyp

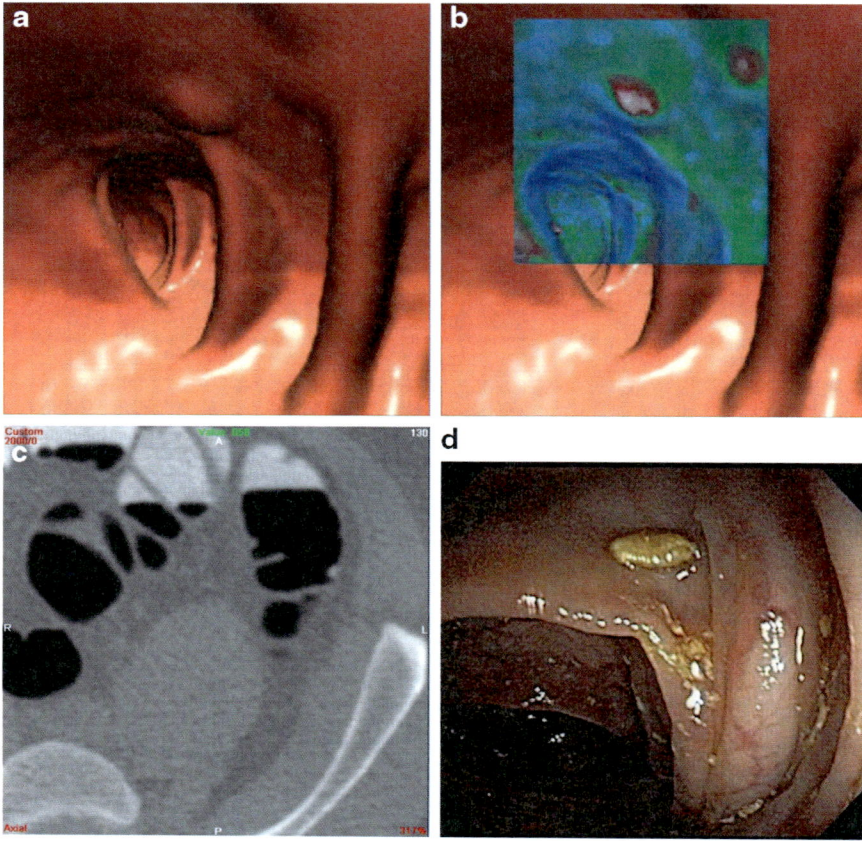

Fig. 8.41 Ingested material that is not removed during the cathartic phase of the bowel prep can present a problem with CTC interpretation. Images (**a**)–(**d**) demonstrate adherent vegetable seeds which can mimic sessile polyps. Ingested material usually changes position with prone and supine imaging

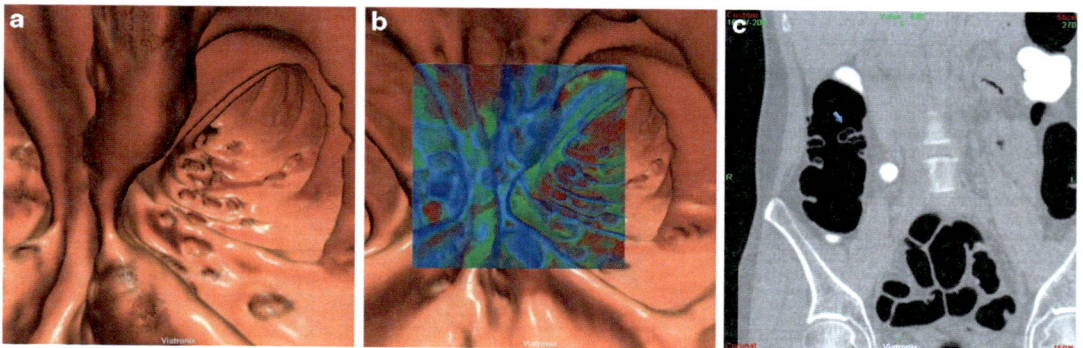

Fig. 8.42 Images (**a**)–(**c**) demonstrate a case of pneumatosis cystoides intestinalis which can mimic sessile polyps on the 3-D images. Density analysis and 2-D correlation easily identify the submucosal air-filled cysts

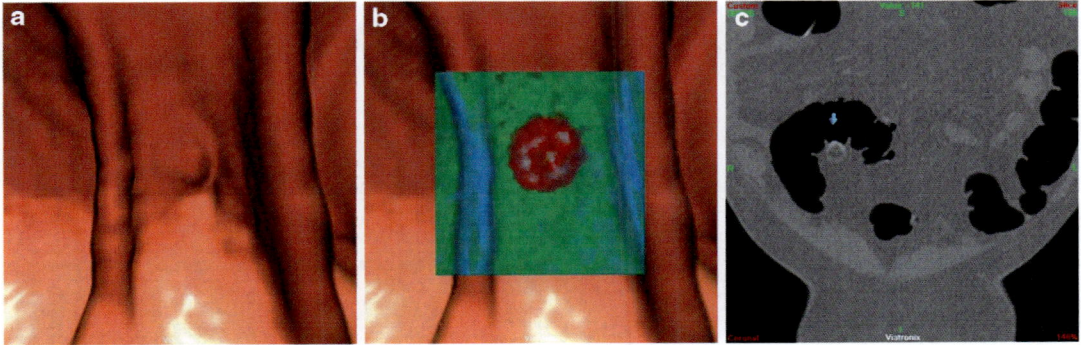

Fig. 8.43 Retained stool in a diverticulum usually contains a mixture of dense contrast, fecal fat, and microbubbles of air. Images (**a**)–(**c**) demonstrate a stool-filled sigmoid colon diverticulum. The heterogeneous makeup of the stool ball is readily apparent on density analysis and the corresponding 2-D source image (image **c**)

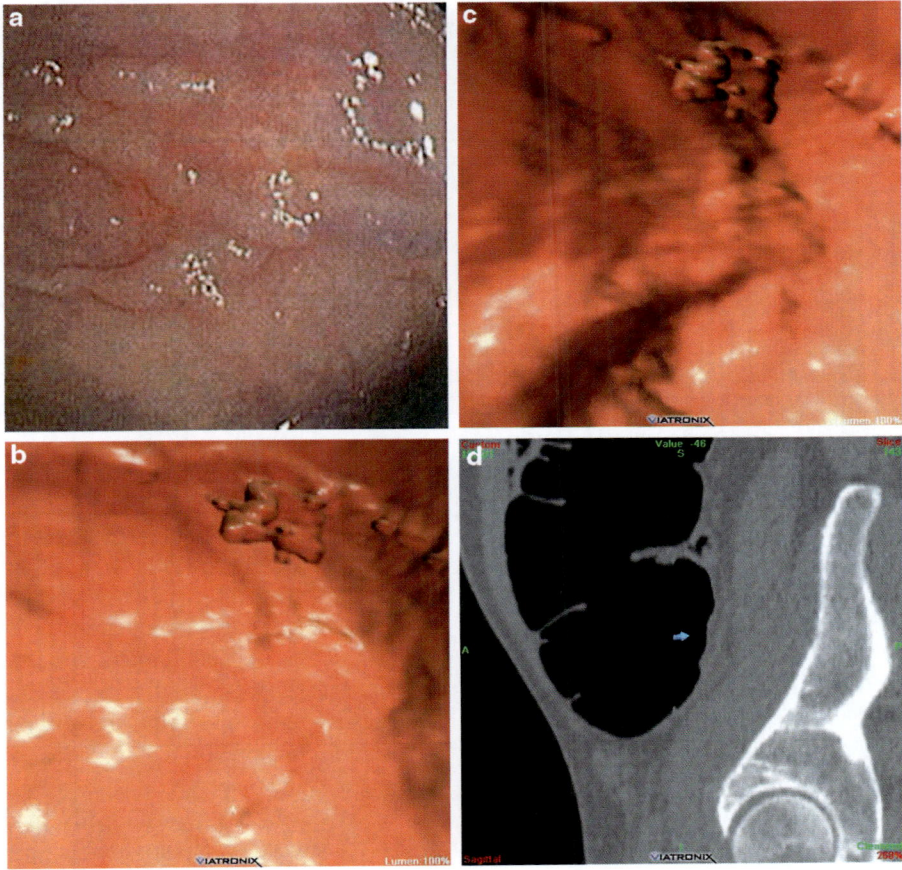

Fig. 8.44 Images (**a**)–(**d**) demonstrate a subtle flat polyp on the medial wall of the cecum. The polyp is not easily seen on the standard 3-D endoluminal view (images **a** and **b**). By varying the position of the artificial light source, the flat lesion becomes more apparent (image **c**). This flat polyp has a subtle appearance on the 2-D source image as well (image **d**)

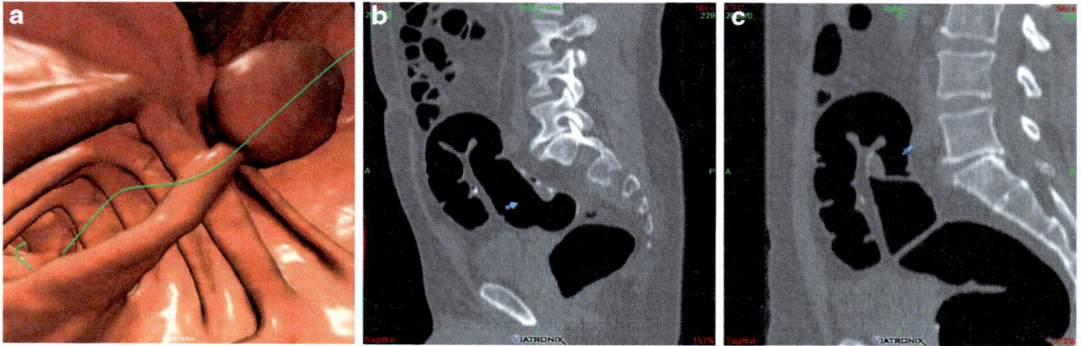

Fig. 8.45 Pedunculated polyps on long stalks can show significant mobility and therefore mimic stool. Images (**a**)–(**c**) demonstrate a pedunculated polyp in the sigmoid colon with a significant change in position on the prone and supine images

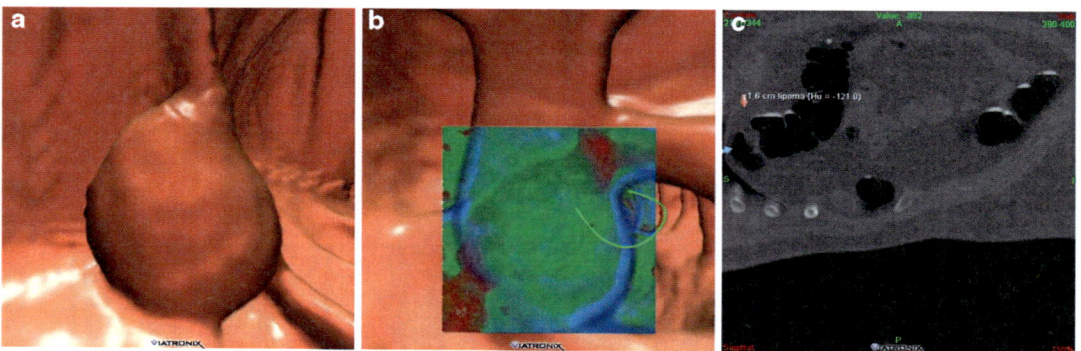

Fig. 8.46 Lipomas are uniform in their fat attenuation with Hounsfield units of −75 to −125. This is easily seen with density interrogation on either the 3-D endoluminal or 2-D source views. Images (**a**)–(**c**) demonstrate a sessile lipoma on a fold in the transverse colon

found around the anus. They can be displayed as linear or polypoid mucosal defects radiating from the anus (Fig. 8.49a, b). Any of these entities, if prominent enough, can mimic a rectal polyp.

The appendix is readily apparent on most CTC studies. In fact, with the present day use of mechanical CO_2 insufflation and stool/fluid tagging, the appendix is usually well distended with gas or contrast. A "mass" involving the appendiceal orifice can represent a multitude of conditions. If the patient has had a prior appendectomy, it may represent an inverted appendiceal stump. Correlation with the patient's surgical history is required when considering this entity (Fig. 8.50a–c). A prolapsing base of the appendix can also produce a mass or pseudopolypoid defect of the appendiceal orifice. This defect is usually self-reducible on the contralateral images (Fig. 8.51a–d). If there is a persistent mass or defect involving the appendiceal orifice, then such entities such as carcinoid, mucocele, adenocarcinoma, and lymphoma must also be considered (Fig. 8.52a, b). Endoluminal visualization of the cecum and appendiceal orifice incompletely evaluates the entire appendix, and analysis of the 2-D source images is required for complete assessment of the appendix.

The ileocecal valve is also readily apparent on most CTC studies. It has a variable appearance between individual patients and also between positioning in the same patient. Ileocecal valve morphology can range from a sessile, fish-mouth appearance to a more bulbous, polypoid appearance. The valve usually takes on a more

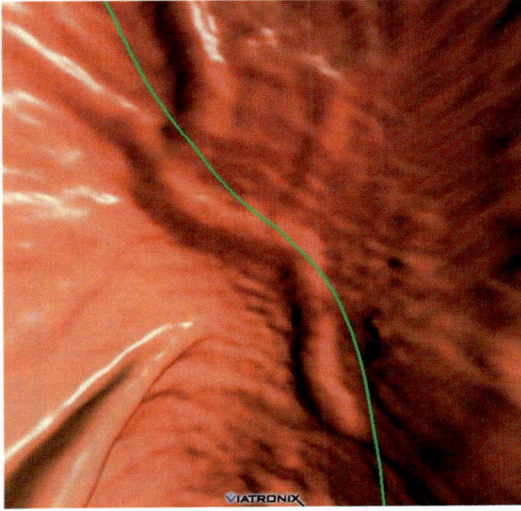

Fig. 8.47 Prominent rectal veins are usually torturous and bifurcating in nature. The image demonstrates an isolated rectal vein with that configuration

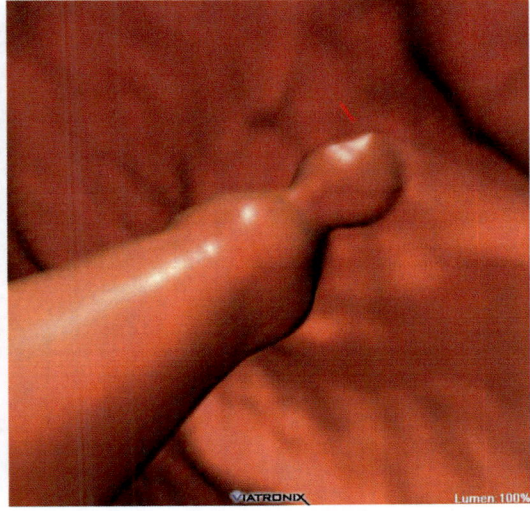

Fig. 8.48 Anal papillae are usually seen as small polypoid soft tissue nodules abutting the rectal catheter as it traverses the anus. The image demonstrates a small anal papilla in its characteristic location

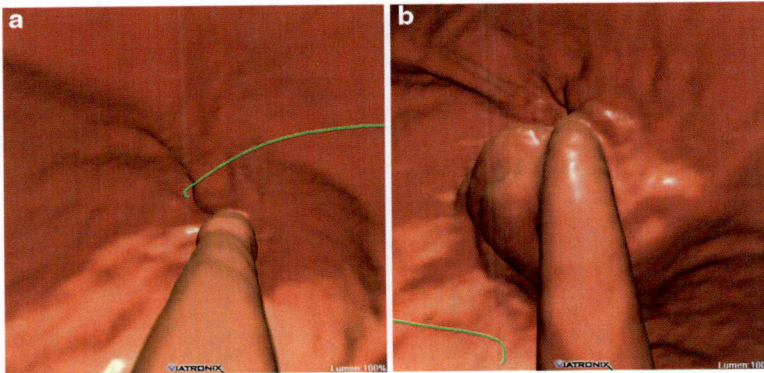

Fig. 8.49 Internal hemorrhoids can be seen as linear or polypoid mucosal masses radiating from the anus. Images (**a**) and (**b**) demonstrate both configurations

bulbous contour when the patient is imaged in the prone position. This is felt to be secondary to increased intraluminal small bowel pressure associated with prone positioning (Fig. 8.53a–c). The ileocecal valve usually demonstrates fat attenuation on the 3-D and 2-D images as well as on color windows and region of interest (ROI) interrogation (Fig. 8.54a–c). Polypoid projec-

tions off of the ileocecal valve are a common finding on CTC. These can represent benign entities such as a drop of barium (Fig. 8.55a–c) or a lipoma (Fig. 8.56a–c). Any polypoid projection off the ileocecal valve that demonstrates soft tissue density, however, must be considered a polyp until proven otherwise (Fig. 8.57a–d). One must also be careful not to assume any polypoid

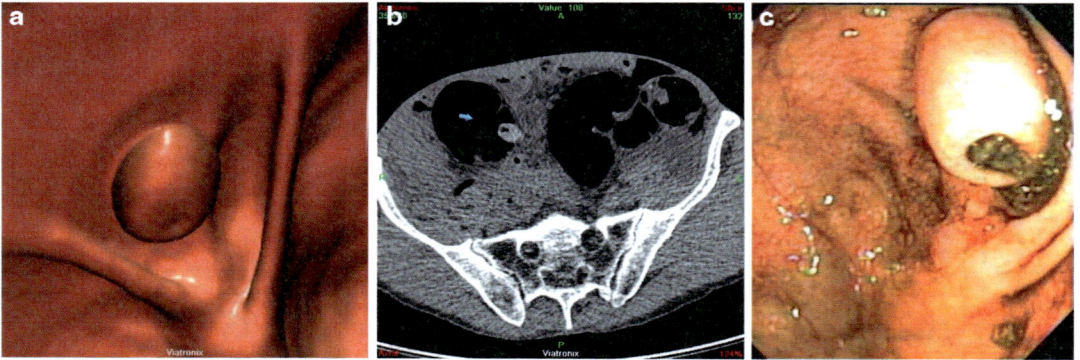

Fig. 8.50 Images (**a**)–(**c**) demonstrate an inverted appendiceal stump in a patient who has had an appendectomy

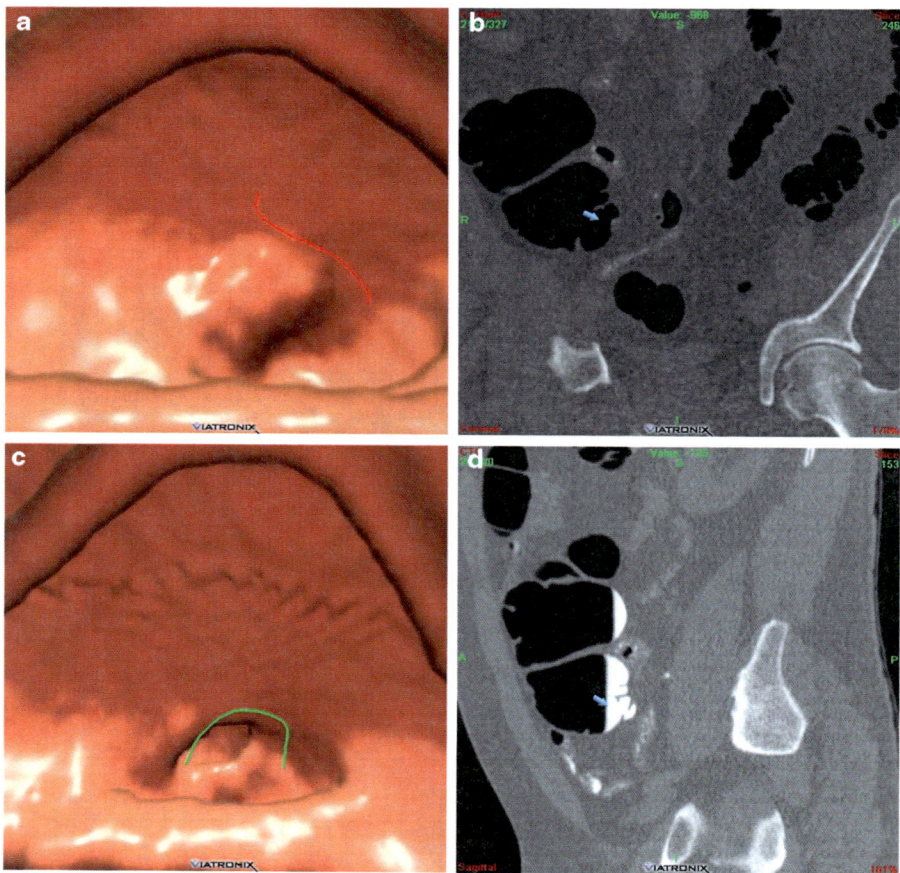

Fig. 8.51 A prolapsing base of the appendix can produce a transient soft tissue mass involving the appendiceal orifice. Images (**a**)–(**d**) demonstrate the reducible nature of the prolapsing base of the appendix on both the 3-D endoluminal and 2-D source images

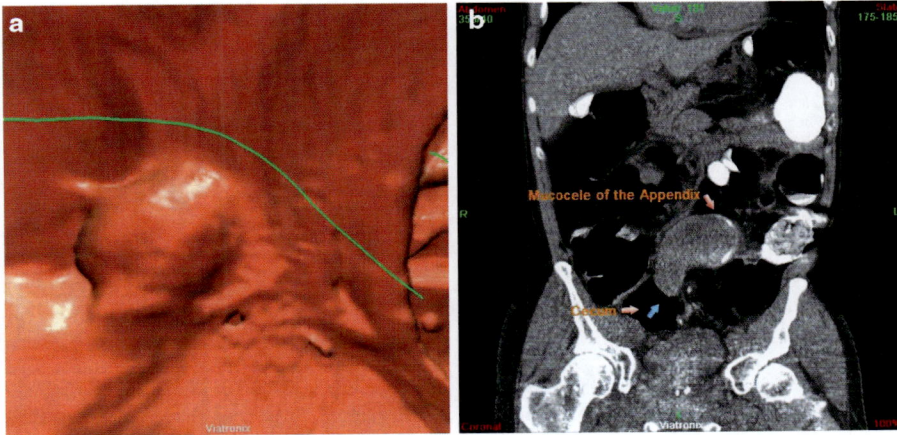

Fig. 8.52 Image (**a**) demonstrates a persistent sessile mass in the appendiceal orifice on the 3-D endoluminal images. The corresponding 2-D source image (image **b**) identifies the defect as the base of a distended, mucous-filled appendix with mural calcifications, consistent with a mucocele

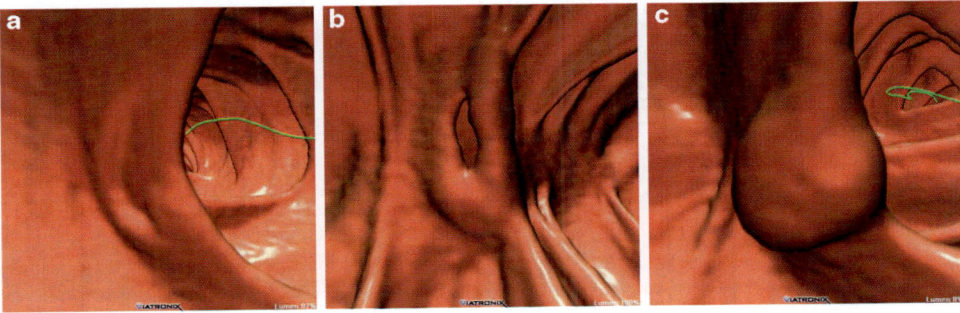

Fig. 8.53 Images (**a**)–(**c**) demonstrate the various configurations a normal ileocecal valve can assume on CTC imaging

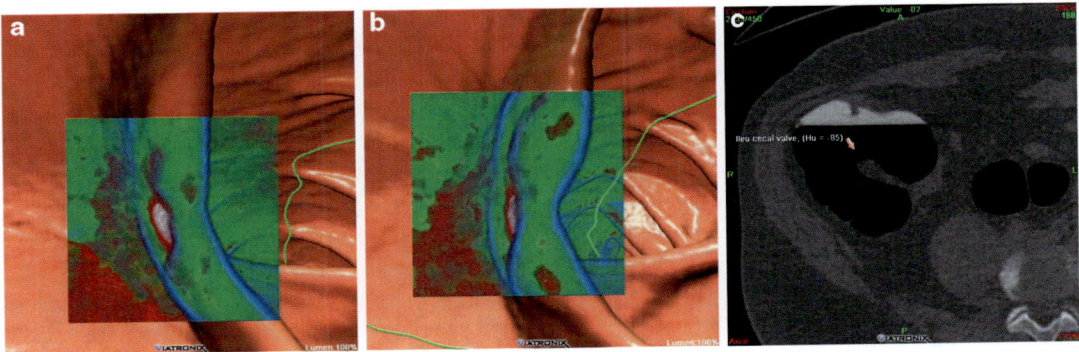

Fig. 8.54 Images (**a**)–(**c**) demonstrate the characteristic fat attenuation of the ileocecal valve on the 3-D and 2-D images

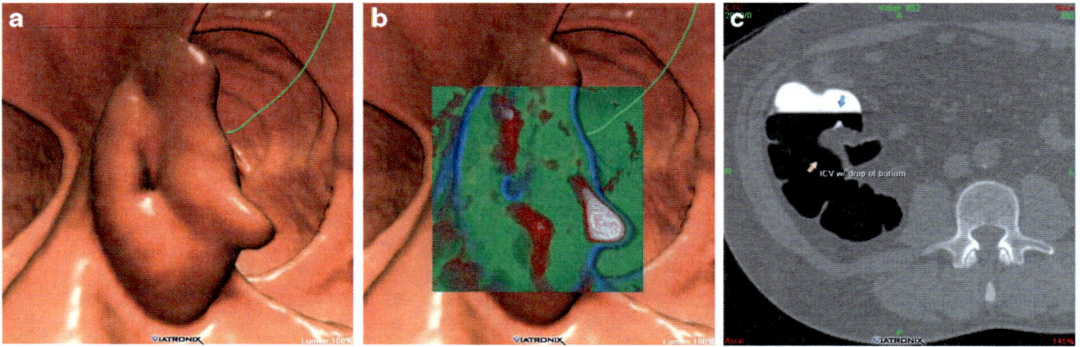

Fig. 8.55 Barium droplets can adhere to the ileocecal valve simulating small polyps on the 3-D endoluminal views. These droplets are easily identified by their increased density. Images (**a**)–(**c**) demonstrate 3-D, color window and 2-D views of a drop of barium on the ileocecal valve

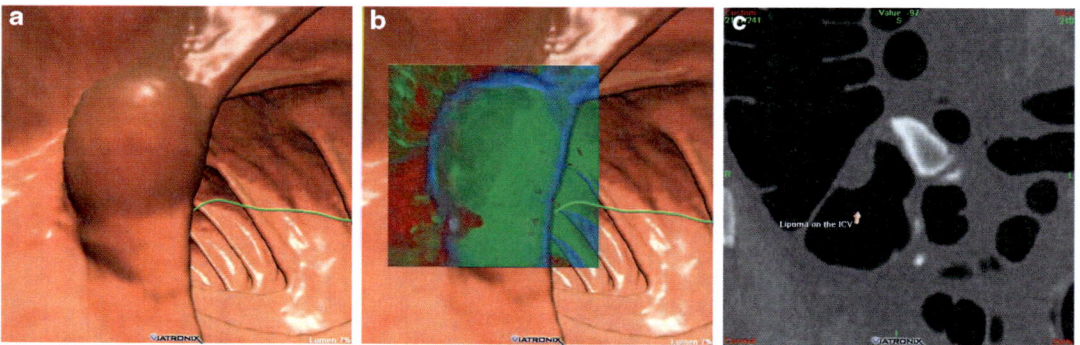

Fig. 8.56 Lipomas of the ileocecal valve are polypoid projections that demonstrate uniform fat attenuation. Images (**a**)–(**c**) demonstrate 3-D, color window and 2-D views of a lipoma on the ileocecal valve

structure in the cecum is simply the ileocecal valve. A cecal mass can be mistaken for the ileocecal valve (Fig. 8.58a–c). Complete assessment of the ileocecal valve must include evaluation of the valve's morphology, attenuation, and position in the cecum on the 3-D and 2-D images.

Conclusion

There are multiple potential pitfalls and artifacts associated with CTC imaging. The reader must be cognizant of these to adequately analyze the study and provide an accurate interpretation. This chapter has provided examples of the most common CTC pitfalls and artifacts, along with techniques for correctly identifying and characterizing these findings. With proper attention to technique in patient preparation, bowel distension, and image acquisition diagnostic quality, high-quality CTC studies can be obtained. Through careful analysis of the 3-D images with 2-D correlation, color windows, and ROI interrogation, the majority of these pitfalls and artifacts can be recognized and adequately managed.

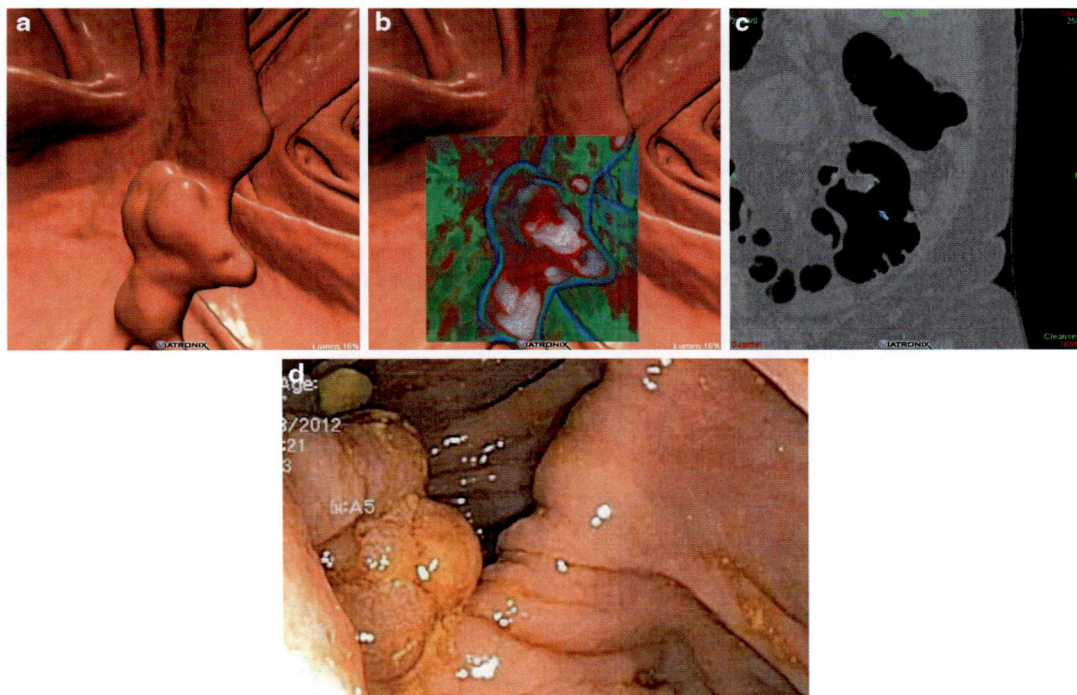

Fig. 8.57 Polyps can also project off the ileocecal valve. Images (**a**)–(**c**) demonstrate 3-D, color window and 2-D views of a large, sessile polyp projecting off the inferior aspect of the ileocecal valve. Image (**d**) shows the endoscopic correlation of this polyp

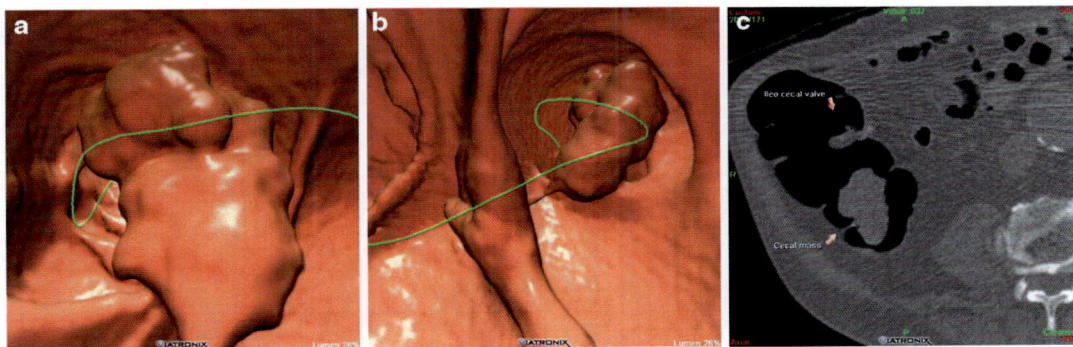

Fig. 8.58 Images (**a**)–(**c**) demonstrate a large mass on a fold deep within the cecum. This mass should not be mistaken for the ileocecal valve, which is seen more proximal in the cecum

Suggested Readings

1. Mang T, et al. Pitfalls in multi-detector row CT colonography: a systematic approach. Radiographics. 2007;27:431–54.
2. Dachman AH, et al. CT colonography: visualization methods, interpretation, and pitfalls. Radiol Clin North Am. 2007;45:347–59.
3. Halligan S, Taylor SA. CT colonography: results and limitations. Eur J Radiol. 2007;61:400–8.
4. Christensen KN, Fidler JL, Fletcher JG, Maccarty R, Johnson CD, et al. Pictorial review of colonic polyp and mass distortion and recognition with the CT virtual dissection technique. Radiographics. 2010. doi:10.1148/rg.e42.
5. Barish MA, et al. Multislice CT colonography: current status and limitations. Radiol Clin North Am. 2005;43:1049–62.
6. Hoon JI, et al. Multislice CT colonography: current status and limitations. Eur J Radiol. 2003;47:123–34.
7. Fletcher JG, Gluecker TM. CT colonography (virtual colonoscopy) for the detection of colorectal polyps and neoplasms: current status and future developments. Eur J Cancer. 2002;38:2070–8.
8. Dachman AH. Atlas of virtual colonoscopy. New York: Springer; 2003.
9. Pickhardt PJ, Kim DH. CT colonography: principles and practice of virtual colonoscopy. Philadelphia, PA: Saunders; 2010.

Future Directions/Innovations with CTC (Prepless CTC, Alternative Displays, Computer-Aided Detection)

9

Farid Dahi and Abraham H. Dachman

In Chap. 5 the routine preparation and methods of colon cleansing were discussed. A common refrain we hear is "the worst thing about colorectal cancer (CRC) screening is the preparation." While reduced cathartic and even so-called "prepless" CTC without any cathartic have been done successfully in published reports, these processes have not yet reached the mainstream for clinical application. A well-known phrase among abdominal radiologists who perform barium enemas was "heaven is a clean colon." The same still holds true for CTC, yet the possibility of routine "prepless" CTC is within the realm of feasibility [1]. Below we will discuss these options.

Issues of training and interpretation of CTC images were also covered in Chap. 5; however, many novel viewing methods have been developed by researchers and commercial vendors. We refer to these generically as "novel" or "alternated display" methods. Some have the potential to make CTC faster or more intuitive to interpret. A variety of names are used, some of which may be vendor specific, but often by common jargon in field they have taken on a more generic meaning. We will discuss and show examples of several of these methods.

Thirdly, computer-aided detection (CAD) to improve the sensitivity and confidence of inter-

pretation of CTC has been studied for years, but now, FDA-approved software has reached the marketplace. We will review and explain the current status of CAD for CTC as well as research combining CAD with prepless CTC.

"Prepless" CTC

Cathartic preparation has been shown to be one of the most unpleasant portions of whole colon CRC screening, and the poor compliance with complex bowel preparation or dietary restrictions contributes to reduce the patient acceptance for CRC screening [1, 2]. The introduction of fecal/fluid tagging gave the advantage to CTC over optical colonoscopy (OC) to reduce or eliminate cathartic preparation and increase patient acceptance. Oral barium or ionized iodinated contrast materials (sodium amidotrizoate and meglumine amidotrizoate; Gastrografin) or the combination of both made it possible to distinguish lesions from fecal residues [3]. However because of potential risk for fatal complications of iodine idiosyncrasy, there have been some concerns around their use for fecal tagging [4]. Conversely, barium has been shown to be safe with minimal side effects, relatively palatable, and effective for tagging solid residue [5]. Another advantage of reduced or noncathartic bowel preparation is avoiding potential complications reported with full-dose cathartic preparations including renal failure, preexisting electrolyte abnormalities, congestive heart failure, ascites, or ileus, which can occur in addition to the discomfort

F. Dahi, M.D. • A.H. Dachman, M.D. (✉)
Department of Radiology, The University of Chicago
Medical Center (UCMC), Chicago, IL, USA
e-mail: adachman@radiology.bsd.uchicago.edu

and inconvenience that patients experience as a result of cathartic preparation [6].

There are number of disadvantages to noncathartic CTC. The laxative-free preparation cannot be considered to be totally "prepless," since in most noncathartic preparations, patients are prescribed a fairly rigorous regimen consisting of dietary restriction and various oral contrast agents. Some contrasts, such as diatrizoate, have a cathartic-like effect. Also, lack of cathartic preparation precludes same-day therapeutic OC. Moreover, the potential negative impact on accuracy can result in missing lesions or overuse of OC [7]. Investigations have mostly focused on the feasibility of different reduced or noncathartic bowel preparation schemes with regard to patient compliance and diagnostic performance of CTC.

Patient Compliance

Patient acceptability is a key factor for any screening test. In recent years there has been a moderate increase in CRC screening adherence rates, reaching 63% in 2008 versus 52% in 2002 [8]. In a study of barriers against CRC screening tests and patient preferences in a nonadherent urban population, 65% of patients who were not adherent to CRC screening recommendations had breast and prostate cancer screening in the past, suggesting that significant barriers, such bowel cleansing preparation, may be specific to CRC screening [9]. Regarding the current conventional CTC bowel preparation, Yoon et al. [4] compared different combinations of laxatives (sodium phosphate and magnesium citrate) and barium-based fecal-tagging agents (Tagitol V and EZ-CAT) on 69 patients who were undergoing CTC. The worst compliance was seen with the combination of sodium phosphate and EZ-CAT. They suggested the combination of magnesium citrate, and a small amount (60 ml) of high concentration (40% wt/vol) of a barium-tagging agent was associated with better compliance and preserved diagnostic accuracy.

The spectrum of studies on patient compliance ranges from limited use of laxatives to laxative-free CTC exams. Neri et al. [3] used a mild laxative, PEG macrogol 3350, which is usually used to treat chronic constipation, together with iodixanol for fluid tagging in a study performed on 130 asymptomatic patients. They did not observe any cathartic effect or laxative-related side effects, and there were no altered lifestyle and habits. Besides optimal fluid tagging, an excellent level of acceptance was achieved (average of 9 on a 10-point scale questionnaire). In another study, a minimal dose of bisacodyl (20 mg) accompanied by a 2-day low-fiber diet and diatrizoate meglumine and barium for fecal tagging provided good image quality and high patient acceptance during CTC exams of 40 increased-risk patients. Increasing the amount of laxative did not lead to higher attenuation of tagging, more homogeneous tagging, or significant improvement in subjective image quality and was associated with a lower patient acceptance. However, regardless of the amount of laxative for CRC screening, the majority of patients preferred the bowel preparation for CTC over cleansing laxative bowel preparation (PEG) for colonoscopy [10].

Taking it one step further, Buccardi et al. omitted any frank laxative drug in 132 average-risk patients prepared for CTC with a laxative-free fecal-tagging (LFT) regimen using a water-soluble iodinated contrast agent (Gastrografin) and compared the results with 132 average-risk control patients prepared with traditional cathartic cleansing(TC) with respect to patient tolerance. Severe abdominal pain was seen in 107/132 of the TC group, while only 25/132 of the LFT group had the same experience. Although Gastrografin is not a frank laxative, it has a mild-strong osmotic laxative effect due to an increased colonic osmotic load. Most papers on fecal-tagging techniques reported very few cases of severe abdominal pain [11]. In another comparison study, patient acceptance and future preference was significantly higher for CTC with dry preparation (combination of dietary restriction and small amount of contrast agent) versus conventional OC [12]. In a study performed by Florie et al. [13] in 61 patients at increased risk of CRC, 81% of patients preferred

CTC without cathartic cleansing compared with 13% who preferred OC and 7% who were indifferent. Their preparation regimen consisted of a low-fiber diet starting 2 days prior the exam, lactulose for stool softening, taken for three mornings prior to the test, and amidotrizoic acid for fecal tagging. Patients rated the limited bowel preparation (prior to CTC) less burdensome than the bowel preparation prior to OC.

Diagnostic Performance

In addition to patient acceptability, diagnostic performance is also a key factor which should be taken into account during simplification of CTC preparation. Several feasibility studies have evaluated the image quality and diagnostic performance of CTC with noncathartic bowel preparation. In a recent study, 80 asymptomatic patients aged 48–72 years old were divided into two groups of 40 patients. The first group underwent CTC with conventional bowel preparation, full cathartic dose, and oral contrast during the 3 days preceding the CTC. The second group had CTC with no cathartic preparation and only residue tagging administered on the test day. There were no significant differences with regard to examination quality and overall CTC accuracy. They found 94.1% true positives in the group with the conventional bowel preparation and very close to that number (92.3%) for the group that underwent noncathartic bowel preparation [14]. Conversely, Dachman et al. [15] did not find favorable results when comparing two groups of patients (14 in each group) who underwent CTC with (prepped) and without (prepless) cathartic preparation. Both groups received 40% barium for residue tagging. They compared multiple factors between the two groups, including percentage of residual stool that was touching or near-touching mucosa, the largest piece of retained stool, effectiveness of tagging, height of residual fluid, degree of distention, ease of interpretation, and reading time. There were no significant differences in degree of distention, percentage of tagged stool, or reading time. However, significant differences were seen in the

amount of stool-covering mucosa, the ease of interpretation, the mean size of largest piece of stool, and the height of residual fluid. Three polyps ≥5 mm in size were found during OC in three patients in the prepless group, none of which were prospectively detected at CTC. They concluded that noncathartic bowel preparation leaves significant residual stool, which is not desirable even if it is well tagged.

Sensitivity of any screening test is very important for high prevalent conditions in order to reduce false-negative results. Although OC has the highest sensitivity for polyp and cancer detection, the sensitivity in elderly patients (at increased risk of CRC) can be reduced due to incomplete examinations or decreased compliance to bowel preparation, mainly because of limiting comorbidities [16–18]. Jensch et al. designed a study to evaluate the sensitivity and specificity of prepless CTC performed on 168 elderly patients (mean age 65 years) [19]. One hundred fourteen patients had histologically proven polyps (56 polyps ≥6 mm and 17 polyps ≥10 mm). The preparation regimen consisted of 80 ml of barium sulfate and 180 ml of diatrizoate meglumine. Bisacodyl was added for stool softening. They reported 76% of sensitivity for patients with lesions ≥6 mm and 82% for lesions ≥10 mm. The specificity was 79% and 97%, respectively. Per-polyp sensitivity was 70% and 82% for lesions ≥6 mm and ≥10 mm, respectively. Another study involving 56 patients with known or suspected colorectal polyps or cancer revealed that the sensitivity for polyp detection in prepless patients who had well-labeled stool approached the published sensitivity for cathartic prepared colon [20]. In this study, preparation consisted of oral administration of dilute barium sulfate (225 ml, 1.2% barium sulfate wt/vol) for seven doses during 48 h prior to CTC.

In a larger study, Iannaccone et al. evaluated diagnostic performance of prepless CTC in 203 patients who had a variety of indications for OC [21]. All patients underwent low-dose multidetector CTC 3–7 days (average 4.2 days) prior to OC. No cathartic was used for CTC bowel preparation. Diatrizoate meglumine and diatrizoate sodium was added to regular meals for fecal tagging. The average per-polyp sensitivity for CTC was 95.5% for polyps≥8 mm while per-patient sensitivity and specificity were 89.9% and 92.2%, respectively. Also the positive predictive value (PPV) and negative predictive value (NPV) of CTC were 88% and 93.5%, respectively. To make CTC more comfortable and increase in patient compliance, Liedenbaum et al. decided to go one step further and not only eliminated cathartic bowel preparation but also omitted the low-fiber diet which is usually prescribed prior to CTC under the assumption that such a diet reduces the bowel content and provides a much homogeneous tagged feces [22]. In this study, 50 patients with positive fecal occult blood test underwent prep-less CTC with iodine fecal tagging: 25 patients used a low-fiber diet and 25 had no special diet. Findings during OC, performed 2 weeks after CTC, were used as reference for estimation of per-polyp sensitivity for polyps 6 mm in diameter and larger. The results showed that use of a low-fiber diet in bowel preparation for CTC resulted in less untagged feces and better residue homogeneity. Since there was no significant difference in patient acceptance between restricted and unrestricted diet, they concluded that low-fiber diet should be used to obtain good image quality in prepless CTC.

Electronic Cleansing

In a prepless (noncathartic prepared) colon, incompletely tagged solid or semisolid stool is distributed on the colonic wall. The distributed tagged residues with various shapes and sizes may obscure lesions that are submerged in or adjacent to the tagged materials or can imitate small lesions and make it difficult to accurately interpret images. Electronic cleansing, as an emerging technique, virtually cleans the colon after image acquisition, by subtracting tagged solid and semisolid fecal materials as well as tagged fluids from CTC images. This is a promising technique that may provide a better approach for prepless CTC [6].

There are some technical barriers for electronic cleansing schemes in that they tend to generate artifacts on cleansed CTC images. One of the major artifacts, called "degradation of soft-tissue structures," is produced by artificial increments of tissue attenuation, which results primarily from beam-hardening effect caused by adjacent high-attenuation tagged materials. This leads electronic cleansing to confuse soft-tissue structures (folds or polyps) with tagged materials and mistakenly remove them [6]. Another artifact, called "pseudo-soft-tissue structure," is caused by partial volume effect at the boundary between the luminal air and the tagged regions (air-tagging boundary), which results in overlap of CT attenuation of voxels at the boundary with soft-tissue structures [23]. Since current electronic cleansing methods recognize tagged fluid as large, flat, and horizontal surfaces, they remove only the horizontal portions of the air-tagging boundary and leave the bumpy portions, which may mimic colonic soft-tissue structures. Moreover, electronic cleansing methods consider homogenous high CT attenuations as tagged materials. However, fecal materials are heterogeneous and composed of a mixture of undigested food, fat, and air bubbles which results in a combination of high and low attenuations. Therefore, electronic cleansing methods may remove only materials with high CT attenuation and leave a low-attenuation tagged material, which is referred to "incomplete cleansing" [6].

To overcome these technical barriers, several image-processing functions have been developed, such as a "structure-analysis cleansing" scheme that uses local morphologic information rather than CT attenuation values, allowing differentiation of submerged colonic soft-tissue structures (polyp-like and fold-like structures) from fecal tagged materials and subtract the latter from CTC images (Fig. 9.1). Application of structure-analysis cleansing in 237 cases undergoing prepless CTC showed promising results [6]. Structure-analysis cleansing along with other cutting-edge image-processing techniques can provide diagnostic-quality cleansed CTC images and make prepless CTC a patient-friendly and highly sensitive tool for detection of colorectal polyps and cancer.

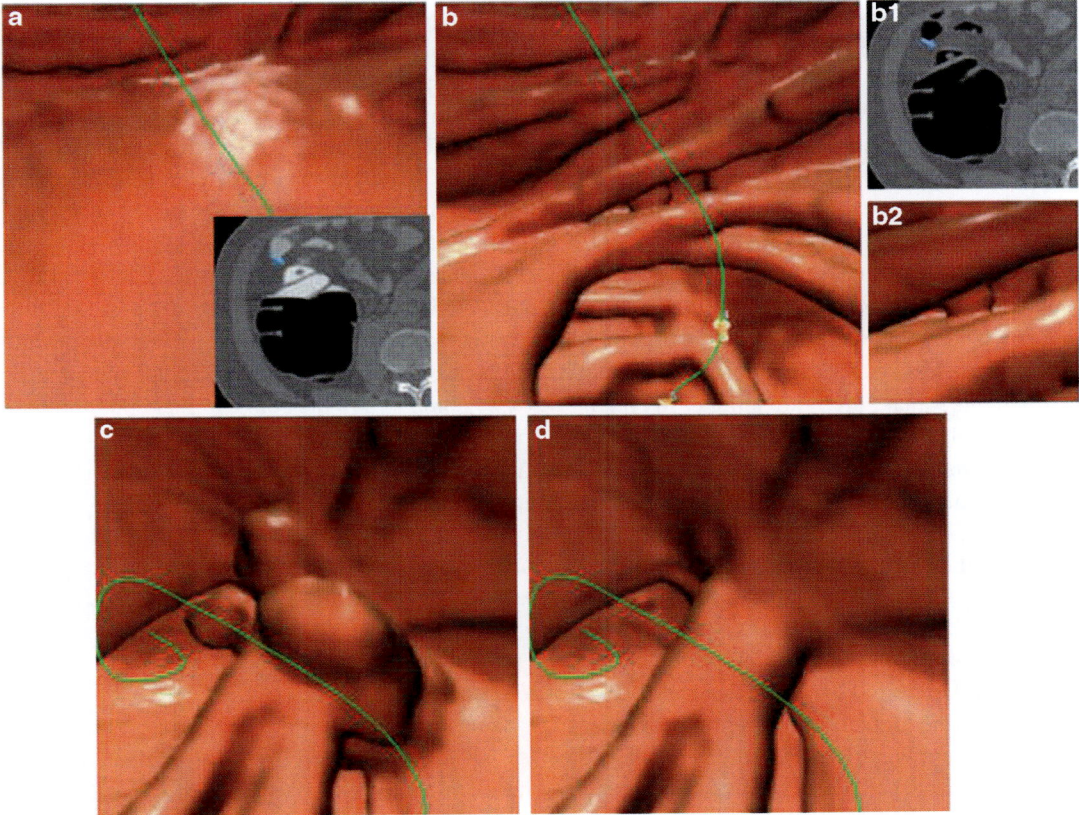

Fig. 9.1 Recovery of submerged polyps and folds. *Green lines* indicate the center line of the colonic lumen, which is used for the fly-through for virtual colonoscopy. (**a**) Three-dimensional endoscopic CT colonographic image and axial CT colonographic image (*insert*) show an 8.2-mm cecal polyp submerged in tagged fecal material (*arrow*). (**b**) On a 3D endoscopic CT colonographic image and axial CT colonographic image obtained after the application of structure-analysis cleansing, the polyp is clearly visible (*arrow* on (**b1**)). Figure (**b2**) shows a magnified 3D endoscopic view of the polyp. (**c**) Three-dimensional endoscopic CT colonographic image shows folds that are partially submerged in semisolid tagged stool. (**d**) On a 3D endoscopic CT colonographic image obtained after the application of structure-analysis cleansing, the submerged portions of the folds have been well recovered and are connected to the nonsubmerged portions without interruption (courtesy of Wenli Cai, PhD, and Hiro Yoshida, PhD, Massachusetts General Hospital and Harvard Medical School, Boston, MA)

Alternative Displays

The data acquired from CT scans can be processed by different commercially available programs that can display the images for analysis by the radiologist in two-dimensional (2D) and three-dimensional (3D) formats. The 2D display consists of either axial images or multiplanar reformatted images (MPR). All readers and current consensus guidelines favor a combined 2D/3D approach for CTC reading [24, 25]. Advantages of the 2D view include better visualization of wall thickness and possibility of extracolonic evaluation (if necessary) and allow a more specific distinction of homogeneous soft-tissue density polyps from more heterogeneous residual stool. It is also easier to recognize other polypoid appearing findings such as inverted diverticula, stool-impacted diverticula, prolapsed appendix, and ingested materials or pills on 2D view. However, greater interobserver variability has been seen in 2D approaches, and the relative constant attention and focus needed for a satisfactory 2D read may result in increased reader fatigue and eye strain [25].

The most common 3D display being used is the endoluminal fly-through technique in which the reader can navigate antegrade and retrograde through a volume-rendered endoscopic view of the colon, with the help of a self-created, semiautomated, or automated path provided by software [24, 26]. The advantages of the 3D endoluminal view include less reader fatigue and eyestrain as well as the fact that polyps are more easily distinguished from adjacent haustral folds when viewed as a 3D rendering, since in a 2D view polyps and a haustral folds may appear identical on a static axial image. However, the 3D view has limitation in visualization of polyps obscured behind folds or situated deeply within a sacculated haustra between high folds [25]. There is a shorter learning curve for endoluminal review; however, 2D correlation is required for characterization of all polypoid filling defects, prolonging interpretation time. Moreover, to increase the percentage of visualized mucosal surface, the reader should evaluate colon with four fly-through examinations, including antegrade and retrograde fly-throughs of supine and prone data sets, which some feel makes the endoluminal review method less time efficient than 2D review [24, 27].

In order to reduce the reading time, and to overcome other limitations of the endoluminal view, new visualization techniques have been developed. As early as the late 1990s, Beaulieu et al. proposed "panoramic viewing," the acquisition of a sequence of unfolded 60° views perpendicular to the central path. The technique resulted in higher sensitivity than 2D and 3D cine loops; however, it may not provide full visibility, since forward and backward viewing directions are not included [28]. In this chapter we discuss more prevalent novel visualization methods including (1) virtual dissection, (2) perspective-filet view, (3) panoramic endoluminal (band view) method, and (4) unfolded cube method.

Although "flattening" or "cutting the colon open" enables viewing of a part or the entire colon, it results in some distortion ("morphing")

of the colonic structures. Some methods cut the colon open in half without laying it flat to avoid the distortion ("split view") (Fig. 9.2) [29]. Lee et al. compared image distortion among different novel visualization methods (virtual dissection, split view, band view, and filet view) and conventional endoluminal view for 10- and 20-mm synthetic polyps [27]. Split view and band view represented the least image distortion index (1.02 and 1.03 for 10-mm polyps and 1.02 and 1.01 for 20-mm polyps, respectively). The distortion index was not significantly different with these views compared to the conventional endoluminal view (1.03 and 1.02 for 10-mm and 20-mm polyps, respectively). However, virtual colon dissection and filet view revealed higher mean image distortion index (3.27 and 1.65 for 10-mm polyps and 3.85 and 1.55 for 20-mm polyps, respectively).

Virtual Dissection

Virtual dissection, referred also as filet view or virtual pathology display, is a 3D visualization method in which the colon is virtually unraveled, dissected open, and flattened. The 360° view of the inner colonic surface is displayed as a series of segmented strips on a single monitor, which the strips' lengths can be adjusted to meet the reader preference. Also, there is overlap at the edges of dissected plane which allows lesions located at the cut surface of colon to be extended into overlapped area (Fig. 9.3) [25, 30]. Comparing with conventional 3D endoluminal view, virtual dissection has the advantage of displaying the entire mucosal surface, in contrast there are blind spots in conventional endoluminal view. Moreover, only a single review is performed with visual dissection method, rather than bidirectional reading approach with traditional fly-through display [31]. Therefore, this method has potentials to provide less evaluation time and reader fatigue than conventional endoluminal view. However, the process of straightening and flattening may cause distortions of normal turns and haustral folds, and lesions may be displayed more than once in some areas or appear elongated

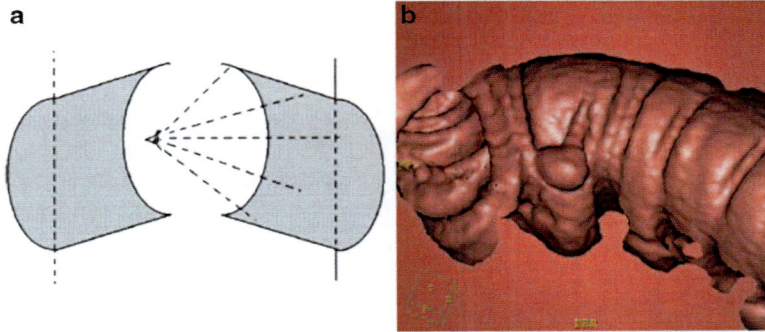

Fig. 9.2 Split view. (**a**) Diagram of the colon split into two cups without flattening the colon. (**b**) View of one-half of the split colon. This technique avoids the morphing and distortion associated with flattening (courtesy of Philips Medical Systems, Inc, Bothell, WA; with permission)

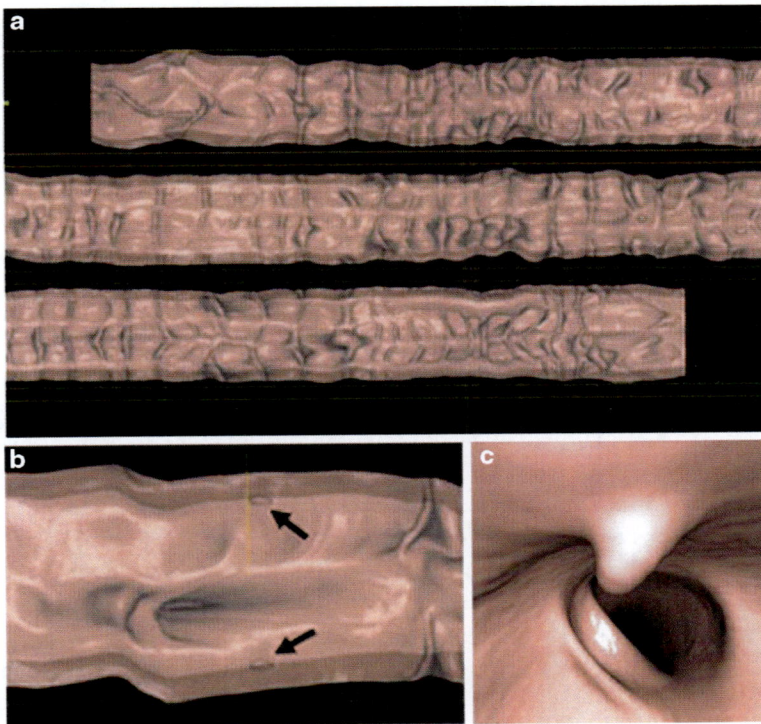

Fig. 9.3 (**a**) Virtual dissection view. The complete colon (divided into three stripes) is displayed in the monitor for inspection and interpretation. (**b**) Overlapping tissue at the plane of dissection in a flattened view. Notice that a small sessile polyp (*arrows*) is displayed on both sides of the plane of dissection, thus ensuring that a potential lesion will not be overlooked because of the dissection. (**c**) The same polyp is well demonstrated on the 3D endoluminal image

or stretched out [25]. Because of possible distortions, it is essential for readers to get familiar with the spectrum of appearances related to this display technique. In a study by Johnson et al. [32], polyp distortion was shown to be related to the underlying morphologic features. Sessile and flat masses appeared as flame- or pea-shaped lesions and pedunculated masses generally appeared as flame- or club-shaped lesions. There were few bizarrely shaped lesions which represented a pedunculated polyp. Generally, it is possible to differentiate areas of distortion from true lesions by performing a real-time comparison of virtual dissection images with the corresponding 2D axial and 3D endoluminal images [31].

Several studies have evaluated the performance of virtual dissection display technique [32–34]. There is a report of 98.7% sensitivity and 79.1% specificity for virtual dissection display in detection of polyps >6 mm, in a large study on over 4,300 subjects [25]. However, Juchems et al. [26] found less detection rate in their study on 21 patients who had either colon polyps or cancer. Overall per-lesion sensitivity using filet view for lesions <5 mm, between 5 and 10 mm, and >10 mm was 47.1%, 56.3%, and 75%, respectively. This was compared with conventional endoluminal and MPR views with an overall per-lesion sensitivity of 35.3%, 81.5%, and 100% for lesions ≤5 mm, 5–10 mm, and >10 mm, respectively. The average total time needed for evaluation was 10 min (5–13 min) using filet view, versus 38 min (23–55 min) using conventional endoluminal and MPR views. Rottgen et el. [34] reported a high sensitivity and specificity for polyp detection as of 94 and 80% with virtual dissection versus 89 and 80% with using conventional endoluminal view. However, by size stratified comparison, they found no significant difference in sensitivity between these two display techniques for polyps ≥5 mm, but the difference was significant for smaller lesions (<5 mm).

Perspective-Filet View

The method is similar to virtual dissection, except that the filet view provides a dynamic display compared with static display in virtual dissection. It creates a movie loop of unrolled colon lumen (along its center axis), and each section is displayed for a short period of time in the center of the screen. Since there is no considerable distortion in the exact center of screen, reader can concentrate on one short segment while still using 2D

and/or traditional endoluminal view. By tilting the projection rays from the eye point as a function of distance from the centerline, it adds a perspective view which provides a better visualization, and the reader can move through the colon and see inside traditional blind spots behind the folds (Fig. 9.4) [25, 35]. The resulted strips (filet) can be rapidly viewed, and there is a significant reduction in reading time. Carrascosa et al. [36] compared the detection rate and reading time of conventional CTC views (axial images and endoluminal views) with perspective-filet view in CTC exams performed on 23 patients with 35 colonic lesions (15 ≤5 mm, 18 between 5 and 9 mm, and 2 ≥9 mm). They found the sensitivity and specificity of 86.67% and 99.12% for conventional visualization versus 82.86% and 98.25%, respectively, for perspective-filet view. Also, there was a significant reduction in reading time using filet view, 8 ± 2 min compared with 15 ± 3 min in conventional visualization.

The main advantages of perspective-filet view is that there is no need for ante- and retrograde review, since almost complete surface is visible in single direction way. Moreover, it provides full circumferential 360° view with additional overlap of 10° at the edges [36]. However distortion at flexure points is still an issue. Polyps may be grossly distorted, or folds may be appear polypoid [30].

Panoramic Endoluminal (Band View) Method

Panoramic endoluminal (band) view is similar to the one described by Beauleau et al. [37]. Both techniques display inner surface of colon in a panoramic way by using perspective rays projected from the central colonic path to the lateral colonic wall. The difference is that in method proposed by Beauleau et al., six 60° field of view (FOV) conventional endoluminal images were placed side by side, taken along the colonic circumference in 60° increments. Therefore there is unnatural wrinkled transition at the border between two adjacent 60° FOV endoluminal images. However, in a band-view technique

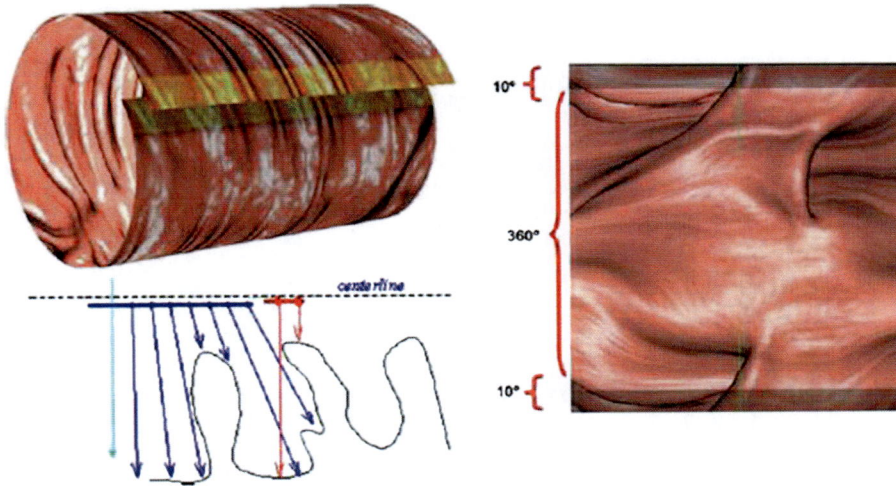

Fig. 9.4 Principles of perspective-filet view. The perspective-filet view presents the colon lumen unrolled along its center axis, with all resampling performed using projection rays perpendicular to the centerline. This method uses a Mercator projection providing a complete 360° view with an additional overlap of 10° at the bottom and the top. The generated image panel is displayed as an enlarged, flattened view of the inner colonic surface (Carrascosa P, et al. Multidetector CT colonoscopy: evaluation of the perspective-filet view virtual colon dissection technique for the detection of elevated lesions. Abdom Imaging. 2007;32(5):582–8)

proposed by Lee et al. [27], it uses a continuous array of radial perspective rays all the way around the entire colonic circumference, which results in a 380° by 120° band-like panoramic endoluminal view, and the entire colon can be sequentially viewed with reduced image distortions with unidirectional navigation. It allows visualization of both sides of haustral fold and the intervening mucosa located between two adjacent folds (Fig. 9.5) [25].

In terms of comparison, band view showed the least image distortion compared with filet and virtual colon dissection views, when they were applied in image processing of a CTC performed on 51-year-old man who had no lesion detected in OC. Ten- and 20-mm electronically generated, completely symmetric, spherical synthetic polyps were added to the supine scan data of the patient. Mean image distortion values were calculated, in which 1 indicated no distortion and the larger number had greater distortion. Band-view method significantly demonstrated the best image quality with the values 1.03 and 1.01 for 10-mm and 20-mm polyps, respectively, while the values of the filet view and virtual colon dis-

section for 10-mm polyps were 1.65 and 3.27, respectively, and for 20-mm polyps were 1.55 and 3.85, respectively. At the same study, detection rate and interpretation time were compared between band view and conventional endoluminal view through study of 52 patients who underwent CTC and OC on the same day. There were no significant difference in sensitivity and specificity for detecting adenomatous polyps≥ 6 mm, but the interpretation time was significantly shorter with band view compared with conventional endoluminal view [27].

Unfolded Cube Method

The unfolded cube projection provides the complete FOV around a point within the lumen by showing the six images (forward and backward views, superior, inferior, and lateral walls) surrounding the point of view in the center of colon. The projections of the six imaginary cube faces, which represent complete FOV, are unfolded on a single plane (Fig. 9.6). The reader can simultaneously view both forward and reverse projections, as well as entire

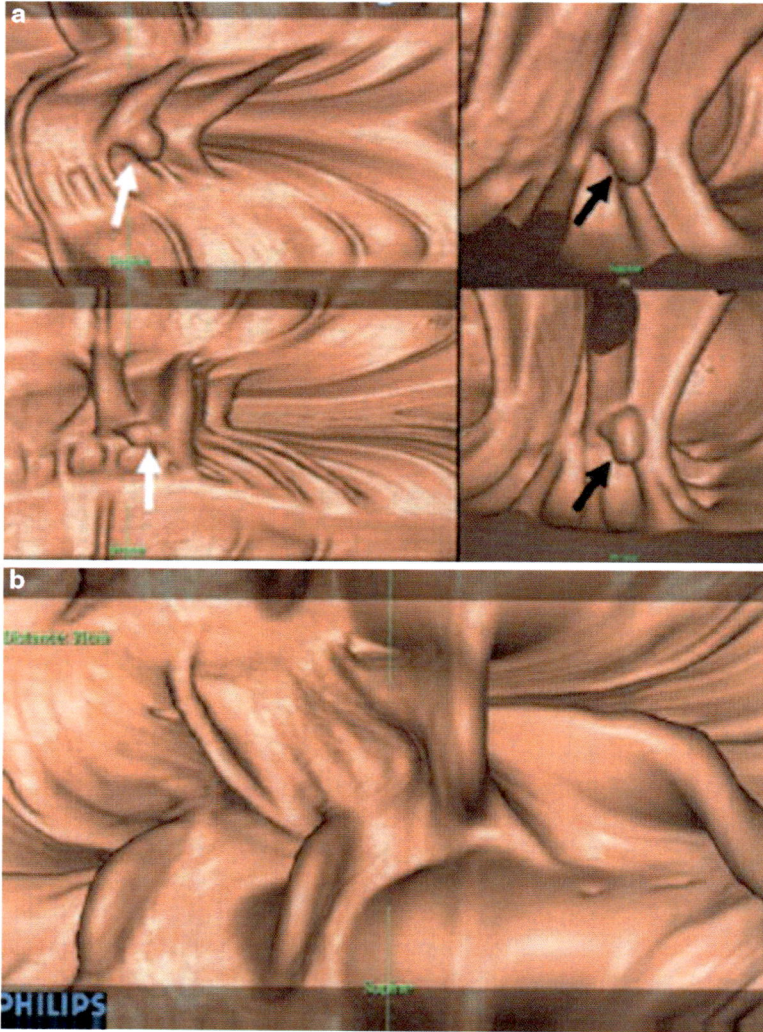

Fig. 9.5 Panoramic endoluminal display ("band view"), supine views on the top and prone views on the bottom (**a**). The segment located in the middle of the screen of the band view shows little to no distortion. However, the folds located proximal and distal to the central segment are markedly distorted. The 8-mm pedunculated polyp is well seen on both band views (*white arrows*) and both 3D endoluminal views (*black arrows*). On the cine display (**b**), as a fold moves through the screen during the movie loop, each side of the fold is well displayed either immediately before or immediately after the fold occupies the center of the screen

surrounding colonic walls in a single pass. If any suspected spot is detected, the cine review can be paused, and further inspection and characterization can be done through 2D- and 3D-reformatted images [25, 30]. Vos et al. [28] demonstrated a better surface visibility by using unfolded cube method, 93.8% of the colon surface came into view; however, by using conventional endoluminal view, 95.5% of the colon surface was visible. Similar to other alternative displays, interpretation time was significantly shorter with unfolded cube method compared to conventional endoluminal view.

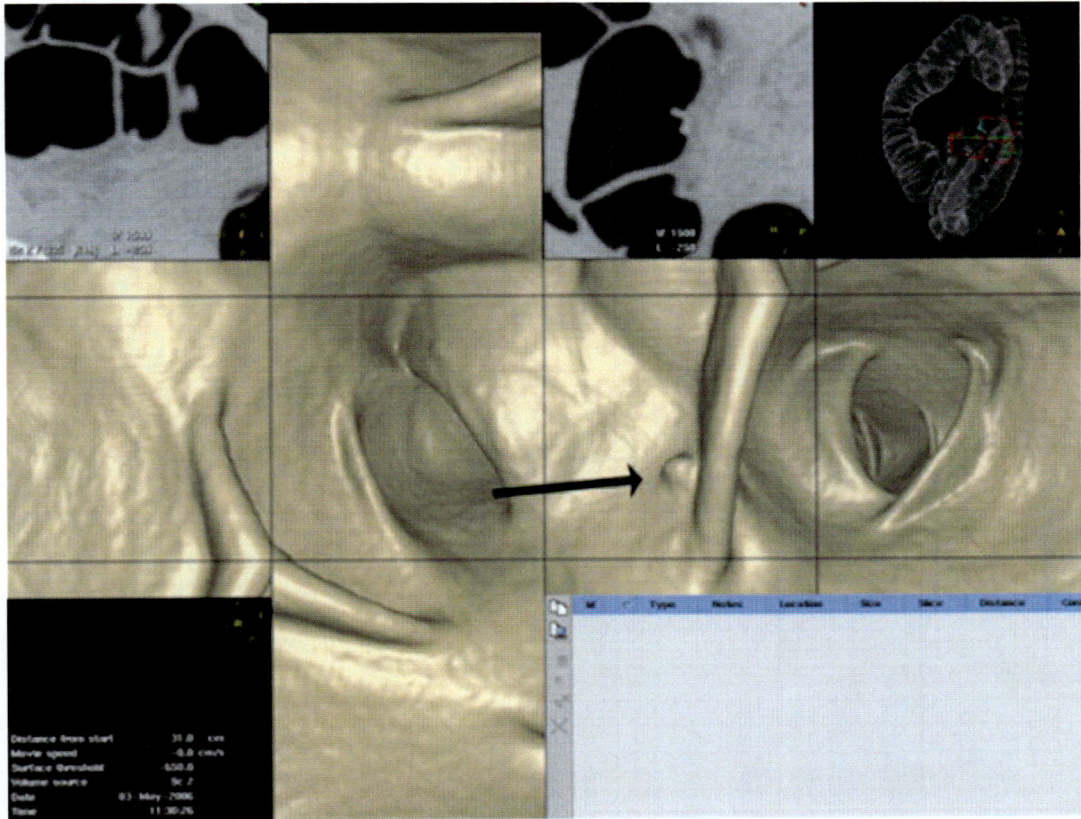

Fig. 9.6 Unfolded cube projection. This display method opens ("unfolds") the segment being evaluated from the center of an imaginary cube. The six images of the unfolded cube include the forward (F) and backward (B) views, as well as the superior (S), inferior (I), and right (R) and left (L) lateral walls. Note the small sessile polyp (*arrow*)

There were no significant difference in sensitivity and specificity between two methods for detection of medium and large polyps (5 mm or larger).

Supine-Prone Image Synchronization

Segments of colon (particularly sigmoid, transverse, and cecum) can move and change their location inside the abdomen as patient's position changes. This makes it hard for readers to interpret lesions located in these segments and decide to consider them as two separate polyps, one relocated polyp, or a mobile fecal residue. Experimental works are undergoing to develop automated methods for matching lesions found on two CTC acquisitions in supine and prone positions. Preliminary work using internal or external topographic features of the colon for co-registration of polyps has been promising [25].

Full Automated CTC with Multiple Views

Gentle Colon [38] is designed and recently introduced as a full automated Colon Engine, which means it process thousands of CTC exams on a server without any mouse click. The aim is to create a solution which permits rapid workflow in a very busy environment, which defines the requirements to the software and offers the option for a standard documentation.

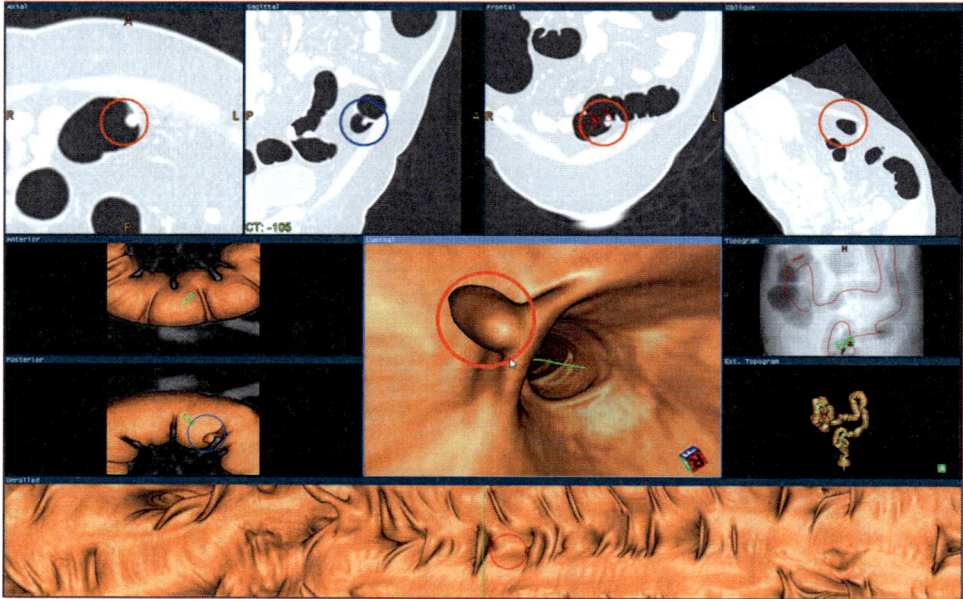

Fig. 9.7 Detected 8-mm polyp shown (*circles*) simultaneously in different views, including multiplanar 2D view, 3D endoluminal view, split view, and virtual dissection view

The software displays full 3D information of the CTC data set (Fig. 9.7). The software operates with full 3D navigation on any Windows operating system. The aim of the layout of the graphical user interface of *Gentle Colon* was to supplement the retrograde flight with a (split) view which enables in one undistorted view, viewing behind folds (without any manual interaction) combined with a 100% colonic mucosa coverage with no blind areas. The idea is to show the "behind-the-wall area" without any unnecessary or redundant information on the folds wall. It is not intended to "read" something on the folds, such as a blackboard which would create too much information. The profile section of the folds allows a quick assessment as to whether a lesion is present. The automatically created split view offers to assess wall thickening in the given cross section. Further, it offers automatic visualization of the adjacent mesenteric fat to assess the infiltration in question of the colon neighborhood. To assess a wall thickening correlated value over the full circumference, one can utilize Rendoscopy's "deep

colorization" view (Fig. 9.8). The deep colorization can be switched on/off for the whole colonic mucosa surface. It creates a color-mapped image of the HU on every perpendicular point on the colonic mucosa in a given depth. The HU density is displayed in a temperature color-mapped scale. The main difference to similar visualization techniques is that the colorization may not be used for assessment purposes of the colonic mucosa to create a diagnosis but to find (flat and small) lesions quicker and more accurate (Fig. 9.9). The adjacent mesenteric fat helps to differentiate the surrounding organs. The deep colorization is not just "opening" the visualization of flat lesions, but it permits excellent depiction of all the surrounding anatomic structures outside the colon. Organs which touch each other are shown as such. More pathophysiologically relevant is the depiction of the vascularity of the colonic mucosa (Fig. 9.10) in the case of a higher cell turnover caused by an inflammatory disease or a cancer. This may have interesting diagnostic potential.

The unrolled view demonstrates the limitations similar to those of a Mercator maps inherent

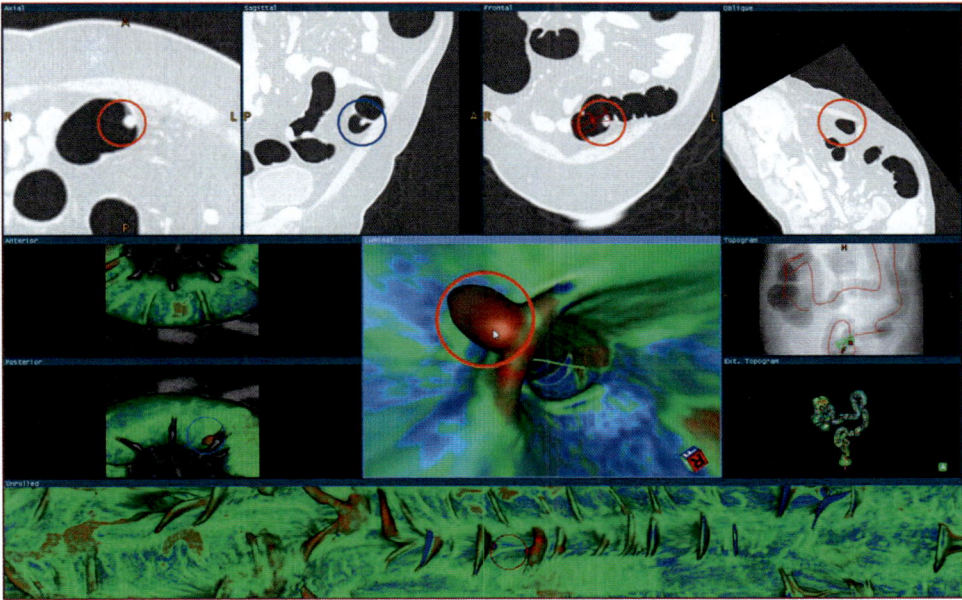

Fig. 9.8 The same 8-mm polyp with Rendoscopy's color-mapped deep colorization information (*circles*). Temperature scale for HU mapping is applied. Color code is as follows: The warmer the color is the more dense material underneath to every perpendicular surface point should be expected. The colorization can be applied to entire colon, not just for a small rectangular area which is done mainly for assessing the mucosa and muscularis. Colorization of the entire colon is intended particularly for lesion detection which reduces over-readings

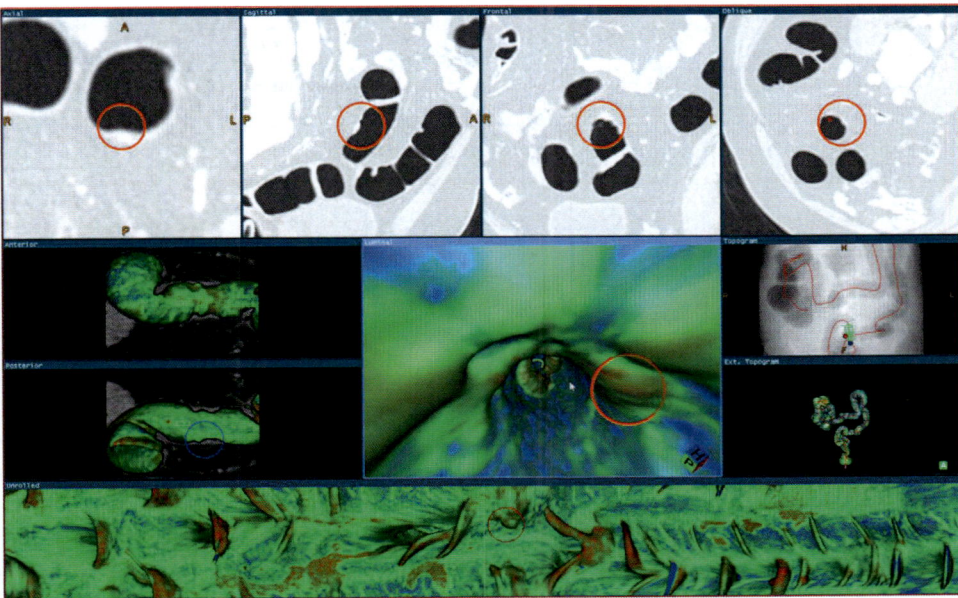

Fig. 9.9 Deep colorization helps to identify flat lesions. A flat lesion (*red circles*) found as a local wall thickening which ousts the mesenteric fat

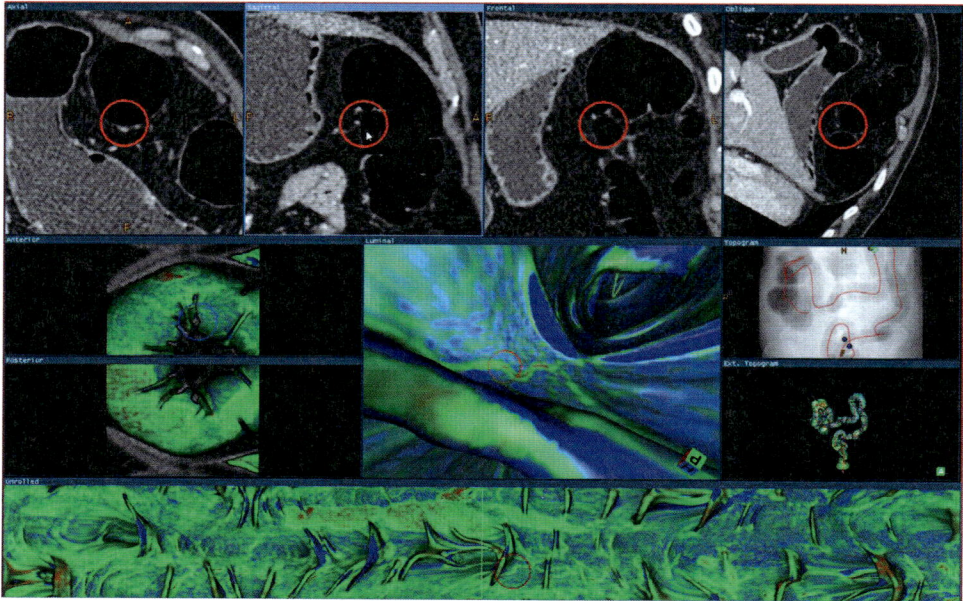

Fig. 9.10 Deep colorization also provides visualization of colon vasculature which is helpful in evaluation of cancer or inflammatory diseases

projection problem which manifests while transferring a 3D object into a 2D object.

Computer-Aided Detection

The concept of computer-aided detection was first introduced by Winsberg et al. [39] and applied for detection of mammographic abnormalities. Since then, there has been extensive research to improve CAD algorithms, and huge number of CAD-assisted mammography procedures has been performed. In 1998, the US Food and Drug Administration (FDA) approved the first CAD system for clinical use in screening mammography. Application of CAD extended to other fields, such as detection of lung cancer with chest X-ray and detection of lung nodules with chest CT. Also, there has been an increasing interest in the use of CAD for colorectal polyp detection [40, 41].

Most errors in CTC interpretation are related to failure to detect a polyp that is visible in retrospect [42]. Computer-aided detection has been proposed to complement CTC by reducing perceptual error and interobserver variance, improve sensitivity, and even reduce interpretation time [43, 44]. Computer-aided detection schemes locate possible abnormal areas on images, and further decision to confirm or dismiss is made by radiologist (Fig. 9.11). In a typical CAD workstation, "CAD marks" are revealed in the form of color-highlighted areas or arrows pointing to polyp candidates on 2D and 3D views. Depending on the software, there may be more options to see the list of suspected areas which user can toggle through and confirm or reject them. Some software also provides the polyp diameter and volume (Fig. 9.12).

Radiologist's approach to the CAD-suggested areas can be categorized in three different reading paradigms (modes), including primary-reader, secondary-reader, and concurrent-reader paradigms. Secondary reader is mostly recommended, due to less bias, and is the classic-implemented reading paradigm. In primary-reader paradigm, CAD hits are shown initially, and the reader reviews all CAD-marked areas and then he/she reads the remaining areas for any additional findings. In secondary-reader paradigm, the CAD

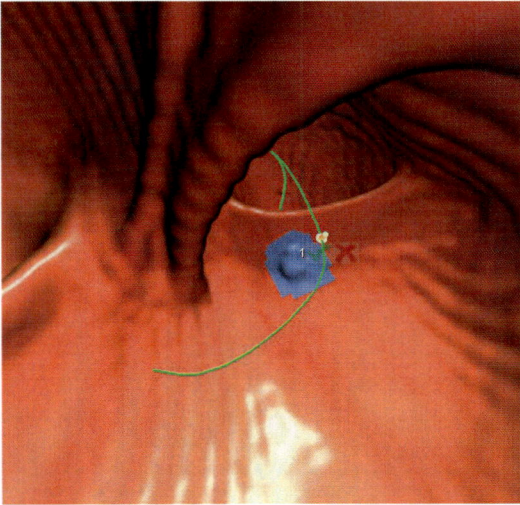

Fig. 9.11 Integration of CAD marks with endoluminal display method. The CAD software correctly identified a sessile poly and is displayed as a blue painting of the surface of the polyp on this 3D endoluminal display mode

hits are turned off initially, and the reader goes through case independently, then CAD hits are revealed, and the reader can look for any missed lesion. Primary-reader mode has the most bias, since CAD-suggested spots make reader to have less vigilance for full evaluation of the case; however, this may also happen in secondary-reader mode since the reader knows that CAD hits will be revealed later. In concurrent-reader paradigm, CAD hits are visible, and the reader reviews the case while CAD-suspected areas are showing. This mode is more time efficient compared with secondary-reader mode and showed similar sensitivity for polyps ≥ 6 mm; however, secondary-reader mode maximizes sensitivity, particularly for smaller lesions [45, 46]. It is recommended to first read the case via 3D fly-through, which is fast and bidirectional, on both supine and prone, and use CAD as secondary reader. Looking at 2D images helps for evaluation of segments not well seen in 3D and for detection of flat lesions or large masses. Next step is turning CAD off and evaluating CAD-suspected areas. Lesion texture, interactive/level adjustment, 2D MPR image comparison, 2D-3D image comparison, and supine-prone comparison may be needed to confirm or ignore suspected areas.

CAD Feasibility Studies

There are several reported studies in literature evaluating CAD performance in polyp detection [47–54]. Some studies (stand-alone studies) evaluate CAD performance, independently, in polyp detection on a set of CTC cases. Other studies compare performance of human readers in both CAD-assisted and CAD-unassisted CTC interpretations. CAD has shown to have positive effect on reading CTC images; however, stand-alone studies demonstrated higher sensitivity than CAD-assisted human readers. This is because radiologists may mistakenly dismiss polyps correctly suggested by CAD. Therefore, there is likely the need for more intelligent CAD systems which have more concentration on those true-positive polyps that are more likely to be ignored as false positive [55].

In a large stand-alone study, Lawrence et al. [56] retrospectively applied CAD to CTC screening data set of 1,638 women and 1,408 men. Per-patient and per-polyp sensitivities for polyps ≥ 6 mm were 93.8% and 90.1%, respectively, and for polyps ≥ 10 mm were 96.5% and 96%, respectively. CAD sensitivities for advanced neoplasia and cancer were 97% and 100%, respectively. The mean false-positive rate was 9.4 per patient. Summer et al. [57] also tested their CAD scheme on 75 patients with 86 adenomas. It resulted to per-patient and per-polyp sensitivities of 82.4% and 82.1%, respectively, for adenomas 6–9 mm, and 97.6% and 91.5%, respectively, for adenomas ≥ 10 mm. The mean false-positive rate was 9.6 per patient. A group at University of Chicago studied their new developed method aimed to reduce false positives (region-based supine-prone correspondence), in CAD performance on CTC database of 121 patients (242 scans), including 42 polyps ≥ 5 mm in 28 patients. Per-polyp sensitivity was reported as 90.5% with the average 2.4 false positives per patient (1.4 false positives per scan) [58]. In general, stand-alone CAD performance studies have reported per-patient sensitivity ranged between 70 and 100%, and per-polyp sensitivity ranged between 60 and 96%, with FP range of 1–31 per patient, for polyps 6 mm and larger [45].

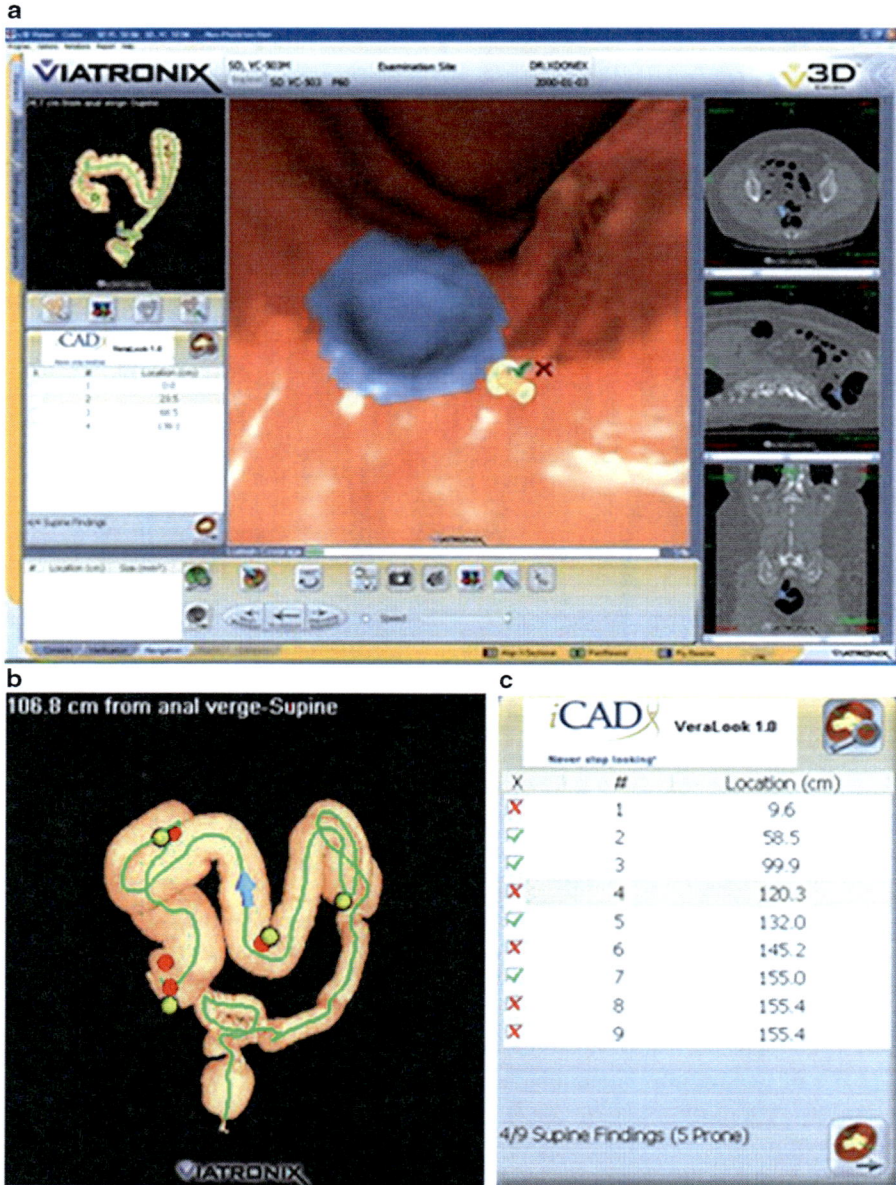

Fig. 9.12 CAD integrated into visualization software. (a) CAD marks displayed as "*blue caps*" on the virtual colon wall in the 3D view. The *green check mark* and *red "X" marks* displayed near each CAD mark in the 3D view enables users to accept or reject CAD marks as polyps. CAD marks are displayed as *yellow circles* on image slices in the 2D views. (b) CAD marks are displayed as *yellow circles* on the "full colon" view. (c) CAD findings are numbered and displayed in a list that indicates the distance from the anal verge and whether or not each CAD mark has been accepted or rejected as a polyp. The icon to the right of the logo enables users to toggle CAD marks on/off (defaulted off), as does the "C" key on the keyboard

In a human reader comparative study, Mang et al. [52] compared CAD assisted with unassisted reading in terms of sensitivity and reading time in a study performed on 52 CTC patient data sets including 37 patients with 55 endoscopically confirmed polyps ≥ 0.5 cm and 7 cancers and 15 patients with no abnormal findings. Four radiologists, two expert and two inexpert in CTC, reviewed cases unassisted and CAD assisted in a second-reader mode. The overall sensitivity before applying CAD for expert readers was 91% each. The number increased to 96% ($p=0.25$) and 93% ($p=1$). However, a significant increase in sensitivity was observed in two inexpert readers, before and after applying CAD, from 76 to 91% ($p=0.008$) and 75 to 95% ($p=0.001$). CAD showed poor performance in detection of stenotic carcinomas which highlighted the need for improvement of CAD algorithm before wide clinical application. Also, there was an increased reading time by average of 2.1 min in CAD-assisted reads. Conversely, Haligan et al. [54] demonstrated that despite the significant effect of using CAD as the reading assistant in improving reader performance, it cannot cover up inadequate CTC training and expertise for polyp detection. Ten readers trained in CT, but inexpert in CTC, reviewed 107 CTC cases (142 polyps overall) with and without CAD aid (reading interval of 2 months). Per-polyp sensitivity increased significantly in CAD-assisted reads. Per-patient sensitivity also increased significantly in 70% of CAD-assisted readers. However, the overall readers performance was relatively poor with detection rate of 51% for polyps 10 mm and larger and 38.2% for polyps ≥ 6 mm. Small (≤ 5 mm)- and medium-sized (6–9 mm) polyps were significantly more likely to be detected when prompted correctly by CAD.

In the largest multicenter, multireader (MRMC) trial [59], 19 readers and 100 colonoscopy-proved cases were involved. Cases included 35 patients with polyps sized ≥ 6 and <10 mm, 17 patients with polyps ≥ 10 mm (4 with one and 1 with two synchronous 6–9 mm polyps), and 48 patients with no abnormal findings. The overall 74 polyps (53 sessile, 13 pedunculated, and 8 flat) were distributed along 65 colon segments. The polyps' size ranged from 6 to 20 mm, and the ratio of small to large polyps was 3:2. Nineteen blinded readers reviewed cases without and with CAD (as a second reader), a total of 200 readings for each reader. The readers' average segment-level area under the curve (AUC) with CAD was significantly higher than the average AUC in unassisted group. Higher reading accuracy was seen in 68% of readers. Readers' per-segment, per-patient and per-polyp sensitivity were higher for all polyps ≥ 6 mm ($p<0.011$, 0.007, 0.005, respectively) in CAD-assisted group compared with unassisted (0.517 vs. 0.465, 0.521 vs. 0.466, and 0.477 vs. 0.422, respectively). CAD provided a higher sensitivity for patients with at least one large polyp ≥ 10 mm (0.777 with CAD versus 0.743 without CAD). The average reader sensitivity improved by >0.08 for small adenomas. Although there was a small reduction of 0.025 in specificity ($p=0.050$) and increase in reading time, the CAD system resulted in a significant improvement in overall reader performance.

CAD Systems Pitfalls

Although CAD is accepted to reduce interobserver variability and improve sensitivity for polyp detection, there are still limitations such as failure to detect difficult lesions which results in false negatives (FN) or confusing normal colon structures, stool, and artifacts with polyps causing false positives (FP). Since CAD techniques consider any cap-like shapes or significantly bulged lesions as polypoid lesion, diminutive (<5 mm), small (5–9 mm), and flat lesions may be missed because of losing their margin (due to partial volume effect). CAD may also be confused when it encounters lesions with significant deviated shape from polypoid or misses polyps located in collapsed region or submerged in untagged fluid [60]. Efforts have been devoted to develop techniques to make CAD systems smarter. Suzuki et al. [61] at University of Chicago developed and compared their CAD scheme, massive-training artificial neural network (MTANN), with conventional CAD scheme with linear discriminant analysis (LDA) for detection of difficult polyps in 24 FN cases who had at least one polyp missed by human reader (23 polyps and one mass). A sensitivity of 58% (14/24) with 8.6 FPs per patient was achieved by MTANN CAD scheme, compared with 25% at the same FP rate for conventional scheme (Fig. 9.13).

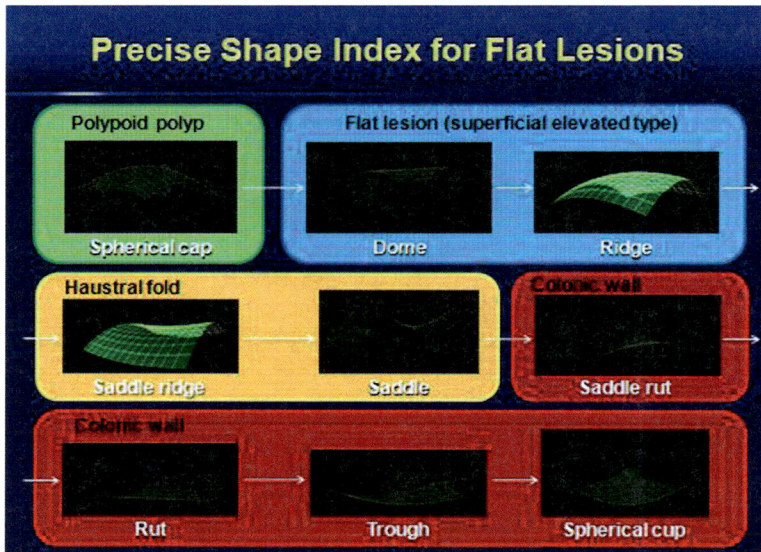

Fig. 9.13 MTANN CAD scheme: shape index (SI) for characterizing five different shapes. Polypoid polyps can be identified with the SI as a cap. Haustral folds can be identified as a saddle or ridge. Colonic walls can be identified as rut or cup

CAD FPs are a major problem which tend to be more than human readers FPs. However, most of them can be easily differentiated from true lesions, and only 10–20% are challenging [60, 62]. A recent analysis of various causes of CAD FPs on 50 cases showed that "colonic fold" is the most common source with the incidence of 42% (in prone view) and 32.9% (in supine view) [59]. Suboptimal colon distention or sigmoid muscular hypertrophy can cause thickened haustral folds and resulted FP. Looking at nearby folds helps to dismiss as FP. Other causes include nodular folds and convergence of two or more normal folds, which in these cases reconciliation between 2D and 3D views is helpful.

Some other sources of CAD FPs include untagged or poorly tagged stool, ileocecal valve, small bumps (<6 mm), rectal tube, poor colonic distention, flexural pseudotumor, extrinsic compression, anal papillae, motion artifacts (such as peristalsis), high-density objects within abdomen (e.g., hip prosthesis), small residual subtraction artifacts after electrical cleansing, diverticular fecaliths, inverted diverticula, and sharp turns or bindings. In most of them, confident differentiation can be done by reconciliation between 2D and 3D views and between different scan views.

Internal mottle texture pattern, irregular angulated contour, internal diffuse gas, and internal positive contrast tagging are clues to dismiss untagged or poorly tagged stool as FP [44, 59]. Several works have been done targeted on developing methods to reduce CAD FPs [58, 63–68].

Summary

In summary, there have been substantial advances in CTC during last decade which resulted in better image quality, higher readers' performance, and increased patient acceptance. However, there are still technical and practical challenges in CTC preparation, acquisition, visualization, and interpretation, which the trend of progress is very promising.

Key Points

- CTC is currently undergoing continued technical improvement through introducing different tools and techniques.
- Studies have shown encouraging results and feasibility of these techniques which resulted

in improvement in detection rate, reading time, and higher patients acceptance.

- Cathartic preparation has shown to be one of the most unpleasant portion of CTC and contributes to reduce the patient acceptance for CRC.
- Noncathartic CTC technique, also known as "prepless CTC," has shown very good level of patient acceptance and diagnostic performance in different studies.
- The method of "electronic cleansing" has been promising for a better approach to prepless CTC by digital subtracting of tagged solid and semisolid materials from CTC images.
- New visualization methods have been developed with the purpose of reducing reading time and overcoming limitations of conventional endoluminal view.
- Most frequent novel displays include virtual dissection, perspective-filet view, panoramic endoluminal (band view) method, and unfolded cube method.
- Computer-aided detection has been proposed to complement CTC by reducing perceptual error and interobserver variance and improve sensitivity and even reduce interpretation time.

References

1. Lenhart DK, Johnston RP, Zalis ME. Patient preparation and tagging. In: Dachman AH, Laghi A, editors. Atlas of virtual colonoscopy. New York: Springer; 2011. p. 79–86.
2. Weitzman ER, Zapka J, Estabrook B, Goins KV. Risk and reluctance: understanding impediments to colorectal cancer screening. Prev Med. 2001;32(6):502–13.
3. Neri E, Turini F, Cerri F, Vagli P, Bartolozzi C. CT colonography: same-day tagging regimen with iodixanol and reduced cathartic preparation. Abdom Imaging. 2008;34(5):642–7.
4. Yoon SH, Kim SH, Kim SG, Kim SJ, Lee JM, Lee JY, et al. Comparison study of different bowel preparation regimens and different fecal-tagging agents on tagging efficacy, patients' compliance, and diagnostic performance of computed tomographic colonography: preliminary study. J Comput Assist Tomogr. 2009;33(5):657.
5. Taylor SA, Slater A, Burling DN, Tam E, Greenhalgh R, Gartner L, et al. CT colonography: optimisation, diagnostic performance and patient acceptability of reduced-laxative regimens using barium-based faecal tagging. Eur Radiol. 2008;18(1):32–42.
6. Cai W, Yoshida H, Zalis ME, Nappi JJ, Harris GJ. Informatics in radiology: electronic cleansing for noncathartic CT colonography: a structure-analysis scheme. Radiographics. 2010;30(3):585–602.
7. Pickhardt PJ. Colonic preparation for computed tomographic colonography: understanding the relative advantages and disadvantages of a noncathartic approach. In: Mayo Clinic Proceedings. 2007. p. 659.
8. Vital signs: colorectal cancer screening among adults aged 50-75 years – United States, 2008. MMWR Morb Mortal Wkly Rep. 2010;59(26):808–12.
9. Ho W, Broughton DE, Donelan K, Gazelle GS, Hur C. Analysis of barriers to and patients' preferences for CT colonography for colorectal cancer screening in a nonadherent urban population. Am J Roentgenol. 2010;195(2):393.
10. Jensch S, de Vries AH, Pot D, Peringa J, Bipat S, Florie J, et al. Image quality and patient acceptance of four regimens with different amounts of mild laxatives for CT colonography. Am J Roentgenol. 2008;191(1):158–67.
11. Buccicardi D, Grosso M, Caviglia I, Gastaldo A, Carbone S, Neri E, et al. CT colonography: patient tolerance of laxative free fecal tagging regimen versus traditional cathartic cleansing. Abdom Imaging [Internet]. 2010 [cited 16 June 2011]. Available from: http://www.springerlink.com/content/572319 5112008747/
12. Bielen D, Thomeer M, Vanbeckevoort D, Kiss G, Maes F, Marchal G, et al. Dry preparation for virtual CT colonography with fecal tagging using water-soluble contrast medium: initial results. Eur Radiol. 2003;13(3):453–8.
13. Florie J, Gelder RE, Schutter MP, Randen A, Venema HW, Jager S, et al. Feasibility study of computed tomography colonography using limited bowel preparation at normal and low-dose levels study. Eur Radiol. 2007;17(12):3112–22.
14. Faccioli N, Foti G, Barillari M, Zaccarella A, Camera L, Biasiutti C, et al. A simplified approach to virtual colonoscopy using different intestinal preparations: preliminary experience with regard to quality, accuracy and patient acceptability. Radiol Med [Internet]. 2011 [cited 16 June 2011]. Available from: http://www.springerlink.com/index/10.1007/s11547-011-0661-1
15. Dachman AH, Dawson DO, Lefere P, Yoshida H, Khan NU, Cipriani N, et al. Comparison of routine and unprepped CT colonography augmented by low fiber diet and stool tagging: a pilot study. Abdom Imaging. 2007;32(1):96–104.
16. Schmilovitz-Weiss H, Weiss A, Boaz M, Levin I, Chervinski A, Shemesh E. Predictors of failed colonoscopy in nonagenarians: a single-center experience. J Clin Gastroenterol. 2007;41(4):388–93.
17. Ness RM, Manam R, Hoen H, Chalasani N. Predictors of inadequate bowel preparation for colonoscopy. Am J Gastroenterol. 2001;96(6):1797–802.
18. Chorev N, Chadad B, Segal N, Shemesh I, Mor M, Plaut S, et al. Preparation for colonoscopy in hospitalized patients. Dig Dis Sci. 2007;52(3):835–9.

19. Jensch S, Bipat S, Peringa J, Vries AH, Heutinck A, Dekker E, et al. CT colonography with limited bowel preparation: prospective assessment of patient experience and preference in comparison to optical colonoscopy with cathartic bowel preparation. Eur Radiol. 2009;20(1):146–56.

20. Callstrom MR, Johnson CD, Fletcher JG, Reed JE, Ahlquist DA, Harmsen WS, et al. CT colonography without cathartic preparation: feasibility study. Radiology. 2001;219(3):693–8.

21. Iannaccone R, Laghi A, Catalano C, Mangiapane F, Lamazza A, Schillaci A, et al. Computed tomographic colonography without cathartic preparation for the detection of colorectal polyps. Gastroenterology. 2004;127(5):1300–11.

22. Liedenbaum MH, Denters MJ, de Vries AH, van Ravesteijn VF, Bipat S, Vos FM, et al. Low-fiber diet in limited bowel preparation for CT colonography: influence on image quality and patient acceptance. Am J Roentgenol. 2010;195(1):W31.

23. Cai W, Yoshida H, Zalis M, Näppi J. Delineation of tagged region by use of local iso-surface roughness in electronic cleansing for CT colonography. In: Proceedings of SPIE. 2007. p. 651409.

24. Christensen KN, Fidler JL, Fletcher JG, MacCarty R, Johnson CD. Pictorial review of colonic polyp and mass distortion and recognition with the CT virtual dissection technique. Radiographics. 2010;30(5):e42.

25. Chang KJ, Soto JA. Computed tomographic colonography: image display methods [Internet]. In: Dachman AH, Laghi A, editors. Atlas of virtual colonoscopy. New York: Springer; 2011. p. 111–32 [cited 16 June 2011]. Available from: http://www.springerlink.com/content/w651282706558kh2/

26. Juchems MS, Fleiter TR, Pauls S, Schmidt SA, Brambs H-J, Aschoff AJ. CT colonography: comparison of a colon dissection display versus 3D endoluminal view for the detection of polyps. Eur Radiol. 2005;16(1):68–72.

27. Lee SS, Park SH, Kim JK, Kim N, Lee J, Park BJ, et al. Panoramic endoluminal display with minimal image distortion using circumferential radial ray-casting for primary three-dimensional interpretation of CT colonography. Eur Radiol. 2009;19(8):1951–9.

28. Vos FM, van Gelder RE, Serlie IWO. Florie J, Nio CY, Glas AS, et al. Three-dimensional display modes for CT colonography: conventional 3D virtual colonoscopy versus unfolded cube projection. Radiology. 2003;228(3):878–85.

29. Dachman AH, Lefere P, Gryspeerdt S, Morin M. CT colonography: visualization methods, interpretation, and pitfalls. Radiol Clin North Am. 2007;45(2):347–59.

30. Pickhardt PJ, Schumacher C, Kim DH. Polyp detection at 3-dimensional endoluminal computed tomography colonography: sensitivity of one-way fly-through at 120 degrees field-of-view angle. J Comput Assist Tomogr. 2009;33(4):631–5.

31. Silva AC, Wellnitz CV, Hara AK. Three-dimensional virtual dissection at CT colonography: unraveling the colon to search for lesions. Radiographics. 2006;26(6):1669–86.

32. Johnson KT, Johnson CD, Fletcher JG, MacCarty RL, Summers RL. CT colonography using 360-degrees virtual dissection: a feasibility study. Am J Roentgenol. 2006;186(1):90.

33. Hock D, Ouhadi R, Materne R, Aouchria A-S, Mancini I, Broussaud T, et al. Virtual dissection CT colonography: evaluation of learning curves and reading times with and without computer-aided detection. Radiology. 2008;248(3):860–8.

34. Röttgen R, Fischbach F, Plotkin M, Lorenz M, Freund T, Schröder RJ, et al. CT colonography using different reconstruction modi. Clin Imaging. 2005;29(3):195–9.

35. Kim SH, Lee JM, Eun HW, Lee MW, Han JK, Lee JY, et al. Two- versus three-dimensional colon evaluation with recently developed virtual dissection software for CT colonography. Radiology. 2007;244(3):852–64.

36. Carrascosa P, Capunay C, Martín López E, Ulla M, Castiglioni R, Carrascosa J. Multidetector CT colonoscopy: evaluation of the perspective-filet view virtual colon dissection technique for the detection of elevated lesions. Abdom Imaging. 2007;32(5):582–8.

37. Beaulieu CF, Jeffrey Jr RB, Karadi C, Paik DS, Napel S. Display modes for CT colonography. Part II. Blinded comparison of axial CT and virtual endoscopic and panoramic endoscopic volume-rendered studies. Radiology. 1999;212(1):203–12.

38. Rust G-F. 3-D postprocessing in virtual endoscopy [Internet]. In: Kramme R, Hoffmann K-P, Pozos RS, editors. Springer handbook of medical technology. Berlin: Springer; 2011. p. 1209–16 [cited 21 Oct 2011]. Available from: http://www.springerlink.com/content/w253q35v50g7131g/

39. Winsberg F, Elkin M, Macy J, Bordaz V, Weymouth W. Detection of radiographic abnormalities in mammograms by means of optical scanning and computer analysis. Radiology. 1967;89(2):211.

40. Morton MJ, Whaley DH, Brandt KR, Amrami KK. Screening mammograms: interpretation with computer-aided detection – prospective evaluation. Radiology. 2006;239(2):375.

41. Bogoni L, Cathier P, Dundar M, Jerebko A, Lakare S, Liang J, et al. Computer-aided detection (CAD) for CT colonography: a tool to address a growing need. Br J Radiol. 2005;78 Suppl 1:S57–62.

42. Doshi T, Rusinak D, Halvorsen RA, Rockey DC, Suzuki K, Dachman AH. CT colonography: false-negative interpretations. Radiology. 2007;244(1):165–73.

43. Dachman AH. Atlas of virtual colonoscopy. New York: Springer; 2003.

44. Näppi JJ, Nagata K. Sources of false positives in computer-assisted CT colonography. Abdom Imaging. 2011;36(2):153–64.

45. Suzuki K, Dachman AH. Computer-aided diagnosis in computed tomographic colonography. In: Dachman AH, Laghi A, editors. Atlas of virtual colonoscopy. New York: Springer; 2011. p. 163–82.

46. Taylor SA, Charman SC, Lefere P, McFarland EG, Paulson EK, Yee J, et al. CT colonography: investigation of the optimum reader paradigm by using computer-aided detection software. Radiology. 2007; 246(2):463–71.

47. Kiss G, Van Cleynenbreugel J, Thomeer M, Suetens P, Marchal G. Computer-aided diagnosis in virtual colonography via combination of surface normal and sphere fitting methods. Eur Radiol. 2002;12(1): 77–81.

48. Nappi J, Frimmel H, Dachman A, Yoshida H. New high-performance CAD scheme for the detection of polyps in CT colonography. In: Proceedings of SPIE. 2004. p. 839.

49. Taylor SA, Halligan S, Burling D, Roddie ME, Honeyfield L, McQuillan J, et al. Computer-assisted reader software versus expert reviewers for polyp detection on CT colonography. AJR Am J Roentgenol. 2006;186(3):696–702.

50. Wang Z, Liang Z, Li L, Li X, Li B, Anderson J, et al. Reduction of false positives by internal features for polyp detection in CT-based virtual colonoscopy. Med Phys. 2005;32(12):3602–16.

51. Okamura A, Dachman AH, Parsad N, Näppi J, Yoshida H. Evaluation of the effect of CAD on observers' performance in detection of polyps in CT colonography. Int Congr Ser. 2004;1268:989–92.

52. Mang T, Peloschek P, Plank C, Maier A, Graser A, Weber M, et al. Effect of computer-aided detection as a second reader in multidetector-row CT colonography. Eur Radiol. 2007;17:2598–607.

53. Petrick N, Haider M, Summers RM, Yeshwant SC, Brown L, Iuliano EM, et al. CT colonography with computer-aided detection as a second reader: observer performance study. Radiology. 2008;246(1):148–56.

54. Halligan S, Altman DG, Mallett S, Taylor SA, Burling D, Roddie M, et al. Computed tomographic colonography: assessment of radiologist performance with and without computer-aided detection. Gastroenterology. 2006;131:1690–9.

55. Taylor SA, Robinson C, Boone D, Honeyfield L, Halligan S. Polyp characteristics correctly annotated by computer-aided detection software but ignored by reporting radiologists during CT colonography. Radiology [Internet]. 2009. Available from: http://www.hubmed.org/display.cgi?uids=19789221

56. Lawrence EM, Pickhardt PJ, Kim DH, Robbins JB. Colorectal polyps: stand-alone performance of computer-aided detection in a large asymptomatic screening population. Radiology [Internet]. 2010. Available from: http://www.hubmed.org/display.cgi?uids=20663973

57. Summers RM, Handwerker LR, Pickhardt PJ, Van Uitert RL, Deshpande KK, Yeshwant S, et al. Performance of a previously validated CT colonography computer-aided detection system in a new patient population. AJR Am J Roentgenol. 2008;191(1):168–74.

58. Näppi J, Okamura A, Frimmel H, Dachman A, Yoshida H. Region-based supine-prone correspondence for the reduction of false-positive CAD polyp candidates in CT colonography. Acad Radiol. 2005;12(6):695–707.

59. Dachman AH, Obuchowski NA, Hoffmeister JW, Hinshaw JL, Frew MI, Winter TC, et al. Effect of computer-aided detection for CT colonography in a multireader, multicase trial. Radiology. 2010;256(3):827–35.

60. Yoshida H, Näppi J. CAD in CT colonography without and with oral contrast agents: progress and challenges. Comput Med Imaging Graph. 2007;31:267–84.

61. Suuzuk K, Rockey DC, Dachman AH. CT colonography: advanced computer-aided detection scheme utilizing MTANNs for detection of "missed" polyps in a multicenter clinical trial. Med Phys. 2010;37(1):12–21.

62. Roehrig J. The manufacturer's perspective. Br J Radiol. 2005;78(Spec No 1):S41–5.

63. Göktürk SB, Tomasi C, Acar B, Beaulieu CF, Paik DS, Jeffrey Jr RB, et al. A statistical 3-D pattern processing method for computer-aided detection of polyps in CT colonography. IEEE Trans Med Imaging. 2001;20(12):1251–60.

64. Näppi J, Yoshida H. Automated detection of polyps with CT colonography: evaluation of volumetric features for reduction of false-positive findings. Acad Radiol. 2002;9(4):386–97.

65. Acar B, Beaulieu CF, Göktürk SB, Tomasi C, Paik DS, Jeffrey Jr RB, et al. Edge displacement field-based classification for improved detection of polyps in CT colonography. IEEE Trans Med Imaging. 2002;21(12):1461–7.

66. Jerebko AK, Summers RM, Malley JD, Franaszek M, Johnson CD. Computer-assisted detection of colonic polyps with CT colonography using neural networks and binary classification trees. Med Phys. 2003;30(1):52–60.

67. Suzuki K, Yoshida H, Näppi J, Dachman AH. Massive-training artificial neural network (MTANN) for reduction of false positives in computer-aided detection of polyps: suppression of rectal tubes. Med Phys. 2006;33(10):3814–24.

68. Suzuki K, Yoshida H, Näppi J, Armato 3rd SG, Dachman AH. Mixture of expert 3D massive-training ANNs for reduction of multiple types of false positives in CAD for detection of polyps in CT colonography. Med Phys. 2008;35(2):694–703.

Index

Printed by Publishers' Graphics LLC
CIMO20121213.19.21.1